DISEASES OF RENAL PARENCHYMA

Edited by **Manisha Sahay**

Diseases of Renal Parenchyma
Edited by Manisha Sahay

Published by InTech
Janeza Trdine 9, 51000 Rijeka, Croatia

Publishing Process Manager Adriana Pecar

Technical Editor Teodora Smiljanic

Cover Designer InTech Design Team

Additional hard copies can be obtained from orders@intechopen.com

Diseases of Renal Parenchyma, Edited by Manisha Sahay
p. cm.
ISBN 978-953-51-0245-8

For EU product safety concerns:
IN TECH d.o.o., Prolaz Marije Krucifikse Kozulić 3, 51000 Rijeka, Croatia,
info@intechopen.com or visit our website at intechopen.com.

Meet the editor

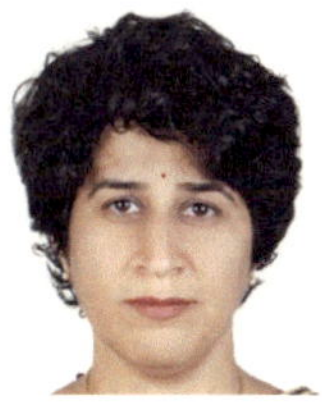

Dr. Manisha Sahay is currently the Professor and Head, Department of Nephrology, Osmania General Hospital & Osmania Medical College and Consultant Nephrologist, Aditya Hospital, Hyderabad, Andhra Pradesh, India. She did her DNB in Nephrology in 2003 under National Board of Examinations, National Academy of Medical Sciences, India in which she secured first rank and gold medal. She acquired her MD in 1998 from Osmania Medical College, Hyderabad and MBBS from SMS Medical College, Jaipur, Rajasthan. She was State topper in 10th Board Examination and has been awarded 12 gold medals till date. She has received the " Tanker – Young Investigator Award" of Indian Society of Nephrology. She has many publications to her credit both in national and international journals. She is the executive committee member of Young nephrologists' committee of International society of nephrology. She is also the governing body member of Indian society of nephrology. She has contributed to several textbooks and is the reviewer for Indian and international journals. She is the Associate editor of Journal of Academy of Medical Sciences and Guest Editor for Indian journal of endocrinology and metabolism - Renal endocrinology.

Contents

Preface

The first section of this book deals with various primary glomerular diseases. It discusses the pathogenic aspects of Alport's syndrome. The second section focuses on tubular diseases. Dent's disease, which is an important tubular disorder, has also been highlighted. The third section gives some insight into the kidney's role in various systemic diseases, as illustrated in the chapters on diabetic kidney disease. The other important systemic disease that has significant renal involvement is systemic lupus erythematosus. The latest developments in the field of SLE which have been incorporated will be of use to the readers in their clinical practice.

The role of uric acid in health and disease is an area of active research. Kidney diseases may be the cause or effect of disturbed uric acid metabolism, which is very well illustrated in the chapter on uric acid and the kidney. The book also provides insight into the effect of pregnancy on the kidney. The kidney is an innocent bystander in various hemolytic anemias and the renal involvement in sickle cell disease highlights this point.

It is widely recognized that obesity contributes to morbidity and mortality from diabetes, heart disease, stroke, and some forms of cancer, yet the important role that it plays in the progression of kidney disease is rarely mentioned. The chapter on obesity and kidney disease aims to raise awareness about the importance of obesity in chronic kidney disease.

This book will contribute to the readers' development of a lifelong interest in nephrology. The aim of this book is to give ample opportunities to the learners as well as masters of the subject.

Dr. Manisha Sahay
Professor and Head, Dept. of Nephrology,
Osmania General Hospital / Osmania Medical College, Hyderabad
Consultant Nephrologist, Aditya Hospital, Tilak Road, Abids
Member of Young Nephrologists Committee - International Society of Nephrology
Executive Committee Member - Indian Society of Nephrology (Central)
Executive Committee Member - Southern Chapter of Indian Society of Nephrology
Ameerpet, Hyderabad
India

Part 1

Glomerular Diseases

1

The Power of Molecular Genetics in Establishing the Diagnosis and Offering Prenatal Testing: The Case for Alport Syndrome

Constantinos Deltas[1*], Konstantinos Voskarides[1], Panagiota Demosthenous[1], Louiza Papazachariou[1], Panos Zirogiannis[2] and Alkis Pierides[3]

[1]*Molecular Medicine Research Center and Laboratory of Molecular and Medical Genetics Department of Biological Sciences, University of Cyprus*

[2]*Athens General Hospital "G. Gennimatas"*

[3]*Department of Nephrology Hippocrateon Hospital, Nicosia*

[1,3]*Cyprus*

[2]*Greece*

1. Introduction

Most Alport cases, 85%, are caused by mutations in the X-linked gene, *COL4A5* that encodes the α5 chain of type IV collagen, the most abundant structural protein in the glomerular basement membrane (GBM). The remaining 15% of cases are caused by autosomal recessive mutations in the genes that encode the α3 and α4 chains of the type IV collagen, *COL4A3/COL4A4* [1,2]. Thin basement membrane nephropathy (TBMN) is reportedly also a genetically heterogeneous condition, caused by heterozygous *COL4A3/COL4A4* mutations in about 40-50% of the cases. No other responsible genes have been identified as yet.

Collagen type IV, as all collagens, is a trimer formed by combinations of three of the six alpha chains, α1-α6. Genes *COL4A1* and *COL4A2* map to chromosome 13q34, *COL4A3* and *COL4A4* map to chromosome 2q36–q37 and *COL4A5* and *COL4A6* map to Xq22-23. All six genes are encoded in nearly 50 exons and close to 1600 aminoacids, and consist of an N-terminal 7S domain, a C-terminal non-collagenous (NC1) domain and a large collagenous domain in between, containing the characteristic Gly-X-Y repeat, common to all collagens. All six alpha chains contain 22-26 natural interruptions of the Gly-X-Y repeats, spread throughout their central collagenous domain. These are presumably regions of specific function and/or ligand binding sequences, of significance to its structural role in the basement membrane. Although there are many possible combinations among the six alpha chains, only three are biologically compatible and found in basement membranes. These are composed of α1α1α2, α3α4α5 and α5α5α6. Type IV collagen participates in forming networks interacting with additional important components of the basement membranes, such as laminin and nidogen [3,4]. As a component of the glomerular filtration barrier, along

* Corresponding Author

with the endothelial cells and the podocytes, basement membranes play a crucial role as a selective filter, based on molecular size and charge. A damage of the basement membrane or inherited defects such as mutations in type IV collagen lead to the abnormal passage of red blood cells in the urine. Mutations in five of the six *COL4A* chains have been linked to specific phenotypes (Table 1).

Chain	Gene	Chromosome	Disease association	References
α1(IV)	COL4A1	13q34	Porencephaly; Brain small vessel disease with hemorrhage; autosomal dominant hereditary angiopathy with nephropathy, aneurysms, and muscle cramps (HANAC syndrome)	20-22
α2(IV)	COL4A2	13q34	None	
α3(IV)	COL4A3	2q36–q37	Autosomal Recessive Alport Syndrome; Autosomal Dominant Alport Syndrome; Benign Familial Hematuria and Thin Basement Membrane Nephropathy; Thin Basement Membrane Nephropathy associated with Focal Segmental Glomerulosclerosis	1, 9, 23, 24
α4(IV)	COL4A4	2q36–q37	Autosomal Recessive Alport Syndrome; Autosomal Dominant Alport Syndrome; Benign Familial Hematuria and Thin Basement Membrane Nephropathy; Thin Basement Membrane Nephropathy associated with Focal Segmental Glomerulosclerosis	1, 9, 25, 26
α5(IV)	COL4A5	Xq22-23	X-liked Alport Syndrome	27
α6(IV)	COL4A6	Xq22-23	X-liked Alport Syndrome with Diffuse Leiomyomatosis (Contiguous Gene Syndrome)	28

Table 1. Type IV collagen chains, genes, chromosomal locations and related diseases.

2. Familial microscopic hematuria

In view of the Case we are presenting in the next section, it is worth discussing the issue of microscopic hematuria as the presenting symptom of patients with TBMN due to heterozygous mutations in the collagen IV genes. According to some older publications, these patients occasionally progress to proteinuria and chronic kidney disease (CKD) while a small percentage reach end-stage kidney disease (ESKD) on long follow-up [5-8]. In a paper we published in 2007, we presented our initial experience in investigating 116 patients of 13 Cypriot families, where 20 renal biopsies had the dual diagnosis of focal segmental glomerulosclerosis (FSGS) and TBMN. These families segregated microscopic hematuria, mild proteinuria and CKD of variable severity, including several patients with ESKD. Initially, we searched with no success, for mutations in genes responsible for primary autosomal dominant FSGS, such as *ACTN4* (α-actinin 4) and *CD2AP* that were known and cloned at the time [9]. After some lengthy molecular investigations and new ideas, we ended up discovering that all patients who had FSGS on biopsy as well as many others in the same families, had heterozygous mutations in the *COL4A3* or *COL4A4* genes, which when inherited in homozygosity or compound heterozygosity cause the classic autosomal form of Alport syndrome. In fact in one of our families, two patients developed classical Alport syndrome, as compound heterozygotes, after they inherited two mutations, one from each parent (G1334E/G871C) [9].

In heterozygous patients, this dual diagnosis of TBMN and FSGS in the presence of CKD could not be easily explained. However this work established that under certain circumstances that are not so uncommon, several such patients do not remain with only familial benign microscopic hematuria that offers excellent renal prognosis but rather after the age of 40-50, some of them progress to CKD and ESKD. Long follow-up is the norm in our setting in Cyprus, where owing to the small population and the limited number of nephrology centers (six in total, including one pediatric nephrology clinic), the patients are attended by a small number of experts over several decades. Our current data of 180 patients reveal that nearly 50% of patients at all ages develop additional proteinuria with some degree of CKD, while 21% progress to ESKD (25% of all patients >50-yo) perhaps owing to the confounding role of modifier gene(s). These data cast doubt on the correctness of the belief that the diagnosis of TBMN, in patients who are heterozygous carriers of mutations in the *COL4A3/COL4A4* genes, is synonymous to "benign familial hematuria" with excellent renal prognosis.

3. Case presentation

In early 2008, a young Greek couple from Athens was referred to our laboratory with a clinical situation summarized as follows: The proband, individual III-2 in Figure 1A, was married and interested in having children. She and her husband asked for appropriate investigations aiming, if possible, to have an antenatal test, in order to avoid having children who might develop ESKD like her father. On her father's side there was no previous easily diagnosed history for a familial renal disease. Her father II-1, had presented in a London hospital in 1991, at age 46 years, with persistent microscopic hematuria, proteinuria 3.3g/day, hypertension on treatment with Enalapril, and with chronic renal failure, as evidenced by elevated serum creatinine and urea levels. The attending nephrologist estimated his creatinine clearance at 40-50 ml/min. A renal biopsy showed early glomerulo-sclerosis and uniform thinning of the GBM on EM that also included focal splitting. In the report, the diagnosis of possible hereditary Alport nephritis was discussed but it was not certain. He reached ESKD, four years later, at 50 and was transplanted at 52-yo, still with no deafness. The proband and her older sister had microscopic hematuria since childhood. In addition to microscopic hematuria, the proband's sister, III-1, had proteinuria. The proband's mother was healthy. The paternal uncle, subject II-3, had proteinuria of 2g/day, reduced GFR and elevated plasma creatinine at 2.8 mg/dl, with normal hearing which remained normal until the age of 54 when the last information is available. He also underwent a renal biopsy at age 45 years, which was compatible with focal and segmental glomerulosclerosis but no EM results were available. The proband's paternal grand-mother, subject I-2, was diagnosed with mild renal failure at age 76-yo, when she was evaluated and was refused to serve as a living kidney donor to her son. Her findings could not be properly evaluated and were attributed at the time to a familial condition or age related. The proband had been a competitive swimmer during adolescence and had studied physical education, something that initially prompted her nephrologist in Greece to attribute her microscopic hematuria to her extreme physical activities. Because of the above uncertain family history, the proband sought professional counselling and inquired about the prospects of molecular genetics helping her reach a correct diagnosis. At the same time she and her husband were interested in undergoing a prenatal diagnosis in order to minimize the likelihood of bearing an affected child.

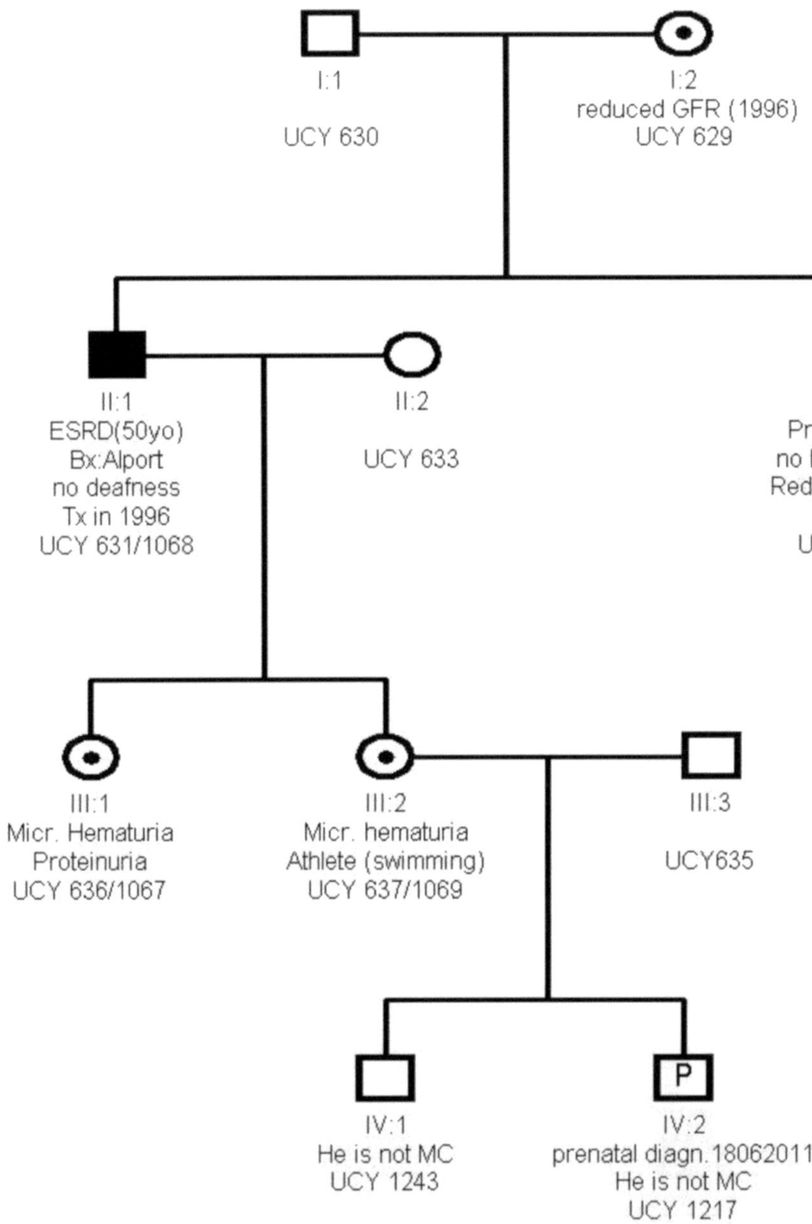

Fig. 1. A: Pedigree with relevant clinical information of the subjects under study. Note that the overall clinical scenario does not support a clear-cut X-linked or autosomal inheritance pattern.

4. Differential diagnosis

Even though the X-linked Alport syndrome was a reasonable suspicion, the attending nephrologist in Greece was not in a position to support this diagnosis unequivocally. The biopsy histological picture and the EM findings of diffuse thinning of the GBM in particular, the absence of deafness as well as the very late age of onset of ESKD of the proband's father were not supportive of the classic adolescence onset X-linked Alport, as known in the early 1990's. This uncertainty was strengthened by the similar and even milder clinical course of his brother. The diagnosis was rather on the borderline between X-linked Alport syndrome and the heterozygous autosomal recessive Alport syndrome that actually presents with TBMN and microscopic hematuria, and then on long follow-up may develop FSGS with progression to CKD and ESKD. This second scenario for TBMN as the primary diagnosis was supported by our recent publication at the time, where we showed that in a large cohort of patients with *COL4A3/COL4A4* heterozygous mutations, a great percentage of patients can progress to CKD and/or ESKD with the need for hemodialysis or kidney transplantation, mostly around or after 50 years of age [9]. Actually, our current data show that 21% of such patients at all ages progress to ESKD, most of them after the age of 50.

The proband was interested in a prenatal diagnosis by molecular means, if possible. Therefore, considering that the molecular analysis of the implicated genes is costly and cumbersome some prerequisites had to be satisfied:

a. Confirmation of the familial nature of the disease,
b. a definite clinical diagnosis,
c. the gene at fault had to be identified unequivocally,
d. the germline mutation or the affected haplotype had to be identified, and
e. a definite and unequivocal molecular test had to be developed.

In view of the uncertainty of the clinical diagnosis, a genetic counseling session took place between the nephrologist, the gynecologist and the parents in Greece, and the geneticist in Cyprus, which resulted in the decision to investigate further the family with molecular tools, with the purpose of satisfying the above necessary criteria before proceeding to pregnancy and a molecular prenatal test. At the time, the only credible symptom that segregated in the family in a dominant fashion was the microscopic hematuria, with three patients in two generations.

5. Molecular investigations

In order to solve the diagnostic dilemma we were faced with and be able to perform a prenatal molecular diagnosis according to the couple's desire, we used the molecular approach. To this end, we first performed classic DNA linkage analysis for the Xq22-23-linked *COL4A5* locus and the chromosome 2q36-37-linked *COL4A3/COL4A4* locus. As shown in Figure 1B, 1C, we used four polymorphic microsatellite markers flanking the *COL4A3/COL4A4* locus and four markers flanking the X-linked locus of *COL4A5*. Under the assumption that the two affected brothers, subject II-1 and subject II-3, had inherited the same disease, we saw that they had inherited from their parents two different haplotypes around the *COL4A3/COL4A4* locus. The probability for this to happen is 25% but this serendipitous event assisted us in excluding this locus as being at fault. Please note that under either an autosomal dominant or autosomal recessive mode of inheritance, if the two brothers had inherited the same disease from their parents we expected them to have at least one haplotype or two haplotypes, respectively, in common. In Figure 1C the analyses with the X-chromosome-linked markers show that both affected brothers, inherited the same haplotype from their mother which, as expected was passed on to the subject's two daughters. Even though this data was not strong enough based on the uncertain clinical diagnosis, we interpreted it as exclusion of the 2q locus and probable linkage to the X-linked locus.

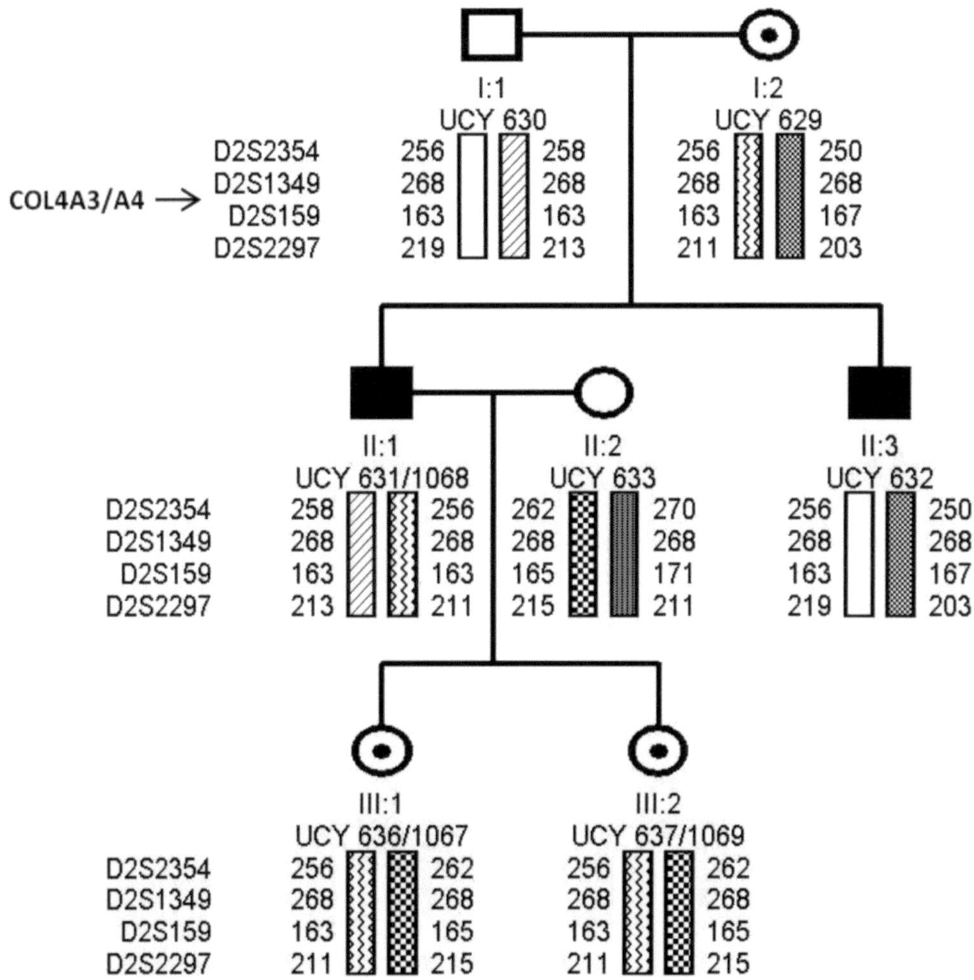

Fig. 1. B: Pedigree with DNA linkage analysis results at locus 2q36-37 (*COL4A3/COL4A4*). Note that the two brothers, II-1 and II-3, have inherited different haplotypes from their parents, hence proving no linkage to this locus.

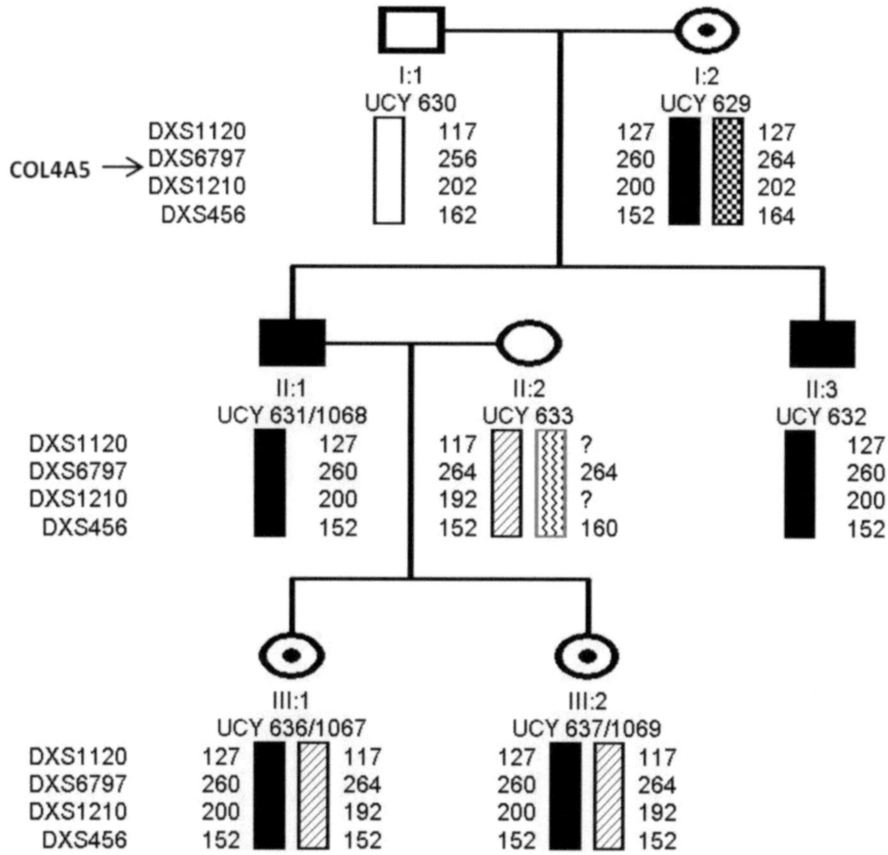

Fig. 1. C: Pedigree with DNA linkage analysis data for locus Xq22-23 (*COL4A5*). Note that these results are compatible with X-linked inheritance.

We then engaged into re-sequencing the *COL4A5* gene in patient II-1 by amplifying and sequencing all exons, including the splicing junctions and around 100 bp of flanking intronic regions. This sequencing revealed several polymorphic sites as well as a collagen mutation at position 624 that resulted in substitution of glycine by aspartic acid, G624D [10]. This mutation had been previously reported by three other groups and it was known to be associated with a milder Alport Syndrome phenotype, something that supported the mild presentation in our family [11-13]. Further molecular analysis for this mutation by polymerase chain reaction and restriction enzyme digestion showed that the two brothers II-1 and II-3 share this identical mutation which they have both inherited from their mother, individual I-2 in the pedigree (Figure 2). As expected, both daughters of subject II-1 inherited this mutation as they both inherited the X chromosome from their father. We now had a definite molecular test we could use for a prenatal diagnosis. We then communicated this information to the doctors and the couple and they went on with a pregnancy and a chorionic villous sampling at around ten weeks of gestation. Molecular testing was performed which showed that the foetus was a mutation-free male. The mother delivered a boy that on testing had no microscopic hematuria. No molecular analysis has been performed on the child yet. Approximately two years later the couple went on for a second pregnancy and a prenatal diagnosis showed again a healthy male. The pregnancy is still in progress.

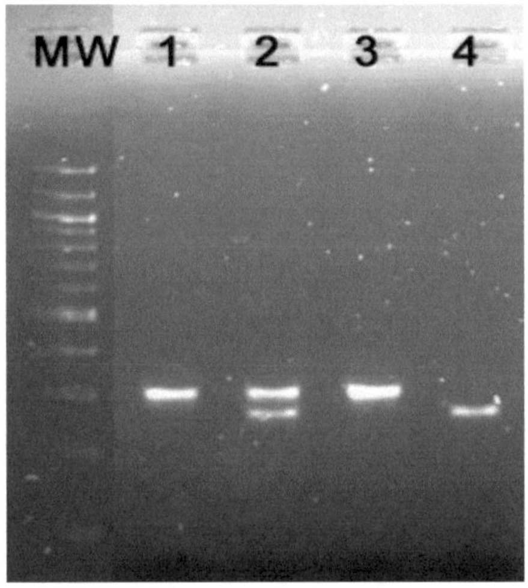

Fig. 2. DNA amplification by polymerase chain reaction, followed by restriction digest with enzyme EcoRV and electrophoresis on 3% agarose gel. The mutation G624D introduces a recognition site for EcoRV. Samples in lanes 1, 3 are from normal subjects, lane 2 is from a heterozygous female and lane 4 is from a hemizygous male. The region amplified encompasses exon 25 where the mutation G624D is located. It is a substitution of aminoacid glycine by aspartate because of a G>A transition at the second position of codon 624.

6. Ethical issues

The issue of prenatal diagnosis is always a difficult one and should be accompanied by proper professional genetic counselling. The classic Alport Syndrome is supposed to be one of the most severe glomerular diseases usually leading to ESKD before 30 years of age. It is true however, that in addition to this so called juvenile onset disease, there is the adult type where patients develop CKD and reach ESKD at older ages [14,15]. Based on current literature, this is certainly published and known by many experts; apparently though it has not become common knowledge to the average practising clinician. In addition to the family presented here we have identified five other families of Hellenic origin who share this same mutation, G624D, with a total of 13 male patients (unpublished results). Although the spectrum of clinical presentation is quite variable, the overall impression is that this mutation is a very mild one that leads to ESKD after the age of 40 years, even close to or after 50 years, in most cases. At the same time the EM studies do not show the classical thickening and lamellation of the usual X-linked Alport but extensive thinning of the GBM. Our findings agree with data presented in previous publications that identified this mutation in families from other populations [10-13]. However, the uncertainty and anxiety that accompany at-risk members belonging to families with conditions like this cannot always be dealt adequately clinically. This anxiety in the family and the uncertainty as to whether they were dealing with an X-linked or autosomal disease and the possibility of bringing to life an affected child, had led them to terminate an earlier pregnancy where the foetus was a male one. We only became aware of this event after the successful birth of their healthy first child. The aborted embryo might have been an affected or a healthy male under the scenario of X-linked inheritance; alternatively the embryo might have been a healthy male carrying no mutation or a heterozygous male, under the scenario of autosomal inheritance.

7. Discussion-concluding remarks

One cannot escape the conclusion that molecular genetics is an extremely powerful tool to use in present day clinical medicine. In another two families we had in Cyprus that segregated *COL4A5* mutation P628L, none of the clinicians that cared for the patients had initially thought of X-linked Alport Syndrome. The variable expression, the very late onset of ESKD and the milder atypical symptoms of male and female patients, even in the presence of older patients with ESKD, did not prompt us to suspect at the beginning X-linked Alport syndrome. A renal biopsy in one patient established the presence of TBMN, thereby suggesting different explanations. Interestingly, the pedigree structure could not give a clear-cut information for X-linked or autosomal inheritance, considering that some females had symptoms of the disease [10]. The symptoms in six female carriers included microscopic hematuria while two of them exhibited additional non-nephrotic proteinuria. Also, a renal biopsy of a 19-year-old female showed TBMN with FSGS. At this setting, perhaps a skin biopsy and immunostaining for collagen IV might be enlightening if the staining came out negative for the alpha 5 chain. No such biopsy was attempted.

Molecular testing for the *COL4A5* was attempted based on the inheritance of microscopic hematuria and exclusion of linkage to the chromosome 2 locus. It was only the molecular approach that established the diagnosis and enabled proper counselling and treatment to the concerned members.

Another issue that complicates matters is the genetic heterogeneity observed in a number of diseases, including inherited kidney conditions. Molecular defects in more than one gene complicate things as it doubles or triples the effort and the cost for a definite diagnosis. Newer tools and more robust methods for gene re-sequencing are clearly making things easier. Next generation sequencing and exome sequencing aimed at analyzing specifically the coding exonic sequences, can accelerate *COL4A3/COL4A4* screening in 1-2 weeks instead of the 8-12 months needed with the conventional methods in small laboratories [16]. However, still not every routine clinical diagnostic or University research laboratory is equipped with or has easy access to this newer generation of technology and machinery.

In conclusion, as regards the Alport Syndrome and mutations in one of the *COL4* genes, one should be aware of a) the rare, milder cases of X-linked *COL4A5,* Alport syndrome that presents with TBMN and delayed ESKD in the 50's and b) the late development of CKD and ESKD in patients with heterozygous *COL4A3/COL4A4* mutations and TBMN, also referred to by some as autosomal dominant Alport. The spectrum of these collagen IV nephropathies extends from vary mild cases with isolated microscopic hematuria for life on one end, and patients reaching ESKD during adolescence on the other end. Professionals involved in offering treatment and genetic counselling should be aware of these wide scenarios and they should offer the best possible advice making use of all available tools of our generation, including molecular approaches. Finally, it should be realized that the aetiology of familial microscopic hematuria is even more heterogeneous genetically. Recently, another inherited glomerulopathy, CFHR5 nephropathy, was described by Gale et al (2010) [17] and Athanasiou et al (2011) [18] that is mainly characterized by isolated C3 deposits in the mesangium and the sub-endothelial GBM area of the glomerulous. This nephropathy presents usually in childhood with persistent microscopic hematuria and 25% of such patients also show episodes of macroscopic hematuria that usually follow upper respiratory tract infections. Mostly affected are the male patients who can also progress to CKD and ESKD at ages over 30-40. Therefore, a useful algorithm is presented as a guideline for molecular testing of patients belonging to families segregating glomerular microscopic hematuria. A kidney or a skin biopsy may be performed before or after the molecular analysis depending on the clinical status or disease progression of the patient, for histological evaluation [19] (Figure 3).

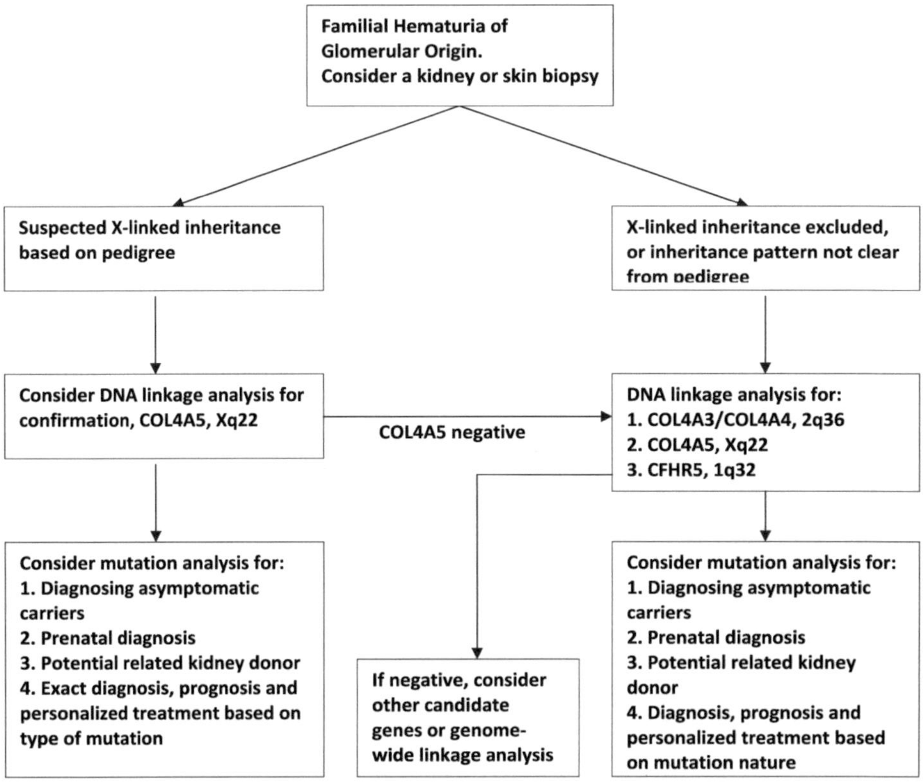

Fig. 3. Algorithm for molecular testing of patients belonging to families segregating microscopic hematuria of glomerular origin. A histological evaluation via a skin or renal biopsy accompanied by immunostaining before or after molecular investigations are performed, may assist in the diagnosis or provide useful clues for the direction of molecular analysis. When a causative germinal mutation is identified, it becomes feasible to offer genetic counseling as well as a reliable molecular diagnosis and prenatal testing with much easier and mush less costly approaches (From ref. 19, with permission from Springer Publisher).

8. Acknowledgements

The authors express their gratitude to all patients and relatives who participated and made this study possible. The authors also thank Dr M. Petersen of Eurogenetica, Greece, for preparing and providing the foetal CVS sample. The work was partly supported from the Cyprus Research Promotion Foundation, through the grants ΠΕΝΕΚ/ΕΝΙΣΧ/0308/08 and NEW INFRASTRUCTURE/STRATEGIC/0308/24 to CD and through the University of Cyprus articles 3/311 and 3/346 (CD).

9. References

[1] Mochizuki T, Lemmink HH, Mariyama M, Antignac C, Gubler MC, Pirson Y, Verellen-Dumoulin C, Chan B, Schröder CH, Smeets HJ, et al: Identification of mutations in

the α3(IV) and α4(IV) collagen genes in autosomal recessive Alport syndrome. *Nat Genet* 8:77–81, 1994.

[2] Hudson BG, Tryggvason K, Sundaramoorthy M, Neilson EG: Alport's syndrome, Goodpasture's syndrome, and type IV collagen. *N Engl J Med* 348:2543–2556, 2003.

[3] LeBleu VS, Macdonald B, Kalluri R: Structure and function of basement membranes. *Exp Biol Med (Maywood)* 232:1121-1129, 2007.

[4] Khoshnoodi J, Pedchenko V, Hudson BG: Mammalian collagen IV. *Microsc Res Tech* 71:357-1370, 2008.

[5] Kashtan CE: Familial hematurias: what we know and what we don't. *Pediatr Nephrol,* 20: 1027-1035, 2005.

[6] Thorner PS: Alport syndrome and thin basement membrane nephropathy. *Nephron Clin Pract,* 106: c82-88, 2007.

[7] Haas M: Alport syndrome and thin glomerular basement membrane nephropathy: a practical approach to diagnosis. *Arch Pathol Lab Med,* 133: 224-232, 2009.

[8] Pierides A, Voskarides K, Athanasiou Y, Ioannou K, Damianou L, Arsali M, Zavros M, Pierides M, Vargemezis V, Patsias C, Zouvani I, Elia A, Kyriacou K, Deltas C: Clinico-pathological correlations in 127 patients in 11 large pedigrees, segregating one of three heterozygous mutations in the COL4A3/ COL4A4 genes associated with familial haematuria and significant late progression to proteinuria and chronic kidney disease from focal segmental glomerulosclerosis. *Nephrol Dial Transplant,* 24: 2721-2729, 2009.

[9] Voskarides K, Damianou L, Neocleous V, Zouvani I, Christodoulidou S, Hadjiconstantinou V, Ioannou K, Athanasiou Y, Patsias C, Alexopoulos E, Pierides A, Kyriacou K, Deltas C: COL4A3/COL4A4 mutations producing focal segmental glomerulosclerosis and renal failure in thin basement membrane nephropathy. *J Am Soc Nephrol,* 18: 3004-3016, 2007.

[10] Demosthenous P, Voskarides K, Stylianou K, Hadjigavriel M, Arsali M, Patsias C, Georgaki E, Zirogiannis P, Stavrou C, Daphnis E, Pierides A, Deltas C: X-linked Alport syndrome in Hellenic families: Phenotypic heterogeneity and mutations near interruptions of the collagen domain in COL4A5. *Clin Genet,* 2011 (doi: 10.1111/j.1399-0004.2011.01647).

[11] Martin P, Heiskari N, Zhou J, Leinonen A, Tumelius T, Hertz JM, Barker D, Gregory M, Atkin C, Styrkarsdottir U, Neumann H, Springate J, Shows T, Pettersson E, Tryggvason K: High mutation detection rate in the COL4A5 collagen gene in suspected Alport syndrome using PCR and direct DNA sequencing. *J Am Soc Nephrol,* 9: 2291-2301, 1998.

[12] Barker DF, Denison JC, Atkin CL, Gregory MC: Efficient detection of Alport syndrome COL4A5 mutations with multiplex genomic PCR-SSCP. *Am J Med Genet,* 98: 148-160, 2001.

[13] Slajpah M, Gorinsek B, Berginc G, Vizjak A, Ferluga D, Hvala A, Meglic A, Jaksa I, Furlan P, Gregoric A, Kaplan-Pavlovcic S, Ravnik-Glavac M, Glavac D: Sixteen novel mutations identified in COL4A3, COL4A4, and COL4A5 genes in Slovenian families with Alport syndrome and benign familial hematuria. *Kidney Int,* 71: 1287-1295, 2007.

[14] Feingold J, Bois E, Chompret A, Broyer M, Gubler MC, Grunfeld JP: Genetic heterogeneity of Alport syndrome. *Kidney Int,* 27: 672-677, 1985.

[15] Gubler MC, Antignac C, Deschenes G, Knebelmann B, Hors-Cayla MC, Grunfeld JP, Broyer M, Habib R: Genetic, clinical, and morphologic heterogeneity in Alport's syndrome. *Adv Nephrol Necker Hosp,* 22: 15-35, 1993.

[16]Artuso R, Fallerini C, Dosa L, Scionti F, Clementi M, Garosi G, Massella L, Carmela Epistolato M, Mancini R, Mari F, Longo I, Ariani F, Renieri R, Bruttini M: Advances in Alport syndrome diagnosis using next-generation sequencing. *Eur J Hum Genet* advanced online publication, September 7, 2011; doi:10.1038/ejhg.2011.164.

[17] Gale DP, Goicoechea de Jorge E, Cook T, Martinez-Barricarte R, Hadjisavvas A, McLean AG, Pusey CD, Pierides A, Kyriacou K, Athanasiou Y, Voskarides K, Deltas C, Palmer A, Frémeaux-Bacchi V, de Cordoba SR, Maxwell PH, Pickering MC: Complement Factor H-Related protein 5 (CFHR5) Nephropathy: an endemic cause of renal disease in Cyprus. *The Lancet* 376(9743):794-801, 2010.

[18]Athanasiou Y, Voskarides K, Gale DP, Damianou L, Patsias C, Zavros M, Maxwell PH, Cook HT, Demosthenous P, Hadjisavvas A, Kyriacou K, Zouvani I, Pierides A, Deltas C: Familial C3 glomerulopathy associated with *CFHR5* mutations: Clinical characteristics of 91 patients in 16 pedigrees. *Clin J Am Soc Nephrol* 6(6):1436-1446, 2011.

[19] Deltas C, Pierides A, Voskarides K: The role of molecular genetics in diagnosing familial hematuria(s). *Pediatr Nephrol.* DOI: 10.1007/s00467-011-1935-5, 2011.

[20] Gould DB, Phalan FC, Breedveld GJ, van Mil SE, Smith RS, Schimenti JC, Aguglia U, van der Knapp MS, Heutink P, John SWM: Mutations in Col4a1 cause perinatal cerebral hemorrhage and porencephaly. *Science* 308: 1167-1171, 2005.

[21] Gould DB, Phalan FC, van Mil SE, Sundberg JP, Vahedi K, Massin P, Bousser MG, Heutink P, Miner JH, Tournier-Lasserve E, John SWM: Role of COL4A1 in small-vessel disease and hemorrhagic stroke. *New Eng J Med* 354: 1489-1496, 2006.

[22] Plaisier E, Gribouval O, Alamowitch S, Mougenot B, Prost C, Verpont MC, Marro B, Desmettre T, Cohen SY, Roullet E, Dracon M, Fardeau M, Van Agtmael T, Kerjaschki D, Antignac C, Ronco P: COL4A1 mutations and hereditary angiopathy, nephropathy, aneurysms, and muscle cramps. *New Eng J Med* 357: 2687-2695, 2007.

[23] van der Loop FTL, Heidet L, Timmer EDJ, van den Bosch BJC, Leinonen A, Antiganc C, Jefferson JA, Maxwell AP, Monnens LAH, Schroder CH, Smeets HJM: Autosomal dominant Alport syndrome caused by a COL4A3 splice site mutation. *Kidney Int* 58:1870–1875, 2000.

[24] Badenas C, Praga M, Tazon B, Heidet L, Arrondel C, Armengol A, Andres A, Morales E, Camacho JA, Lens X, Davila S, Mila M, Antignac C, Darnell A, Torra R: Mutations in the COL4A4 and COL4A3 genes cause familial benign hematuria. *J Am Soc Nephrol* 13: 1248–1254, 2002.

[25] Ciccarese M, Casu D, Wong FK, Faedda R, Arvidsson S, Tonolo G, Luthman H, Satta A. Identification of a new mutation in the a4(IV) collagen gene in a family with autosomal dominant Alport syndrome and hypercholesterolaemia. *Nephrol Dial Transpl* 16:2008–2012, 2001.

[26] Lemmink HH, Nillesen WN, Mochizuki T, Schroder CH, Brunner HG, van Oost BA, Monnens LA, Smeets HJ: Benign familial hematuria due to mutation of the type IV collagen _4 gene. *J Clin Invest* 98: 1114–1118, 1996.

[27] Barker DF, Hostikka SL, Zhou J, Chow LT, Oliphant AR, Gerken SC, Gregory MC, Skolnick MH, Atkin CL: Identification of mutations in the COL4A5 collagen gene in Alport syndrome. *Science* 248:1224–1227, 1990.

[28] Zhou J, Mochizuki T, Smeets H, Antignac C, Laurila P, de Paepe A, Tryggvason K, Reeders ST: Deletion of the paired alpha 5(IV) and alpha 6(IV) collagen genes in inherited smooth muscle tumors. *Science* 261:1167-1169, 1993.

Part 2

Tubular Disorders

2

Dent's Disease

Elena Levtchenko[1], Arend Bökenkamp[2], Leo Monnens[3] and Michael Ludwig[4]
[1]*University Hospitals Leuven*
[2]*VU University Medical Center, Amsterdam*
[3]*Radboud University Medical Centre Nijmegen*
[4]*University of Bonn*
[1]*Belgium*
[2,3]*The Netherlands*
[4]*Germany*

1. Introduction

Dent's disease (MIM #300009) is a rare X-linked disorder characterized by various degrees of proximal tubular (PT) dysfunction, nephrocalcinosis and nephrolithiasis. The exact prevalence is unknown. The disease was first reported by Dent and Friedman, who described two males with vitamin D resistant rickets, hypercalciuria and low molecular weight proteinuria (LMWP) (Dent & Friedman, 1964). Based on these data and another 13 patients with a similar phenotype, Wrong et al. coined the term "Dent's disease" for the combination of X-linked low molecular weight proteinuria, hypercalciuria, nephrocalcinosis, metabolic bone disease and progressive renal failure (Wrong et al., 1994). With the advent of molecular genetics it has become clear that the phenotypically similar disorders *X-linked recessive nephrolithiasis with renal failure* (MIM #310468) and *X-linked recessive hypophosphatemic rickets* (MIM #300554) are also due to mutations in the *CLCN5* gene (Lloyd et al., 1996). Familial idiopathic LMW proteinuria with hypercalciuria in Japanese patients (MIM #308990) – also referred to as Dent's Japan disease (Igarashi et al., 1995) - is a fourth clinical entity resulting from *CLCN5* mutations (Nakazato et al., 1997). Therefore, Scheinman proposed to summarize *CLCN5*-associated renal disease under the term "X-linked hypercalciuric nephrolithiasis" (Scheinman, 1998). The same clinical phenotype has been observed with some mutations in the oculo-cerebrorenal syndrome of Lowe (*OCRL*) gene and is referred to as Dent-2 disease (MIM #300555) (Hoopes et al., 2005; Utsch et al., 2006).

2. Clinical manifestations

The clinical presentation of Dent's disease is frequently subtle with the majority of patients being asymptomatic during childhood. Therefore, many patients are identified through urine screening for hematuria and proteinuria as it is done systematically in Japanese school children (Lloyd et al., 1997).
A summary and the frequency of the major clinical and biochemical characteristics of Dent's disease are presented in table 1. Hereby it should be noted that the manifestations of Dent's

disease are highly variable even within the same family and there is no genotype-phenotype correlation (Ludwig et al., 2006).

	Dent 1 (*CLCN5*)	Dent 2 (*OCRL*)
LMWP	100% (212/212)	100% (28/28)
Hypercalciuria	90% (180/200)	86% (24/28)
Nephrocalcinosis	75% (137/182)	39% (11/28)
Aminoaciduria	41% (31/75)	52% (11/21)
Renal tubular acidosis	3% (2/68)	4% (1/27)
Phosphate wasting	22% (35/156)	24% (6/25)
Potassium wasting	15% (10/67)	6% (1/18)
Glycosuria	17% (18/108)	11% (3/28)
Renal failure	30% (60/203)	32% (8/25)

Table 1. Spectrum of renal dysfunction in Dent's disease due to *CLCN5* (Dent 1) and *OCRL* (Dent 2) mutations (adapted from Bökenkamp et al., 2009).

Although nephrocalcinosis and hypercalciuria are characteristic findings in Dent's disease, it is the presence of LMWP, which distinguishes patients with *CLCN5* mutations from other hypercalciuric stone-formers (Scheinman et al., 2000). Protein excretion in Dent's disease is around 0.5 to 1 g per day, with LMWP accounting for 50 to 70% of the total protein (Scheinman et al., 1998). LMWP can be detected by means of SDS-PAGE urine electrophoresis, or by measurement of marker proteins such as alpha-1 microglobulin, beta-2-microglobulin, cystatin C, lysozyme or retinol-binding protein in the urine. As albumin absorption by endocytosis in the proximal tubule is also impaired, albuminuria is present as well and can be detected by urine dipstick analysis. Recently, two papers reported asymptomatic nephrotic-range proteinuria of up to 50 $mg/m^2/h$ in 6 patients with *CLCN5* mutations (Frishberg et al., 2009; Copelovitch et al., 2007). Of note, serum albumin was normal in all these patients and urine protein consisted largely of low molecular proteins, which underscores the need to measure low molecular proteins in patients with unexplained proteinuria.

The majority of patients have nephrocalcinosis, while nephrolithiasis is observed in some 40% of patients (Claverie-Martin et al., 2011). The kidney stones are composed of calcium phosphate, calcium oxalate or a combination of both (Wrong et al., 1994; Scheinman, 1998). Nephrolithiasis and nephrocalcinosis are also observed in the absence of hypercalciuria (Ludwig et al., 2006), which may be explained by a defect in the clearance of microcrystals in the collecting duct as demonstrated in *CLCN5*-disrupted collecting duct cells (Sayer et al.,

2003, 2004). Urinary excretion of citrate and oxalate is normal in the majority of cases (Wrong et al., 1994; Scheinman et al., 1998), while urinary acidification may become impaired with progressive nephrocalcinosis (Ludwig et al., 2006).

Mild to moderate hypercalciuria of 4 to 6 mg/kg per day is characteristic for Dent's disease, with higher calcium excretion being found in childhood (Scheinman, 1998). In about 10% of patients with *CLCN5* mutations, hypercalciuria is missing, in particular in patients with renal failure because calcium excretion diminishes with decreasing GFR (Ludwig et al., 2006). Half of the patients are reported to have fasting hypercalciuria and almost all have an exaggerated calciuric response after an oral calcium load (Reinhart et al., 1995). Serum parathyroid hormone levels are usually low, while levels of 1,25-dihydroxyvitamin D are frequently high (Scheinman, 1998). This reflects the complex balance between the loss of 25-hydroxyvitamin D along with vitamin D binding protein and the stimulation of 1,25-dihydroxyvitamin D synthesis by increased luminal parathyroid hormone delivery (Günther et al., 2003).

Kidney function is normal during childhood in most patients with a slowly progressive decline during adulthood leading to end-stage renal failure in 30 to 80% of affected patients in the 3rd to 5th decade (Wrong et al., 1994; Bökenkamp et al., 2009). Histological studies may be normal or show tubular atrophy and interstitial fibrosis, foci of calcinosis and non-specific glomerular changes as hyalinosis, sclerosis and periglomerular fibrosis (Wrong et al., 1994). Recently, two papers reported focal segmental glomerulosclerosis with asymptomatic nephrotic range proteinuria associated with *CLCN5* mutations (Frishberg et al., 2009; Copelovitch et al., 2007). As pointed out by Wrong et al., the progressive decline in renal function is more severe than would be expected as a result of nephrocalcinosis alone (Wrong et al., 1994), but is characteristic for various forms of the renal Fanconi syndrome (Norden et al., 2001). Norden et al. demonstrated increased concentrations of potentially bioactive hormones and chemokines such as parathyroid hormone, insulin, insulin-like growth factor 3, growth hormone and monocyte chemoattractant protein 1 in the urine of patients with Dent's disease, autosomal dominant Fanconi syndrome and Lowe syndrome which may be involved in the pathogenesis of the progressive tubulointerstitial damage (Norden et al., 2001).

The proximal-tubular defect in Dent's disease may lead to hypophosphatemia. However, there is no clear correlation between the degree of hypophosphatemia and the presence of rickets, which can be observed in about 1/3 of Dent's patients (Scheinman, 1998). Renal potassium wasting - although relatively infrequent - may be exacerbated by the use of thiazide diuretics as reported by Blanchard et al. (Blanchard et al., 2008). Another finding in patients with Dent's disease as well as in other conditions with proximal tubular dysfunction is the decreased uptake of ^{99mc}Tc-DMSA (dimercaptosuccinic acid) in renal parenchyma with rapid excretion of the tracer into the urine (Lee et al., 2009).

Depending on the degree of lionization, female carriers display a milder phenotype. LMWP is seen in 60 to 90%, while hypercalciuria was observed in around 30% (Reinhart et al., 1995). Although abnormal, the amount of LMWP is 10 to 100 times lower than in males (Scheinman, 1998). Nephrolithiasis and nephrocalcinosis are infrequently seen, and there is only 1 case of end stage renal disease in a female carrier reported so far (Devuyst & Thakker, 2010).

The diagnosis of Dent's disease is based on the presence of low molecular weight proteinuria, hypercalciuria, nephrocalcinosis/nephrolithiasis and various degrees of generalized proximal dysfunction and decreased GFR in otherwise phenotypically healthy males.

Differential diagnosis should include other inherited and acquired causes of proximal tubular dysfunction such as cystinosis, Lowe syndrome, mitochondrial nephropathy or ifosfamide nephropathy.

3. Underlying genetic causes

3.1 *CLCN5* gene (Dent 1, MIM #300008)

The *CLCN5* gene, affected in patients with Dent 1 disease, was initially identified in a family with a microdeletion on the X-chromosome (Fisher et al., 1995). The inheritance is X-linked with ~10% of the mutations being *de novo* (Devuyst & Thakker, 2010). *CLCN5* encodes an electrogenic Cl^-/H^+ antiporter (ClC-5) (Picollo & Pusch, 2005; Scheel et al., 2005) with a transport stoichiometry of 2 Cl^- / 1 H^+ (Zifarelli & Pusch 2009). ClC-5 contains two phosphorylation and one N-glycosylation sites and comprises 18 helices (A - R), which show an internally repeated pattern (helices B - I and J - Q, respectively) forming two roughly repeated halves that span the membrane in opposite (antiparallel) orientations (Dutzler et al., 2002) (Fig.1). The selective flow of chloride ions across cell membranes is catalyzed by a ClC-5 homodimer, with each channel subunit forming its own chloride pore (Dutzler et al., 2002; Jentsch, 2002).

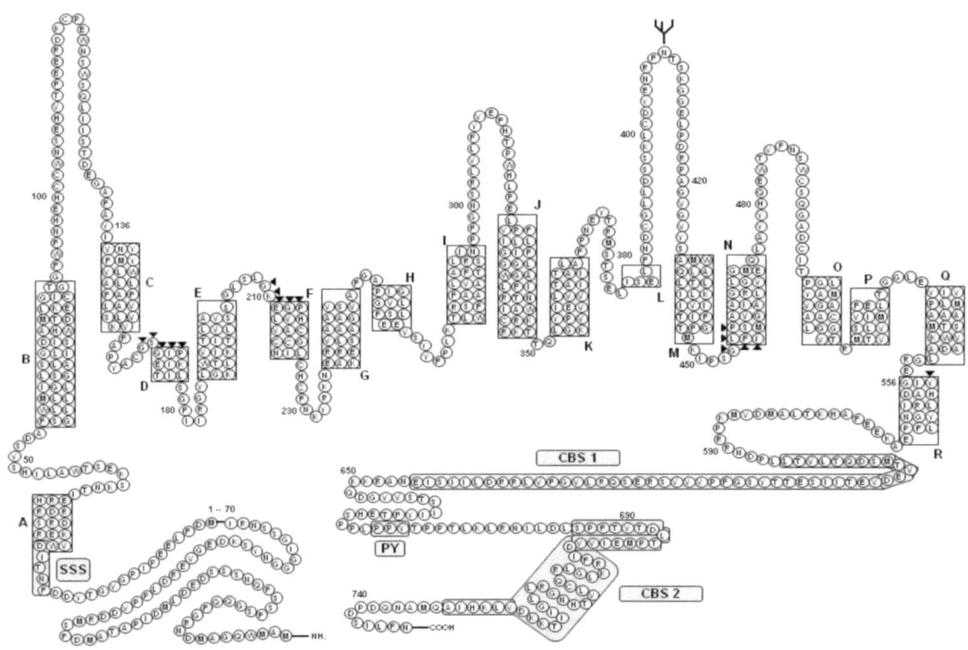

Fig. 1. Topology diagram of the ClC-5 protein adopted from Dutzler et al. (2002, 2003) and Wu et al. (2003). Boxed areas depict helices A-R with the extracellular region shown above, and the cytoplasmic region shown below. Amino acids (helices D, F, N, and R) involved in chloride selectivity filter formation are indicated by black triangles; helices H, I, P, and Q are involved in formation of the dimer interface. Further regions of functional significance are boxed in light gray: SSS, sorting signal sequence (Schwappach et al., 1998); CBS1 and CBS2, cystathionine-β-synthase sequences forming the so-called Bateman domain (Bateman, 1997) that binds ATP (Scott et al., 2004); PY, proline/tyrosine-like internalization signal motif (Schwake et al., 2001). The additional 70 aminoterminal residues in the enlarged ClC-5 isoform (Ludwig et al., 2003) are shown with overall numbering starting with the methionine of the short variant (from Ludwig et al., 2005 printed with kind permission of Springer Science and Business Media).

The *CLCN5* gene spans ~170 kb on chromosome Xp11.23/p11.22 and comprises 17 exons with transcription initiating from at least four different start sites. Transcripts including the untranslated exon 1a (Hayama et al., 2000) or 1b (Fisher et al., 1995) are spliced to exon 2 containing the start-ATG, whereas a third mRNA comprises a larger exon 1b and retains intron 1 (Forino et al., 2004). Two further transcripts (harbouring additional exons I-IV), arise due to alternative splicing of exon II, and are also spliced to exon 2 (Ludwig et al., 2003). Both transcripts carry the start-ATG in exon III, thereby coding for a longer isoform of the ClC-5 protein with additional 70 amino acids at the intracellular amino terminus. Since these two mRNAs maintain the reading frame, the start-codon of the shorter form (746 amino acids) here resides at position 71. So far, the longer variant has only been detected at mRNA but not at protein level (Ludwig et al., 2003).

More than 140 distinct *CLCN5* mutations, distributed along the entire gene, have been reported in patients with Dent 1 disease and no major mutational hot spots have been observed (Wu et al., 2009). There is also no evidence for a genotype-phenotype correlation. Various mutations were found to be associated with quite different clinical phenotypes ranging from 'classic' Dent 1 disease to very slight urinary abnormalities, not only in unrelated patients, but even within the same family (Ludwig et al., 2006).

Dysfunction of mutant ClC-5 channels may be caused by various mechanisms and a lot of the mutations observed are predicted to result in a truncated or absent protein. Complete loss of antiporter function might be caused by impaired homodimerization, altered current kinetics, altered ion selectivity, or defective intracellular trafficking. Heterologous expression of various *CLCN5* mutants, in either *Xenopus laevis* oocytes or HEK293 cells, determined a loss of Cl- conductance in the majority of mutations tested (Lloyd et al., 1996; Ludwig et al., 2005). Further consequences of *CLCN5* mutations were (i) improper N-glycosylation with endoplasmic reticulum retention and degradation of ClC-5 (ii) defective endosomal acidification, (iii) altered endosomal distribution of ClC-5 but not defective endosomal acidification (IV) delayed processing with reduced stability and lower cell surface expression, or impaired internalization (Ludwig et al., 2005; Smith et al., 2009; Grand et al., 2011). The majority of missense mutations cluster at the dimer interface and have been shown to disrupt the assembly of the homodimers (Wu et al., 2003; Smith et al., 2009).

ClC-5-deficient mice recapitulate the human phenotype of Dent's disease with LMWP, generalized aminoaciduria, glycosuria, hypercalciuria and renal calcium deposits. Proximal tubular endocytosis is severely impaired in ClC-5-deficient mice, proving a role for ClC-5 in endosomal uptake of low molecular weight proteins (Wang et al., 2000).

3.2 OCRL gene (Dent 2, MIM #300555)

Recent investigations have revealed defects in the *OCRL* gene in about 15% of patients with a Dent's phenotype (Hoopes et al., 2005; Böckenhauer et al., 2011). This gene, located at Xq26.1 comprises 24 exons occupying 52 kb, and alternative splicing of exon 18a enlarges the resultant 893 amino acids-long protein by eight (in frame) additional amino acids (Nussbaum et al., 1997). *OCRL* encodes a phospatidylinositol 4,5-bisphosphate 5-phosphatase and mutations herein were initially found to cause Lowe syndrome (MIM #309000), a pleiotropic disease, characterized by the triad of congenital cataracts, mental retardation and incomplete renal Fanconi syndrome (Böckenhauer et al., 2008). In the OMIM database, Dent's disease associated with *OCRL* mutations is now termed Dent 2 disease (MIM #300555) to distinguish these patients from the more severe Lowe phenotype. Except a lower prevalence of nephrocalcinosis, the renal phenotype is comparable to Dent 1 cases harbouring a *CLCN5* mutation (Table 1). Dent 2 may present with (mild) extra-renal Lowe symptoms (peripheral cataracts, stunted growth, mild retardation, elevation of serum CK/LDH), implying that Dent 2 disease actually represents a mild form of Lowe syndrome (Bökenkamp et al., 2009; Böckenhauer et al., 2011).

By now, 44 Dent 2 patients having *OCRL* mutations have been reported (Böckenhauer et al., 2011; Hichri et al., 2011). Whereas frame shift mutations or splice defects leading to a premature stop codon in Dent 2 patients all cluster in exons 1-7, they exclusively affect exons 8-23 in Lowe syndrome. Dent 2 was also observed with several missense mutations in exons 9-19, exons typically implicated in Lowe syndrome. Initially, none of the mutations observed in Dent 2 cases had been found in association with classic Lowe syndrome and there was no explanation why the phenotypic consequences of premature termination mutations, expected to cause classic Lowe syndrome, led to the milder form of Dent 2. Most recently, however, Hichri et al. (2011) reported two different *OCRL* mutations (p.Ile274Thr, p.Arg318Cys) each causing both phenotypes even in the same family. Moreover, a patient showing the complete phenotypic Lowe spectrum but absence of any ocular involvement harboured an exon 8 termination mutation (p.Gln199X) (Ludwig et al., 2011), thereby presenting the most severe clinical intermediate between Dent disease and Lowe syndrome.

Given these observations, there exists a phenotypic continuum between patients with Dent 2 disease and Lowe syndrome, not only between patients harbouring different *OCRL* mutations but also between family members affected by the same *OCRL* defect. Nonetheless, the reason(s) why different *OCRL* mutations manifest with the respective phenotype remain(s) to be elucidated. This may be related to the expression profile of inositol polyphosphate 5-phosphatase (INPP5B), which has been shown to compensate for Ocrl deficiency in a mouse model (Jänne et al., 1998). Mice deficient in Ocrl or Inpp5b show little or no phenotype, whereas deficiency of both genes leads to death before implantation. Interestingly, mouse *Inpp5b* and human *INPP5B* differ in expression and splice-site choice (Bothwell et al., 2010). Most recently a mouse model for Lowe syndrome and Dent 2 disease tubulopathy was established by expressing human *INPP5B* in the *Ocrl-/-* mice (Bothwell et al., 2011). These mice showed reduced postnatal growth, LMWP, and aminoaciduria and suggest that human *INPP5B* genotype may influence the clinical manifestation of Dent 2/Lowe syndrome.

It has also been speculated that the use of alternative initiation codons (methionine at position 158, 187, and 206) in exons 7 and 8 will allow the synthesis of truncated OCRL proteins. Indeed, Hichri et al. (2011) have detected two smaller proteins (around 80 kDa) instead of the 104 kDa full-length protein in a Dent 2 case lacking the normal initiator ATG in exon 1. Hence, some residual activity of these smaller products might contribute to the phenotypic differences observed.

3.3 Dent's disease and other candidate genes

Molecular analyses provided evidence for genetic heterogeneity in Dent's disease as in around 25% of patients with typical features of Dent's disease no *CLCN5* or *OCRL* mutations could be detected (Böckenhauer et al., 2011). These patients may carry a *CLCN5/OCRL* mutation undetectable by the common PCR analysis (e.g. in the promoter or an intron, thereby leading to a decrease in expression or a cryptic splice product). On the other hand, a defect in another gene phenocopying Dent's disease might be responsible. Four candidate genes (*CLCN4, CFL1, SLC9A6, TMEM27*) have been investigated so far.

CLCN4, the gene encoding ClC-4 has been analyzed (Ludwig and Utsch, 2004; Hoopes et al. 2005; Wu et al., 2009), since it is located on Xp22.3 and mutations herein would consequently show an X-linked mode of inheritance. ClC-4 (i) is also a member of the ClC-family of chloride channels, giving rise to strongly outwardly rectifying anion currents closely resembling those of ClC-5 (Friedrich et al., 1999), (ii) alike ClC-5, contributes to endosomal acidification and trafficking by epithelial cells of the renal proximal tubule (Mohammad-Panah et al., 2003), and (iii) could be co-immunoprecipitated with ClC-5, indicating that both channels may interact *in vivo* (Mohammad-Panah et al., 2003). In a total of 30 unrelated cases no defect was observed.

Hoopes et al. (2005) investigated the *SLC9A6* gene in a panel of 13 patients that met the strict criteria for Dent's disease. *SLC9A6*, located at Xq26.3, encodes the Na+/H+ exchanger 6 (NHE6; Numata et al., 1998). This sodium-proton exchanger localizes to early recycling endosomes and may contribute to the maintenance of the unique acidic pH values of Golgi and post-Golgi compartments (Nakamura et al., 2005). The X-linked *TMEM27* gene has also been suggested a good candidate since it codes for collectrin, a transmembrane glycoprotein expressed on the apical membrane of proximal tubuli that was shown to be essential for renal amino acid transport (Danilczyk et al., 2006). However, mutation analysis was negative in 26 Dent-like patients as well (Tosetto et al., 2009) as was the case in 10 patients analyzed for defects in *CFL1* (Wu et al., 2009). This autosomal gene locates on chromosome 11q13.1 and encodes cofilin, a protein shown to interact with ClC-5 in regulating albumin uptake in the proximal tubule (Hryciw et al., 2003).

Given these negative results, a further causative gene still awaits identification. Moreover, effects of (a) modifier locus(i) may influence the phenotype in Dent's patients. This would explain the heterogeneity in the clinical features observed among non-related patients sharing the same mutation or even between family members affected by the same defect (Ludwig et al., 2006).

4. Pathophysiology of Dent's disease

4.1 Localisation of ClC-5 in the kidney

In the kidney ClC-5 is found predominantly expressed in the proximal tubule and in α-intercalated cells of the distal nephron. A small fraction may be present at the cell surface of the medullary thick ascending limb of Henle's loop. In the proximal tubule ClC-5 is mainly located in the intracellular subapical endosomes, where it is co-expressed with the proton pump (V-type H^+ ATPase).

4.2 Role of ClC-5 in endosomal acidification

Along the endocytic pathway a successively decreasing pH from 6.3 to 4.7 is detected in early endosomes, late endosomes and lysosomes with a change in the ionic composition along the endocytic pathway (Casey et al., 2010; Scott et al., 2010). The acidification is mainly due to vacuolar H^+ ATPase, mediating ATP-dependent transport of protons. The movement of H^+ across the endosomal membrane results in a net charge translocation, which has to be neutralized by a passive influx of counter ions such as chloride or by efflux of another cation. Na^+ entry increases the membrane potential and limits acidification.

TRPML3 belongs to the mucolipin family of the TRP ion channels and is present in the early endosomes (Puertollano et al., 2009). Shortly after internalisation of the endosomes there is rapid release of Ca^{2+} from early endosomes through TRPML3 that is necessary for allowing

acidification of this compartment. Once late endosomes or lysosomes become highly acidic, the low pH inhibits TRPML3 channel activity, stopping Ca^{2+} exit and preventing further acidification (Martina et al., 2009; Lelouvier et al., 2010) (Fig.2).
In a study in isolated endosomes performed by Saito et al. (2007) the presence of two poor channels (TPC), releasing Ca^{2+} from the endosome, was demonstrated. Ca^{2+} release was inhibited by the endosome luminal Cl^- with a K50 of 82 mM. Reduction of Cl^- activated Ca^{2+} release, which in turn stimulates H^+ transport to the lumen (Fig.2).
There is ample evidence that ClC-5 has an essential role in the acidification of the endosomes (Plans et al., 2009; Wellhouser et al., 2010; Smith & Lippiat, 2010). Two research groups demonstrated that ClC-5 functions as a voltage-dependent electrogenic chloride/proton exchanger (Picollo et al., 2005; Scheel et al., 2005). In their studies the currents required 20-40 mV voltages, which are not observed *in vivo*. When transposed to endosomal membranes, it means a movement of a positive charge (H^+) into and of negative charge (Cl^-) out of the endosome. Sonawane et al. (2009) showed that within 60 s Cl^- concentration in the lumen is decreased from 120 to 20-30 mmol. Zifarelli and Pusch (2009) determined the absolute proton fluxes using *Xenopus* oocytes from the extracellular proton gradient using a pH sensitive dye. A transport stochiometry of $2Cl^-/1H^+$ was demonstrated. Smith and Lippiat (2010) demonstrated using a targeted pH sensitive fluorescent protein in opossum proximal tubular cells that endosomal acidification was only partially sensitive to the inhibitor of V-ATPase bafilomycin-A1. In the presence of bafilomycin-A1, the acidification was almost fully ablated by the knockdown of endogenous ClC-5 by siRNA. Contrasting previous assumption, these authors suggested that ClC-5 exchanges two Cl^- ions from the endosomal lumen for a proton from the cytoplasm. This leads to endosomal acidification directly by ClC-5 in parallel with V-ATPase (Fig.2).

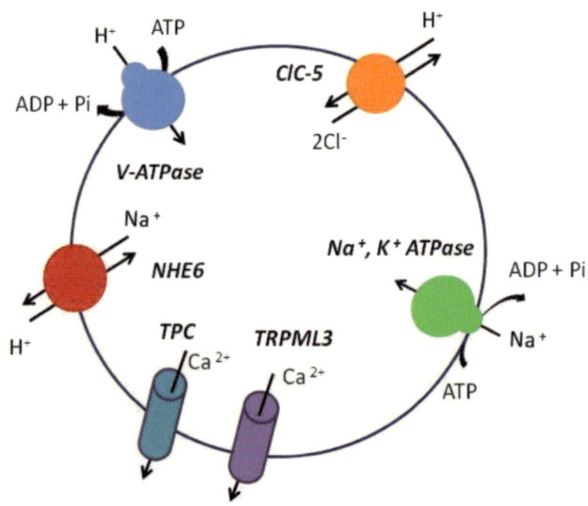

V-ATPase; vacuolar ATPase. ClC-5; chloride channel 5 mutated in Dent 1 disease. NHE6; Na^+/H^+ exchanger 6. TRPML3; mucolipin 3. TPC; two poor channel.

Fig. 2. Major classes of transporters in the early endosome; protons can enter endosome via V-ATPase, ClC-5 and NHE6. Ca^{2+} exit via TRPM3 and via TPC counteracting net charge translocation facilitating endosomal acidification. Na^+ entry increases endosomal membrane potential and limits acidification.

4.3 Role of decreased endosomal acidification in the disturbed proximal tubule transport

A remarkable study was performed by Novarino et al. (2010). They generated mice with a mutation that converted ClC-5 exchanger into a pure Cl^- conductor. In these conditions ATP-dependent acidification of renal endosomes was normal however, proximal tubular endocytosis was impaired. Because the mutation was introduced into the intramembraneous part of the protein, this study made it unlikely that a disturbed interaction between ClC-5 and other partners is involved in the pathogenesis of Dent's disease (Reed et al., 2010). The impaired reabsorption in the proximal tubule is still presumably due to the failure to recycle specific transporters, released by the low endosomal pH, to the apical membrane. A definite pathogenetic concept, however, is still lacking.

4.4 Consequences of ClC-5 dysfunction for the α-intercalated cells

As the acidifying capacity after ammonium chloride loading is normal in the initial phase of Dent's disease, normal H^+ ATPase has to be present at the apical surface of the α-intercalated cells. Carr et al. (2006) demonstrated in a collecting duct cell line, in which ClC-5 was disrupted, a marked increase in annexin A2, a crystal-binding molecule at the plasma membrane. This leads to an accumulation of crystal binding molecules at this site and might underlie nephrocalcinosis in patients with Dent's disease. Interestingly, aquaporin 6 co-localizes with H^+ ATPase in α-intercalated cells and functions as an anion channel, facilitating Cl^- transport (Yasui et al., 1999). The physiological role of aquaporin 6 and its relation to ClC-5 in α-intercalated cells remains to be established.

4.5 Role of OCRL in endosomal trafficking

Detailed description of the cellular phenotype caused by *OCRL* mutations is beyond the scope of this chapter. OCRL protein belongs to a type II polyphosphate 5-phosphatases and is ubiquitously expressed in the Trans-Golgi Network (TGN), endosomes and plasma membrane. OCRL interacts with a broad range of small Rab GTPases, a family of proteins, which together with phosphatidylinositols regulate cellular vesicle trafficking (Vicinanza et al., 2008). Other OCRL interactors include clathrin and adaptor proteins AP1 and AP2. Some mutations detected in patients with Lowe syndrome disturb interaction between OCRL-protein and several Rab GTPases (Hou et al., 2011), however, functional consequences of the other mutations found in Lowe syndrome or in Dent 2 disease are unknown and a mechanistic explanation of differences between the two phenotypes remains to be clarified.

5. Treatment of Dent's disease

At this moment there is no curative treatment of Dent's disease. Supportive therapy is focused on preventing renal stone formation and slowing down the deterioration of renal function. Increased fluid intake and administration of hydrochlorothiazide (HCT) decrease urinary calcium concentrations (Raja et al., 2002), however, hypovolemia and hypokalemia can complicate thiazide treatment (Blanchard et al., 2008). High citrate diet has a positive effect on renal stone formation in the ClC-5 knockout mice (Chebotaru et al., 2005), but its efficiency has not been proven in humans. Inhibition of the renin-angiotensin-aldosterone system (RAAS) might be of potential benefit by reducing proteinuria, but its effect in Dent's disease patients has not been studied. Treatment of rickets with vitamin D and phosphate

supplementation should be performed with caution as it can enhance hypercalciuria and nephrocalcinosis.
Smith et al. (2009) reported that some ClC-5 missense mutants are retained in the endoplasmatic reticulum. The authors suggested that the export of mutant channels might be improved by exposure to chaperones improving forward trafficking by allosteric means. Therefore, the identification of allosteric modulators, specific for ClC-5, may provide a therapy for Dent 1 disease at least caused by this type of mutation.

6. Conclusions

Dent's disease is a rare X-linked disorder characterized by various degrees of proximal tubular dysfunction, nephrocalcinosis and nephrolithiasis. The disease leads to progressive loss of kidney function and causes end stage renal failure (ESRD) mostly in the 3rd to 4th decades of life. Dent's disease mostly affects males, however, female carries can develop mild proximal tubular dysfunction and more rarely nephrolithiasis. Approximately 60% of all Dent's patients (i.e. Dent 1 patients) have inactivating mutations in the *CLCN5* gene encoding the electrogenic Cl-/H+ exchanger ClC-5, which is extensively expressed on the early endosomes in renal PT and is involved in the receptor-mediated endocytosis.
About 15% of Dent's patients have mutations in the *OCRL* gene and are classified as having Dent 2 disease. *OCRL* gene, encoding phosphatidyl-inositol phosphate 5-phosphatase, is known to cause Lowe syndrome, a severe form of X-linked mental retardation associated with proximal tubular dysfunction and congenital cataract.
Studying the pathogenesis of Dent's has elucidated the crucial role of the ClC-5 protein in endosomal acidification required for the progression along the endocytotic machinery. Recent studies demonstrated that ClC-5 functions as a 2Cl-/H+ exchanger, which is directly involved in the acidification of early endosomes.
Treatment of patients with Dent's disease is supportive and focused on preventing renal stone formation and slowing down the deterioration of their renal function. Increased fluid intake and cautious administration of HCT can decrease urinary calcium concentrations. Inhibition of RAAS might be of potential benefit by reducing proteinuria.

7. References

Bateman, A. (1997). The structure of a domain common to archaebacteria and the homocystinuria disease protein. *Trends Biochem Sci* 22, pp. 12-13, ISSN 0968-0004

Blanchard A, Vargas-Poussou R, Peyrard S, Mogenet A, Baudouin V, Boudailliez B, Charbit M, Deschesnes G, Ezzhair N, Loirat C, Macher MA, Niaudet P, Azizi M. (2008). Effect of hydrochlorothiazide on urinary calcium excretion in Dent disease: An uncontrolled trial. *Am J Kidney Dis,* 52, pp. 1084-1095, ISSN 0272-6386

Bockenhauer D, Bokenkamp A, van't Hoff W, Levtchenko E, Kist-van Holthe JE, Tasic V, Ludwig M. (2008). Renal phenotype in Lowe syndrome: A selective proximal tubular dysfunction. *Clin J Am Soc Nephrol,* 3, pp. 1430-1436, ISSN 1046-6673

Böckenhauer D, Bökenkamp A, Nuutinen M, Unwin R, van't Hoff W, Sirimanna T, Vrljicak K, Ludwig M. (2011). Novel *OCRL* mutations in patients with Dent-2 disease. *J Pediatr Genet, in press*

Bökenkamp A, Böckenhauer D, Cheong HI, Hoppe B, Tasic V, Unwin R, Ludwig M. (2009). Dent-2 disease: A mild variant of Lowe Syndrome. *J. Pediatr,* 155, pp. 94-99, ISSN 0022-3476

Bothwell SP, Farber LW, Hoagland A, Nussbaum RL. (2010). Species-specific difference in expression and splice-site choice in Inpp5b, an inositol polyphosphate 5-phosphatase paralogous to the enzyme deficient in Lowe syndrome. *Mammal Genome,* 21, pp. 458-66, ISSN 1432-1777

Bothwell SP, Chan E, Bernardini IM, Kuo YM, Gahl WA, Nussbaum RL. (2011). Mouse model for Lowe syndrome/Dent disease 2 renal tubulopathy. *J Am Soc Nephrol,* 3, pp. 443-8, ISSN 1046-6673

Carr G, Simmons NL, Sayer JA. (2006). Disruption of clc-5 leads to a redistribution of annexin A2 and promotes calcium crystal agglomeration in collecting duct epithelial cells. *Cell Mol Life Sci,* 63, pp. 367-377, ISSN 1420-682X

Casey JR, Grinstein S, Orlowski J. (2010) Sensor and regulators of intracellular pH. *Nat Rev Mol Cell Biol,* 11, pp. 50-61, ISSN 1471-0072

Cebotaru V, Kaul S, Devuyst O, Cai H, Racusen L, Guggino WB, Guggino SE. (2005). High citrate diet delays progression of renal insufficiency in the ClC-5 knockout mouse model of Dent's disease. *Kidney Int,* 68, pp. 642–652, ISSN 0085-2538

Claverie-Martin F, Ramos-Trujillo E, Garica-Nieto V. (2011). Dent's disease: clinical features and molecular basis. *Pediatr Nephrol* , 26, pp. 693-704, ISSN 0391-6510

Copelovitch L, Nash MA, Kaplan BS. (2007). Hypothesis: Dent disease is an underrecognized cause of focal glomerulosclerosis. *Clin J Am Soc Nephrol,* 2, pp. 914-918, ISSN 1046-6673

Danilczyk U, Sarao R, Remy C, Benabbas C, Stange G, Richter A, Arya S, Pospisilik JA, Singer D, Camargo SM, Makrides V, Ramadan T, Verrey F, Wagner CA, Penninger JM. (2006). Essential role for collectrin in renal amino acid transport. *Nature,* 444, pp. 1088-1091, ISSN 0028-0836

Dent CE, Friedman M. (1964). Hypercalciuric rickets associated with renal tubular damage. *Arch Dis Child,* 39, pp. 240-249, ISSN 0003-9888

Devuyst O, Thakker RV. (2010). Dent's disease. *Orphanet J Rare Dis,* 5, pp. 28, ISSN 1359-2998

Dutzler R, Campbell EB, Cadene M, Chait BT, MacKinnon R. (2002). X-ray structure of a ClC chloride channel at 3.0 Å reveals the molecular basis of anion selectivity. *Nature,* 415, pp. 287-294, ISSN 0028-0836

Dutzler R, Campbell EB, MacKinnon R. (2003). Gating the selectivity filter in ClC chloride channels. *Science,* 300, pp. 108-112, ISSN 0036-8075

Fisher SE, van Bakel I, Lloyd SE, Pearce SH, Thakker RV, Craig IW. (1995). Cloning and characterization of CLCN5, the human kidney chloride channel gene implicated in Dent disease (an X-linked hereditary nephrolithiasis). *Genomics,* 29, pp. 598-606, ISSN 0888-7543

Forino M, Graziotto R, Tosetto E, Gambaro G, D'Angelo A, Anglani F. (2004). Identification of a novel splice site mutation of CLCN5 gene and characterization of a new alternative 5' UTR end of ClC-5 mRNA in human renal tissue and leukoctes. *J Hum Genet,* 49, pp. 53-60, ISSN 1018-4813

Friedrich T, Breiderhoff T, Jentsch TJ. (1999). Mutational analysis demonstrates that ClC-4 and ClC-5 directly mediate plasma membrane currents. *J Biol Chem,* 274, pp. 896-902, ISSN 0021-9258

Frishberg Y, Dinour D, Belostotsky R, Becker-Cohen R, Rinat C, Feinstein S, Navon-Elkan P, Ben-Shalom E. (2009). Dent's disease manifesting as focal glomerulosclerosis: Is it the tip of the iceberg? *Pediatr Nephrol,* 24, pp. 2369-2373, ISSN 0391-6510

Grand T, L'Hoste S, Mordasini D, Defontaine N, Keck M, Pennaforte T, Genete M, Laghmani K, Teulon J, Lourdel S. (2011). Heterogeneity in the processing of *CLCN5* mutants related to Dent disease. *Hum Mutat,* 32, pp. 476-483, ISSN 1059-7794

Günther W, Piwon N, Jentsch TJ. (2003). The ClC-5 chloride channel knock-out mouse - an animal model for Dent's disease. *Pflügers Arch,* 445, pp. 456-462, ISSN 1432-2013

Hayama A, Uchida S, Sasaki S, Marumo F. (2000). Isolation and characterization of the human ClC-5 chloride channel gene promoter. *Gene,* 261, pp. 355-364, ISSN 0378-1119

Hichri H, Rendu J, Monnier N, Coutton C, Dorseuil O, Poussou RV, Baujat G, Blanchard A, Nobili F, Ranchin B, Remesy M, Salomon R, Satre V, Lunardi J. (2011). From Lowe syndrome to Dent disease: Correlations between mutations of the OCRL1 gene and clinical and biochemical phenotypes. *Hum Mutat,* 32, pp. 379-388, ISSN 1059-7794

Hoopes RR Jr, Shrimpton AE, Knohl SJ, Hueber P, Hoppe B, Matyus J, Simckes A, Tasic V, Toenshoff B, Suchy SF, Nussbaum RL, Scheinman SJ. (2005). Dent disease with mutation in *OCRL1. Am J Hum Genet,* 76, pp. 260-267, ISSN 0002-9297

Hou X, Hagemann N, Schoebel S, Blankenfeldt W, Goody RS, Erdmann KS, Itzen A. (2011). A structural basis for Lowe syndrome caused by mutations in the Rab-binding domain of OCRL1. *EMBO J,* 30, pp. 1659-1670, ISSN 0261-4189

Hryciw DH, Wang Y, Devuyst O, Pollock CA, Poronnik P, Guggino WB. (2003). Cofilin interacts with ClC-5 and regulates albumin uptake in proximal tubule cell lines. *J Biol Chem,* 278, pp. 40169-40176, ISSN 0021-9258

Igarashi T, Hayakawa H, Shiraga H, Kawato H, Yan K, Kawaguchi H, Yamanaka T, Tsuchida S, Akagi K. (1995). Hypercalciuria and nephrocalcinosis in patients with idiopathic low-molecular-weight proteinuria in Japan: Is the disease identical to Dent's disease in the United Kingdom? *Nephron,* 69, pp. 242-247, ISSN 0028-2766

Jänne PA, Suchy SF, Bernard D, MacDonald M, Crawley J, Grinberg A, Wynshaw-Boris A, Westphal H, Nussbaum RL. (1998). Functional overlap between murine Inpp5b and Ocrl1 may explain why deficiency of the murine ortholog for OCRL1 does not cause Lowe syndrome in mice. *J Clin Invest,* 101, pp. 2042-2053, ISSN 0021-9738

Jentsch TJ. (2002). Chloride channels are different. *Nature,* 415, pp. 276-277, ISSN 0028-0836

Lee BH, Lee SH, Choi HJ, Kang HG, Oh SW, Lee DS, Ha IS, Choi Y, Cheong HI. (2009). Decreased renal uptake of (99m)Tc-DMSA in patients with tubular proteinuria. *Pediatr Nephrol,* 24, pp. 2211-2216, ISSN 0391-6510

Lelouvier B, Puertollano R. Mucolipin-3 regulates luminal calcium, acidification, and membrane fusion in the endosomal pathway. (2011). *J Biol Chem,* 286, 11, pp. 9826-32, ISSN 40169-40176

Lloyd SE, Pearce SH, Fisher SE, Steinmeyer K, Schwappach B, Scheinman SJ, Harding B, Bolino A, Devoto M, Goodyer P, Rigden SP, Wrong O, Jentsch TJ, Craig IW, Thakker RV. (1996). A common molecular basis for three inherited kidney stone diseases. *Nature,* 379, pp. 445-449, ISSN 0028-0836

Lloyd SE, Pearce SH, Günther W, Kawaguchi H, Igarashi T, Jentsch TJ, Thakker RV. (1997). Idiopathic low molecular weight proteinuria associated with hypercalciuric nephrocalcinosis is due to mutations of the renal chloride channel (CLCN5). *J Clin Invest*, 99, pp. 967-974, ISSN 0021-9738

Lloyd-Evans E, Waller-Evans H, Peterneva K, Platt FM. (2010). Endolysosomal calcium regulation. *Biochem Soc Trans*, 38, pp. 1458-1464, ISSN 0300-5127

Ludwig M, Waldegger S, Nuutinen M, Bökenkamp A, Reissinger A, Steckelbroeck S, Utsch B. (2003). Four additional *CLCN5* exons encode a widely expressed novel long ClC-5 isoform but fail to explain Dent's phenotype in patients without mutations in the short variant. *Kidney Blood Press Res*, 26, pp. 176-184, ISSN 1420-4096

Ludwig M, Utsch B. (2004). Dent disease-like phenotype and the chloride channel ClC-4 (*CLCN4*) gene. *Am J Med Genet A*, 128A, pp. 434-435, ISSN 0148-7299

Ludwig M, Doroszewicz J, Seyberth HW, Bökenkamp A, Balluch B, Nuutinen M, Utsch B, Waldegger S. (2005). Functional evaluation of Dent's disease-causing mutations: implications for ClC-5 channel trafficking and internalization. *Hum Genet*, 117, pp. 228-237, ISSN 1018-4813

Ludwig M, Utsch B, Balluch B, Fründ S, Kuwertz-Bröking E, Bökenkamp A. (2006). Hypercalciuria in patients with *CLCN5* mutation. *Pediatr Nephrol*, 21, pp. 1241-1250, ISSN 0391-6510

Ludwig M, Utsch B, Monnens LAH. (2006) Recent advances in understanding the clinical and genetic heterogeneity of Dent's disease. *Nephrol Dial Transplant*, 21, pp. 2708-2717, ISSN 0931-0509

Ludwig M, Refke M, Draaken M, Pasternack S, Betz RC, Reutter H (2011). `Full-blown´ Lowe syndrome without congenital cataracts in a patient with an *OCRL* p.Gln199X mutation and a silent variant, p.Arg35Arg. *Poster presented at the European Human Genetics Conference (ESHG)*, Amsterdam, (2011)

Martina JA, Lelouvier B, Puertollano R. (2009). The calcium channel mucolipin-3 is a novel regulator of trafficking along the endosomal pathway. *Traffic*, 10, pp. 1143-1156, ISSN 1600-0854

Mohammad-Panah R, Harrison R, Dhani S, Ackerley C, Huan LJ, Wang Y, Bear CE. (2003). The chloride channel ClC-4 contributes to endosomal acidification and trafficking. *J Biol Chem*, 278, pp. 29267-29277, ISSN 40169-40176

Nakamura N, Tanaka S, Teko Y, Mitsui K, Kanazawa H. (2005). Four Na+/H+ exchanger isoforms are distributed to Golgi and post-Golgi compartments and are involved in organelle pH regulation. *J Biol Chem*, 280, pp. 1561-1572, ISSN 40169-40176

Nakazato H, Hattori S, Furuse A, Kawano T, Karashima S, Tsuruta M, Yoshimuta J, Endo F, Matsuda I. (1997). Mutation in the CLCN5 gene in Japanese patients with familial idiopathic low molecular weight proteinuria. *Kidney Int*, 52, pp. 895-900, ISSN 0085-2538

Norden AG, Lapsley M, Lee PJ, Pusey CD, Scheinman SJ, Tam FW, Thakker RV, Unwin RJ, Wrong O. (2001). Glomerular protein sieving and implication for renal failure in Fanconi syndrome. *Kidney Int*, 60, 5, pp. 1885-92, ISSN 0085-2538

Novarino G, Weinert S, Rickheit G, Jentsch TJ. (2010). Endosomal chloride-proton exchange rather than chloride conductance is crucial for renal endocytosis. *Science*, 328, pp. 1398-1401, ISSN 0036-8075

Numata M, Petrecca K, Lake N, Orlowski J. (1998). Identification of a mitochondrial Na+/H+ exchanger. *J Biol Chem*, 273, pp. 6951-6959, ISSN 40169-40176

Nussbaum RL, Orrison BM, Jänne PA, Charnas L, Chinault AC. (1997). Physical mapping and genomic structure of the Lowe syndrome gene OCRL1. *Hum Genet*, 99, pp. 145-150, ISSN 1018-4813

Picollo A, Pusch M. (2005). Chloride/proton antiporter activity of mammalian ClC proteins ClC-4 and ClC-5. *Nature*, 436, pp. 420-423, ISSN 0028-0836

Plans V, Rickheit G, Jentsch TJ. (2009). Physiological roles of ClC CL^{-}/H^{+} exchangers in renal proximal tubules. *Eur J Physiol*, 458, pp. 23-37, ISSN 0301-5548

Puertollano R, Kiselyov K. (2009). TRPMLs: in sickness and in health. *Am J Physiol Renal Physiol*, 296, pp. 1245-1254, ISSN 0363-6127

Raja KA, Schurman S, D'mello RG, Blowey D, Goodyer P, Van Why S, Ploutz-Snyder RJ, Asplin J, Scheinman SJ. (2002). Responsiveness of hypercalciuria to thiazide in Dent's disease. *J Am Soc Nephrol*, 13, pp. 2938–2944, ISSN 1046-6673

Reed AA, Loh NY, Terryn S, Lippiat JD, Partridge C, Galvanovskis J, Williams SE, Jouret F, Wu FT, Courtoy PJ, Nesbit MA, Rorsman P, Devuyst O, Ashcroft FM, Thakker RV. (2010). ClC-5 and KIF3B interact to facilitate ClC-5 plasma membrane expression, endocytosis, and microtubular transport: relevance to pathophysiology of Dent's disease. *Am J Physiol Renal Physiol*, 298, p. F365-F380, ISSN 0363-6127

Reinhart SC, Norden AG, Lapsley M, Thakker RV, Pang J, Moses AM, Frymoyer PA, Favus MJ, Hoepner JA, Scheinman SJ. (1995). Characterization of carrier females and affected males with X-linked recessive nephrolithiasis. *J Am Soc Nephrol*, 5, pp. 1451-1461, ISSN 1046-6673

Saito M, Hanson PI, Schlesinger P. (2007). Luminal chloride-dependent activation of endosome calcium channels. Patch clamp study of enlarged endosomes. *J Biol Chem*, 282, pp. 27327-27333, ISSN 0021-9258

Sayer JA, Carr G, Pearce SH, Goodship TH, Simmons NL. (2003). Disordered calcium crystal handling in antisense ClC-5-treated collecting duct cells. *Biochem Biophys Res Commun*, 300, pp. 305-310, ISSN 0006-291X

Sayer JA, Carr G, Simmons NL. (2004). Calcium phosphate and calcium oxalate crystal handling is dependent upon ClC-5 expression in mouse collecting duct cells. *Biochem Biophys Acta*, 1689, pp. 83-90, ISSN 0006-3002

Scheel O, Zdebik AA, Lourdel S, Jentsch TJ. (2005). Voltage-dependent electrogenic chloride/proton exchange by endosomal ClC proteins. *Nature*, 436, pp. 424-427, ISSN 1471-0072

Scheinman SJ. (1998) X-linked hypercalciuric nephrolithiasis: clinical syndromes and chloride channel mutations. *Kidney Int*, 53, pp. 3-17, ISSN 0085-2538

Scheinman SJ, Cox JP, Lloyd SE, Pearce SH, Salenger PV, Hoopes RR, Bushinsky DA, Wrong O, Asplin JR, Langman CB, Norden AG, Thakker RV. (2000). Isolated hypercalciuria with mutation in CLCN5: Relevance to idiopathic hypercalciuria. *Kidney Int*, 57, pp. 232-239, ISSN 0085-2538.

Schwake M, Friedrich T, Jentsch TJ. (2001). An internalization signal in ClC-5, an endosomal Cl^{-} channel mutated in Dent's disease. *J Biol Chem*, 276, pp. 12049-12054, ISSN 0021-9258

Schwappach B, Stobrawa S, Hechenberger M, Steinmeyer K, Jentsch TJ. (1998). Golgi localization and functionally important domains in the NH_2 and COOH terminus of the yeast CLC putative chloride channel Gef1p. *J Biol Chem*, 273, pp. 15110-15118, ISSN 0021-9258

Scott CC, Gruenberg J. (2010). Ion flux and the function of endosomes and lysosomes: pH is just the start. *Bioessays*, 33, pp. 103-110, ISSN 0265-9247

Scott JW, Hawley SA, Green KA, Anis M, Stewart G, Scullion GA, Norman DG, Hardie DG. (2004). CBS domains form energy-sensing modules whose binding of adenosine ligands is disrupted by disease mutations. *J Clin Invest*, 113, pp. 274-284, ISSN 0021-9738

Smith AJ, Reed AA, Loh NY, Thakker RV, Lippiat JD. (2009). Characterization of Dent's disease mutations of CLC-5 reveals a correlation between functional and cell biological consequences and protein structure. *Am J Physiol Renal Physiol*, 296, pp. 390-397, ISSN 0363-6127

Smith AJ, Lippiat JD. (2010). Direct endosomal acidification by the outwardly rectifying CLC-5 $Cl^{(-)}/H^{(+)}$ exchanger. *J Physiol*, 588, pp. 2033-2045, ISSN 0022-3751

Sonawane ND, Thiagarajah JR, Verkman AS. (2002). Chloride concentration in endosomes measured using a rationable fluorescent Cl^- indicator. *J Biol Chem*, 277, pp. 5506-5513, ISSN 0021-9258

Tosetto E, Addis M, Caridi G, Meloni C, Emma F, Vergine G, Stringini G, Papalia T, Barbano G, Ghiggeri GM, Ruggeri L, Miglietti N, D Angelo A, Melis MA, Anglani F. (2009). Locus heterogeneity of Dent's disease: *OCRL1* and *TMEM27* genes in patients with no *CLCN5* mutations. *Pediatr Nephrol*, 24, pp. 1967-1973, ISSN 0391-6510

Utsch B, Bökenkamp A, Benz MR, Besbas N, Dötsch J, Franke I, Fründ S, Gok F, Hoppe B, Karle S, Kuwertz-Bröking E, Laube G, Neb M, Nuutinen M, Ozaltin F, Rascher W, Ring T, Tasic V, van Wijk JA, Ludwig M. (2006). Novel *OCRL1* mutations in patients with the phenotype of Dent disease. *Am J Kidney Dis*, 48, 942, pp. 1-14, ISSN 0272-6386

Vicinanza M, Angelo G D, Di Campli A, De Matteis MA (2008). Phosphoinositides as regulators of membrane trafficking in health and disease. *Cell. Mol. Life Sci.* 65, pp. 2833 - 2841, ISSN 1420-682X

Wang SS, Devuyst O, Courtoy PJ, Wang XT, Wang H, Wang Y, Thakker RV, Guggino S, Guggino WB. (2000). Mice lacking renal chloride channel, CLC-5, are a model for Dent's disease, a nephrolithiasis disorder associated with defective receptor-mediated endocytosis. *Hum Mol Genet*, 9, pp. 2937-45, ISSNISSN 0964-6906

Wang Y, Bartlett MC, Loo TW, Clarke DM. (2006). Specific rescue of cystic fibrosis transmembrane conductance regulator processing mutants using pharmacological chaperones. *Mol Pharmacol*, 70, pp. 297-302, ISSN 0026-895X

Wellhauser LD, Ántonio C, Bear CE. (2010) CLC transporters: discoveries and challenges in defining the mechanisms underlying function and regulation of CLC-5. *Pflugers Arch.*, 460, pp. 543-557, ISSN 0301-5548

Wrong OM, Norden AG, Feest TG. (1994). Dent's disease; a familial proximal renal tubular syndrome with low-molecular-weight proteinuria, hypercalciuria, nephrocalcinosis, metabolic bone disease, progressive renal failure and a marked male predominance. *Q J Med*, 87, pp. 473-493, ISSN 1460-2725

Wu F, Reed AA, Williams SE, Loh NY, Lippiat JD, Christie PT, Large O, Bettinelli A, Dillon MJ, Goldraich NP, Hoppe B, Lhotta K, Loirat C, Malik R, Morel D, Kotanko P, Roussel B, Rubinger D, Schrander-Stumpel C, Serdaroglu E, Nesbit MA, Ashcroft F,

Thakker RV. (2009). Mutational analysis of CLC-5, cofilin and CLC-4 in patients with Dent's disease. *Nephron Physiol,* 112, pp. 53-62, ISSN 1660-8151

Wu F, Roche P, Christie PT, Loh NY, Reed AA, Esnouf RM, Thakker RV. (2003). Modeling study of human renal chloride channel (hCLC-5) mutations suggests a structural-functional relationship. *Kidney Int,* 63, pp. 1426-1432, ISSN 0085-2538

Yasui M, Hazama A, Kwon TH, Nielsen S, Guggino WB, Agre P. (1999). Rapid gating and anion permeability of an intracellular aquaporin. *Nature,* 402, pp. 184-187, ISSN 0028-0836

Zifarelli G, Pusch M. (2009). Conversion of the 2 Cl-/1 H+ antiporter ClC5 in a NO3-/H+ antiporter by a single point mutation. *EMBO J,* 28, pp. 175-182, ISSN 0261-4189

Part 3

Systemic Diseases of Kidney

3

Plasma Concentration of Adipokines, Obstructive Sleep Apnea Syndrome and Chronic Kidney Disease in Patients with Metabolic Syndrome and Non-Alcoholic Fatty Liver Disease

Mariya Severova et al.*
I. M. Sechenov First Moscow Medical State University
Russian Federation

1. Introduction

It is widely accepted that manifestation of target organs damage in patients with metabolic syndrome (MS) often has simultaneous and rapid pattern. Non-alcoholic fatty liver disease (NAFLD) has been described as one of metabolic syndrome-induced target organ damage. NAFLD clinical manifestations vary from ultrasonographically detected liver steatosis to non-alcoholic steatohepatitis (NASH) (Sowers, 2008). Detailed analysis of NAFLD relationship with other organs impairment in MS patients is particularly important for diagnostic procedures adjustment and optimization of treatment.

Different experimental and clinical research data demonstrate strict relation between NAFLD and chronic kidney disease (CKD). In a population study including more than 8,000 healthy men, recruited in South Korea, NAFLD with elevated serum gamma-glutamyltransferase (GGT) concentration was associated with an increased CKD risk among nondiabetic, nonhypertensive men, irrespective of metabolic syndrome. The association was evident even after adjustment for age, glomerular filtration rate (GFR), triglycerides, and high-density lipoprotein cholesterol (Chang et al., 2008). Another study data suggested that NAFLD is associated with an increased prevalence of CKD in type 2 diabetic individuals independent from numerous baseline confounding factors (Targher et al., 2008).

Presence of association between NAFLD and CKD revealed similar risk factors and rate of their coexistence in MS patients and could be explained by similar development mechanisms. Multiple mediators known as adipokines expressed are secreted by adipocytes and play an important role in the induction of endothelial dysfunction, tissue hypertrophy and fibrosis even at an early stage of target organ damage (Antuna-Puente et al., 2008). Pair

* Evgeniya Saginova[1], Marat Galliamov[2], Nickolay Ermakov[3], Alla Rodina[1,3], Mikhail Severov[1], Andrey Pulin[1], Viktor Fomin[1] and Nikolay Mukhin[1]
[1]*I.M. Sechenov First Moscow Medical State University*
[2]*Lomonosov Moscow State University*
[3]*Moscow Scientific Research Institute of Medical Ecology*
Russian Federation

of adipokines - leptin and adiponectin are physiological antagonists. Combination of leptin hyperproduction and peripheral tissues resistance to it in patients with abdominal type of obesity is paired with protector insufficiency - adiponectin. It leads to progression of dysmetabolism, particularly insulin resistance development and organ remodeling intensification (Anubhuti & Arora, 2008; Han et al., 2009). Obstructive sleep apnea syndrome (OSAS) could be integral pathogenetic chain in CKD and NAFLD (Tokuda et al., 2008). Investigation of correlation between plasma leptin and adiponectin concentrations, OSAS and CKD development in NAFLD patients gives opportunity to get closer to mechanisms of target organs damage in MS with subsequent optimization of prophylactic strategy.

2. Materials and methods

Research involved 86 patients (64 males and 22 females) with MS diagnosed according to standard criteria (Alberti et al., 2006) and NAFLD (ultrasonic proven liver steatosis in combination with elevated transaminases, GGT and/or alkaline phosphatase level increase without signs of viral hepatitis or other diseases with hepatic manifestation).

All the patients had abdominal obesity (waist circumference (WC) >94 cm in males and >80 cm in females (Alberti et al., 2006)). Mean age was 44.0±11.0.

Along with general investigation all patients were tested for common risk factors presence and severity (Mancia et al., 2009). Blood pressure was measured using a standard mercury sphygmomanometer under standard conditions as mentioned in cardiovascular survey methods. Each person was examined for height, weight and WC without shoes with minimal clothing as per cardiovascular survey methods. Body mass index (BMI) was calculated by formula of weight in kg/height m^2. All patients underwent biochemical tests: concentrations of HDL cholesterol, LDL cholesterol, VLDL cholesterol, total cholesterol and triglycerides (Biosystems S.A. kit, Spain) were measured on automatic analyzer Beckman Synchron Clinical System CX5delta; also atherogenic index was calculated using equation: atherogenic index = (total cholesterol - HDL cholesterol) / HDL cholesterol.

Presence and grade of insulin resistance and disturbances of carbohydrates metabolism related to it were estimated by fasting serum glucose level (Biosystems S.A. kit, Spain), C-peptide (DPC kit, USA), fasting insulin serum concentration (DPC kit, USA) and HOMA-index calculation (fasting glucose (mmol/L) x insulin (IU/mL) / 22.5).

Plasma concentration of adipokines - leptin and adiponectin were measured by immune-enzyme analysis ("Human Adiponectin ELISA" (BioVendor GmbH, Germany), "Leptin (Sandwich) Elisa" (DRG, USA)).

Signs of target organs damage were registered according to standard recommendations (Alberti et al., 2006): left ventricular hypertrophy was diagnosed echocardiographically using Sokolow-Lyon criteria and left ventricular mass index (Acuson Sequoia 512 (Siemens Acuson, USA)); atherosclerotic involvement of carotid artery was diagnosed by ultrasonic investigation of carotid artery intima-media thickness (CIMT) and/or by detection of atherosclerotic plaque in its wall (ESAOTE (Technos MPX, Italy)); albuminuria was estimated using nephelometric assay (Immage Immunochemistry Systems, Beckman Coulter, USA), GFR was estimated using MDRD formula.

For statistical processing data were analysed by STATISTICA 8.0 (StatSoft, Russia). Various numbers are given as mean value and standard deviation (for normal distribution); median value and interquartile range (for asymmetric distribution). Categorical variables have been compared by parametric and nonparametric methods. The Pvalue < 0.05 was considered as significant.

3. Results

Patients were divided into two groups depending on stage of NAFLD: 48 subjects with clinically unsuspected liver steatosis detected only by ultrasonic investigation and 38 subjects with signs of NASH. Transaminases and G-GT serum levels were comparatively higher in patients with NASH (Table 1), whereas De Ritis ratio was comparatively higher in patients with liver steatosis.

	NASH(n=38)	Liver steatosis (n=48)
AST, IU/mL	54±31*	24±8
ALT, UI/mL	99±73*	32±17
De Ritis ratio	0.6±0.2*	0.8±0.2
G-GT, IU/mL	97±65*	47±30

Table 1. Serum AST, ALT, G-GT levels and De Ritis ratio in patients with MS and NAFLD (n=86). * P<0.001

Comparison of CKD and NASH prevalence rate according to number of damaged target organs revealed that both CKD and NASH prevalence was significantly higher in group of patients with ≥3 target organ damage (Table 2) and lower in other groups (patients with 1 or 2 target organ damage). The patients with 2 and ≥3 target organ damage showed significant increase in albuminuria level. There was no significant difference in plasma concentrations of adiponectin and leptin in all the groups, but ratio leptinemia/adiponectinemia increased significantly in concordance with number of damaged target organ and reached maximum in patients with ≥3 target organ damage.

	1 target organ damage (n=18)	2 target organ damage (n=39)	≥3 target organ damage (n=18)
CKD rate, %	17% P<0.05 vs 2 и ≥3	44%	67%
NASH rate, %	39% P<0.05 vs ≥3	44%	78% P<0.05 vs 2
Albumiuria, mg/24h	6.0 (4.3 - 9.0) P<0.05 vs 2 and ≥3	12.6 (8.0 - 38.0)	30.2 (17.3 - 48.0)
Leptin, ng/mL	23.6±23.4	31.6±27.3	31.2±26.0
Adiponectin, μg/mL	31.3±17.5	22.9±20.2	11.8±5.5
Leptin/Adiponectin	1.0±0.8 P<0.05 vs 2 and ≥3	1.7±1.4	3.1±1.6 P<0.05 vs 2

Table 2. CKD and NASH prevalence, albuminuria and adipokines plasma concentration in patients with MS and NAFLD (n=86).

Among all patients with MS and NASH 37.2% (32 patients) were diagnosed CKD, 26 of them had microalbuminuria, 6 subjects had urinary albumin excretion over 300 mg/24h. Five patients had CKD III stage (GFR <60 mL/min/1.73m^2), all of them also had signs of NASH. Patients with MS, NAFLD and CKD showed marked insulin resistance: fasting insulinemia level, HOMA index and plasma C-peptide concentration in this type of patients were higher than in patients with NAFLD without CKD (Table 3). Moreover in patients with MS, NAFLD and CKD registered significantly higher plasma leptin level.

	Patients with CKD (n=32)	Patients without CKD (n=54)
Insulin, µU/mL	16.8±9.2	11.5±5.6**
HOMA index	4.2±2.2	2.9±1.5**
C-peptide, pmol/L	1326±411	999±341***
Leptin, ng/mL	38.2±28.8	21.6±19.8*
Adiponectin, µg/mL	23.7±19.5	18.1±14.8
Leptin/Adiponectin	2.15±1.58	1.71±1.52

Table 3. Comparison of insulin resistance and plasma adipokines levels in patients with MS and NAFLD in case of CKD presence or absence. *-P=0.003; **-P=0.002; ***-P<0.001.

Correlation analysis showed direct correlation of leptin concentration and BMI, systolic blood pressure, adiponectin level and albumiuria (Table 4). Adiponectin level correlated directly with leptin level, serum HDL cholesterol concentration and De Ritis ratio. Inverse correlation was registered between atherogenic index, CIMT and serum level of adiponectin.

Parameter	Leptin	Adiponectin
BMI	r = 0.27*	r = 0.29
WC	r = 0.21	r = 0.33
Systolic blood pressure	r = 0.24*	r = 0.10
Atherogenic index	r = -0.14	r = -0.43*
HDL cholesterol	r = 0.18	r = 0.43*
CIMT	r = -0.04	r = -0.38*
HOMA index	r = 0.32*	r = -0.18
C-peptide	r = 0.29*	r = -0.02
Insulin	r = 0.35*	r = -0.10
De Ritis ratio	r = 0.13	r = 0.36*
Leptin	-	r = 0.39*
Adiponectin	r = 0.39*	-
Albuminuria	r = 0.28*	r = 0.19

Table 4. Correlation of plasma adipokines concentration with MS criteria and target organs damage in patients with MS and NAFLD (n=86). * - significant correlations

OSAS was diagnosed in 20 (24%) patients (Table 5). These patients had significantly higher blood pressure, BMI, WC, fasting insulin serum concentration and C-peptide. Obese patients with OSAS demonstrated significantly marked target organs damage signs (higher level of albuminuria and lower GFR) in comparison with obese patients without OSAS. Also obese patients with CKD developed OSAS more frequent than obese patients without CKD (38% and 15% respectively, P=0.018).

Index	OSAS	
	Presence (n=20)	Absence (n=66)
Male/female	17/3	47/19
Mean age, years old	45±10	43±11
Mean blood pressure, mm/Hg	106±9	100±9
BMI, kg/m^2	39.8±7.9**	31.5±4.3
WC, cm	125±17**	108±11
HOMA-index	4.1±1.9*	3.1±1.9
C-peptide, pmol/L	1337±422*	1092±384
Leptin, ng/mL	36.7±29.9	25.3±23.0
Adiponectin, µg/mL	20.4±10.8	21.2±19.1
Insulin, µU/mL	16.9±7.8*	12.7±7.3
Albuminuria, mg/24h	21.0 (12.0;38.4)*	10.3 (6.3;19.4)
GFR, mL/min/$1.73m^2$	81±17*	95±24

Table 5. Clinical and laboratory characteristics of patients with MS and NAFLD (n=86) in case of OSAS presence or absence. *-P<0.05; **-P<0.001

4. Discussion

According to our data an increase of target organs damage in patients with MS and NAFLD leads to an increase of CKD and NASH development rate and albuminuria level. Relationship of NAFLD and albuminuria was also shown in other clinical invetigations. Hwang S.T. et al. examined 1361 patients with type 2 diabetes mellitus and prediabetes (Hwang et al., 2010).

The patients with NAFLD had higher prevalence rates of microalbuminuria (6.3% vs 19%; P=0.001 in prediabetes, 4.5% vs 32.6%; P<0.001 in diabetes) and also had a greater albumin-to-creatinine ratio (14.6 +/- 52.0 µg/mg Cr vs 27.7 +/- 63.9 µg/mg Cr; P=0.051 in prediabetes, 11.4 +/- 21.4 µg/mg Cr vs 44.7 +/- 76.4 µg/mg Cr; P<0.001 in diabetes) than those without NAFLD. NAFLD was associated with 3.66 (P=0.013) times higher rate of microalbuminuria in prediabetes patients and 5.47 (P=0.048) times higher in diabetes patients. Our patients with MS and NAFLD showed highest albuminuria level in the group with highest NASH prevalence rate. Leptin/adiponectin ratio raised significantly in observed by our team patients with MS and NAFLD when albuminuria level and NASH prevalence rate increased. It probably indicates that increased expression of tissue-destructive adipokine - leptin is not combined with adequate plasma concentration increase of protective adipokine - adiponectin. It was shown that the increase of leptin/adiponectin ratio is associated with increase of visceral fat mass, MS prevalence (Kumagai et al., 2005) and severity of insulin resistance (Oda et al., 2008).

Both insufficient adiponectin effect and leptin hyperproduction predetermine the increase of insulin resistance. It reaches maximum level in the group of patients with NAFLD and CKD demonstrating highest values of fasting insulin serum concentration, C-peptide and HOMA-index. Evidently insulin resistance in such patients is caused mainly by leptin excess (Anubhuti & Arora, 2008), which maximal plasma concentration registered in patients with NAFLD and CKD. Leptin contribution to insulin resistance of peripheral tissues intensification is more evident as NAFLD progresses and CKD develops, adiponectin plasma concentration and its tissue protective effect gradually decrease (this is also evidenced by our observation of significant leptin/adiponectin ratio increase). It should be noted that leptin mainly shows properties similar to insulin excess and hereby comes into synergic effect with it, in particular by inducing expression of profibrogenic chemokines in target tissues (e.g. transforming growth factor beta (TGF-β)) leading to tissue fibrosis development. Currently, the role of leptin in kidney tissue firosis development is clear (Wolf & Ziyadeh, 2006), pathogenetic role of obesity as CKD risk factor in general population determined in several epidemiological investigations (Foster et al., 2008; Kramer et al., 2005) could be explained by consequences of hyperleptinemia (similar as adiponectin insufficiency). It was also shown that leptin directly increases fibrogenesis in liver tissue in patients with NAFLD. Ikejima K. et al. demonstrated leptin key role in stimulation of TGF-β mRNA expression in Kupffer cells and sinusoidal endothelial cells in rodents with genetically determined leptin and leptin receptor deficiency (Ikejima et al., 2005). Moreover, leptin augmented platelet derived growth factor-dependent proliferation of hepatic stellate cells by enhancing downstream intracellular signaling pathways. Hereby NAFLD and CKD progression in patients with MS is determined mainly by profibrogenic effect of leptin and excess of insulin.

Along with indicated above, leptin and insulin induced endothelial dysfunction could stand as another common mechanism of NAFLD and CKD development. Increasing albuminuria– is a local kidney marker of endothelial dysfunction. It was proved, that hyperleptinemia directly related to microalbuminuria in patients with abdominal obesity (Ikee et al., 2008). Close associations of NAFLD with global impairment of endothelial function were estimated. Thus, examination of 250 obese children showed that presence of NAFLD entails more severe functional and anatomic changes in the arterial wall. Flow-mediated vasodilatation of brachial artery (one of the signs of endothelial dysfunction) was remarkably reduced and CIMT was increased in obese subjects with confirmed MS and NAFLD (Pacifico et al., 2010). Hypertensive patients with NAFLD have a reduced endothelium-dependent vasodilation and highest insulin resistance in comparison with hypertensive patients without NAFLD. In keeping with this, it is possible to hypothesize that liver steatosis may be considered a marker of vascular damage in essential hypertension (Sciacqua et al., 2010). Integrally, NAFLD presence in patients with MS is always combined with the most pronounced endothelial dysfunction, which mainly predetermines intensity of other target organs remodeling, including kidney. The role of hepatic endothelial cells impaired function, related to hyperleptinemia, insulin resistance and insufficient effects of adiponectin, in progression of NAFLD could not be completely excluded. Development of specific laboratory investigation methods is necessary to evaluate their contribution.

Relationships between NAFLD and CKD revealed in this research in patients with MS could be explained by an imbalanced action of antagonistic adipokines – leptin and adiponectin – and combined with it the intensification of insulin resistance. Taking into consideration our correlation analysis data leptin plasma concentration directly correlates with body mass; in parallel with it - insulin resistance and albuminuria. In addition hyperleptinemia is associated with an increased blood pressure. Hypertensive effect of leptin was confirmed in general population. During one of the phases of prospective population investigation - Copenhagen City Heart Study - new-onset hypertension was examined in 620 women and 300 men who were normotensive in the previous examination, which was performed in 1991-1994 (Asferg et al., 2010). Leptin plasma concentration was significantly associated with new-onset hypertension (odds ratio of 1.28 (1.08-1.53; $P < 0.005$) for 1 s.d. higher level of log-transformed leptin), whereas adiponectin was not significantly associated with new-onset hypertension. Adiponectin plasma concentration directly correlated with concentration of HDL cholesterol, and correlated inversely with CIMT and atherogenic index. Our data matches generally accepted conception of adiponectin antiatherogenic properties and its ability to withstand intensification of metabolic disorders, particularly insulin resistance in patients with MS (Han et al., 2009).

Direct correlation between adiponectinemia and De Ritis ratio demonstrated in our study shows inhibitory action of adiponectin on NAFLD progression rate. In case of NASH onset in such patients adiponectin plasma concentration and level of its expression by liver tissue significantly decrease (Jiang et al., 2009; Ma et al., 2009). Thereby leptin/adiponectin imbalance may be regarded as one of the most important mechanisms of organ damage including CKD and NAFLD in patients with MS.

OSAS had a special place among other independent risk factors of CKD severity and progression in patients with MS and NAFLD examined by our team. Patients with OSAS showed maximum levels of insulin resistance markers and exactly those subjects demonstrated the highest albuminuria level and a lower level of estimated GFR in comparison with groups of patients with MS without OSAS. Recently OSAS has been considered as one of "most malignant" variant of MS, during which both target organ damage rate and severity of metabolic impairments could reach maximal intensity. Highest expression levels of adipokines with tissue-destructive effect, in particular - leptin were registered in patients with OSAS. Presence of direct significant correlation between leptin plasma concentration and apnea/hypopnea index was evaluated in patients with OSAS (Tokuda et al., 2008). Stepwise multiple regression analysis showed that BMI ($r=0.807$, $p<0.0001$), the percentage of time with less than 90% hemoglobin saturation level in total sleep time (%T<90)($r=0.399$, $p<0.001$) and apnea/hypopnea index ($r=0.552$, $p<0.001$) were determinant factors for serum leptin levels. Thus, hyperleptinemia raised as OSAS severity and BMI increased. Among the patients who had successful surgical correction of OSAS (uvulopalatopharyngoplasty; or uvulopalatopharyngoplasty and tonsillectomy; or uvulopalatopharyngoplasty, tonsillectomy and radiofrequency ablation of the base of the tongue) leptin and other adipokines with similar effect (interleukin-6. tumor necrosis factor-alfa) plasma concentration dramatically decreased, whereas adiponectin plasma concentration significantly increased after surgery (Adeseun & Rosas, 2010).

Typical for OSAS adipokines hyperproduction leads to the enhancement of target organ damage development. It was confirmed in multiple clinical and epidemiological investigations. In this way OSAS is considered as one of CKD risk factors (Eun et al., 2010). Patients with OSAS demonstrate significantly lower estimated GFR in comparison with patients without OSAS (84.57 and 94.67 mL/min/1.73m^2 respectively, $P=0.037$) (Fleischmann et al., 2010). Patients with estimated GFR <60 mL/min/1.73m^2 show 6 times higher frequency of central apnea episodes in comparison with group of patients with estimated GFR >60 mL/min/1.73m^2. Presence of OSAS as concomitant condition in our patients with NAFLD was associated with significant decrease of estimated GFR which was calculated using MDRD formula. Thereby this category of patients should be subjected to medical examination at first visit for detection of early stages of CKD (assessment of albuminuria level, estimated GFR, including new markers for GFR estimation, particularly cystatin C).

5. Conclusion

The results of our study indicate that in patients with MS a relationship exists between NAFLD and CKD: NASH development is closely related to increase in albuminuria levels. Association of NAFLD and CKD in patients with MS may be explained by mutual mechanisms of onset and progression, among which should be mentioned hyperleptinemia, lack of adiponectin effects and related to it increase of insulin resistance. From this point of view all the patients with MS and NAFLD must be checked for CKD signs (albuminuria, serum creatinine, estimated GFR). Dynamical changes of these markers could play the role of efficacy indicators of integral therapeutic approaches, e.g. medications for treatment of obesity (orlistat), oral hypoglycemic agents (metformin), antihyperlipidemic agents (statins, fenofibrate) and also several antihypertensive drugs (angiotensin receptor blockers).

6. References

Adeseun, G.A. & Rosas, S.E. (2010). The impact of obstructive sleep apnea on chronic kidney disease. *Curr. Hypertens. Rep.*, Vol.12, No.5, (October 2010), pp. 378-383, ISSN 1522-6417

Alberti, K.G.; Zimmet, P. & Shaw, J. (2006). Metabolic syndrome - a new world-wide definition. A Consensus Statement from the International Diabetes Federation. *Diabet. Med*, Vol.23, No.5, (May 2006), pp. 469-480, ISSN 1464-5491

Antuna-Puente, B.; Feve, B.; Fellahi, S. & Bastard J.P. (2008). Adipokines: the missing link between insulin resistance and obesity. *Diabetes Metab.*, Vol.34, No.1, (February 2008), pp. 2-11, ISSN 1878-1780

Anubhuti & Arora, S. (2008). Leptin and its metabolic interactions: an update. *Diabetes Obes. Metab.*, Vol.10, No.11, (November 2008), pp. 973-993, ISSN 1463-1326

Asferg. C.; Møgelvang, R.; Flyvbjerg, A.; Frystyk, J.; Jensen, J.S.; Marott, J.L.; Appleyard, M.; Jensen, G.B. & Jeppesen, J. (2009). Leptin, not adiponectin, predicts hypertension in the Copenhagen City Heart Study. *Am. J. Hypertens.*, Vol.23, No.3, (March 2010), pp. 327-333, ISSN 0895-7061

Chang, Y.; Ryu, S.; Sung, E.; Woo, H.Y.; Oh, E.; Cha, K.; Jung, E. & Kim, W.S. (2008). Nonalcoholic fatty liver disease predicts chronic kidney disease in nonhypertensive and nondiabetic Korean men. *Metabolism,* Vol.57, No.4, (April 2008), pp. 569-576, ISSN 1532-8600

Eun, Y.G.; Kim, M.G.; Kwon, K.H.; Shin, S.Y.; Cho, J.S. & Kim, S.W. (2010). Short-term effect of multilevel surgery on adipokines and pro-inflammatory cytokines in patients with obstructive sleep apnea. *Acta Otolaryngol.*, Vol.130, No.12, (December 2010), pp. 1394-1398, ISSN 0001-6489

Fleischmann, G.; Fillafer, G.; Matterer, H.; Skrabal, F. & Kotanko, P. (2009). Prevalence of chronic kidney disease in patients with suspected sleep apnoea. *Nephrol. Dial. Transplant.*, Vol.25, No.1, (January 2010), pp. 181-186, ISSN 0931-0509

Foster, M.C.; Hwang, S.J.; Larson, M.G.; Lichtman, J.H.; Parikh, N.I.; Vasan, R.S.; Levy, D. & Fox, C.S. (2008). Overweight, obesity, and the development of stage 3 CKD: the Framingham Heart Study. *Am J Kidney Dis.*, Vol.52, No.1, (July 2008), pp. 39-48, ISSN 0272-6386

Han, S.H.; Sakuma, I.; Shin, E.K. & Koh, K.K. (2009). Antiatherosclerotic and anti-insulin resistance effects of adiponectin: basic and clinical studies. *Prog Cardiovasc Dis*, Vol.52, No.2, (September-October 2009), pp. 126-140, ISSN 1532-8643

Hwang, S.T.; Cho, Y.K.; Yun, J.W.; Park, J.H.; Kim, H.J.; Park, D.I.; Sohn, C.I.; Jeon, W.K.; Kim, B.I.; Rhee, E.J.; Oh, K.W.; Lee, W.Y. & Jin, W. (2010). Impact of non-alcoholic fatty liver disease on microalbuminuria in patients with prediabetes and diabetes. *Intern. Med. J.*, Vol.40, No.6, (June 2010), pp. 437-442, ISSN 1444-0903

Ikee, R.; Hamasaki, Y.; Oka, M.; Maesato, K.; Mano, T.; Moriya, H.; Ohtake, T. & Kobayashi, S. (2008). Glucose metabolism, insulin resistance, and renal pathology in non-diabetic chronic kidney disease. *Nephron Clin Pract.*, Vol.108, No.2, (February 2008), pp. c163-c168, ISSN 1660-2110

Ikejima, K.; Okumura, K.; Lang, T.; Honda, H.; Abe, W.; Yamashina, S.; Enomoto, N.; Takei, Y. & Sato N. (2005). The role of leptin in progression of non-alcoholic fatty liver disease. *Hepatol. Res.*, Vol.33, No.2, (October 2005), pp. 151-154, ISSN 1386-6346

Jiang, L.L.; Li, L.; Hong, X.F.; Li, Y.M. & Zhang, B.L. (2009). Patients with nonalcoholic fatty liver disease display increased serum resistin levels and decreased adiponectin levels. *Eur. J. Gastroenterol. Hepatol.*, Vol.21, No.6, (June 2009), pp. 662-666, ISSN 0954-691X

Kramer, H.; Luke, A.; Bidani, A.; Cao, G.; Cooper, R. & McGee, D. (2005). Obesity and prevalent and incident CKD: the Hypertension Detection and Follow-Up Program. *Am J Kidney Dis.*, Vol.46, No.4, (October 2005), pp. 587-594, ISSN 0272-6386

Kumagai, S.; Kishimoto, H.; Masatakasuwa; Zou, B. & Harukasasaki. (2005). The leptin to adiponectin ratio is a good biomarker for the prevalence of metabolic syndrome, dependent on visceral fat accumulation and endurance fitness in obese patients with diabetes mellitus. *Metab. Syndr. Relat. Disord.*, Vol.3, No.2, (Summer 2005), pp. 85-94, ISSN 1540-4196

Ma, H.; Gomez, V.; Lu, L.; Yang, X.; Wu, X. & Xiao S.Y. (2008). Expression of adiponectin and its receptors in livers of morbidly obese patients with non-alcoholic fatty liver disease. *J. Gastroenterol. Hepatol.*, Vol.24, No.2, (February 2009), pp. 233-237, ISSN 0815-9319

Mancia, G.; Laurent, S.; Agabiti-Rosei, E.; Ambrosioni, E.; Burnier, M.; Caulfield, M.J.; Cifkova, R.; Clément, D.; Coca, A.; Dominiczak, A.; Erdine, S.; Fagard, R.; Farsang, C.; Grassi, G.; Haller, H.; Heagerty, A.; Kjeldsen, S.E.; Kiowski, W.; Mallion, J.M.; Manolis, A.; Narkiewicz, K.; Nilsson, P.; Olsen, M.H.; Rahn, K.H.; Redon, J.; Rodicio, J.; Ruilope, L.; Schmieder, R.E.; Struijker-Boudier, H.A.; van Zwieten, P.A.; Viigimaa, M. & Zanchetti, A. (2009). Reappraisal of European guidelines on hypertension management: a European Society of Hypertension Task Force document. *J. Hypertens.*, Vol.27, No.11, (November 2009), pp. 2121-2158, ISSN 0263-6352

Oda, N.; Imamura, S.; Fujita, T.; Uchida, Y.; Inagaki, K.; Kakizawa, H.; Hayakawa, N.; Suzuki, A.; Takeda, J.; Horikawa, Y. & Itoh, M. (2008). The ratio of leptin to adiponectin can be used as an index of insulin resistance. *Metabolism.*, Vol.57, No.2, (February 2008), pp. 268-273, ISSN 1532-8600

Pacifico, L.; Anania, C.; Martino, F.; Cantisani, V.; Pascone, R.; Marcantonio, A. & Chiesa, C. (2010). Functional and morphological vascular changes in pediatric nonalcoholic fatty liver disease. *Hepatology,* Vol.52, No.5, (November 2010), pp. 1643-1651, ISSN 0270-9139

Sciacqua, A.; Perticone, M.; Miceli, S.; Laino, I.; Tassone, E.J.; Grembiale, R.D.; Andreozzi, F.; Sesti, G. & Perticone, F. (2010). Endothelial dysfunction and non-alcoholic liver steatosis in hypertensive patients. *Nutr. Metab. Cardiovasc. Dis.*, Vol.21, No.7, (July 2011), pp. 485-491, ISSN 0939-4753

Sowers, J.R. (2008). The cardiomethabolic syndrome and liver disease. *J. Cardiomethab. Syndr.,* Vol.3, No.1, (Winter 2008), pp. 7-11, ISSN 1559-4572

Targher, G.; Bertolini, L.; Rodella, S.; Zoppini, G.; Lippi, G.; Day, C. & Muggeo, M. (2008). Non-alcoholic fatty liver disease is independently associated with an increased prevalence of chronic kidney disease and proliferative/laser-treated retinopathy in type 2 diabetic patients. *Diabetologia,* Vol.51, No.3, (March 2008), pp. 444-450, ISSN 1432-0428

Tokuda, F.; Sando, Y.; Matsui, H.; Koike, H. & Yokoyama, T. (2008). Serum levels of adipocytokines, adiponectin and leptin, in patients with obstructive sleep apnea syndrome. *Intern. Med,* Vol.47, No.21, (November 2008), pp. 1843-1849, ISSN 1349-7235

Wolf, G. & Ziyadeh, F.N. (2006). Leptin and renal fibrosis. *Contrib Nephrol.*, Vol.151, (2006), pp. 175-183, ISSN 0302-5144

4

The Obesity Epidemic and Kidney Disease: A Literature Review

Veeraish Chauhan, Megha Vaid, Nishtha Chauhan and Akhil Parashar
Drexel University College of Medicine, Hahnemann University Hospital, Philadelphia, PA USA

1. Introduction

It is a fact we are all too well aware of. The world, as we know it, continues to grow fat. The popular press has done an excellent job of educating the lay person about the link between obesity and heart disease, hypertension, etc. However, despite scientific evidence to the contrary, the effect of obesity on the kidneys' function is less well-known. Kidney disease from obesity can progress to End Stage Renal Disease (ESRD), which mandates the use of dialysis to keep the patient alive. It is hence a huge risk factor for morbidity and mortality. Last, but not the least, it puts a tremendous economic and social strain on the healthcare resources of nations around the world.

2. The alarming statistics

The World Health Organization (WHO) considers obesity an international epidemic, stating in 1997 that "obesity's impact is so diverse and extreme that it should now be regarded as one of the greatest neglected public health problems of our time with an impact on health which may well prove to be as great as that of smoking." A quick look at the WHO's statistics paints a scary picture of what we are up against. It is hard to imagine that in 2008 almost one-quarter of humanity, or 1.5 billion people, were reported to be overweight (a body mass index greater than or equal to 25). Of these, over 200 million men and 300 million women were obese (body mass index greater than or equal to 30). Obesity, in combination with diabetes, is the largest epidemic the world has ever faced. It is also the fifth leading cause of deaths worldwide, killing 2.8 million people every year. The prevalence of obesity currently ranges from less than 5% in rural China, Japan and some African countries, to levels as high as 75% of the adult population in urban Samoa. 68% of U.S. adults are either overweight or obese. With this enormous health burden worldwide, the deleterious effects of obesity on kidney function are being increasingly recognized.

2.1 Obesity and kidney disease: The weight of the evidence

There now is a well established risk between obesity and the development of kidney disease. The Framingham Offspring data reported obesity as a major risk factor for the development of kidney disease. This was a large study that followed 1223 men and 1362 women (who were initially free of preexisting kidney disease) for a mean period of 18.5 years. At the end of this follow up period, 244 participants (9.4 percent) had developed

kidney disease (defined as estimated glomerular filtration rate (GFR) of less than 64 and 59 mL/min per 1.73 m2 for men and women, respectively). The researchers also reported a 23% increase in the odds of development of kidney disease for each standard deviation increase in the Body Mass Index (BMI). This risk was present even after adjustment for age, sex, smoking, diabetes, and baseline glomerular filtration rate (GFR). Another study by Hsu et al showed that there is a greater relative risk of development of end-stage renal disease (ESRD) necessitating dialysis, with each gradient increase in BMI. Higher BMI was a risk factor for ESRD in multivariable models that adjusted for age, sex, race, education level, smoking status, history of myocardial infarction, serum cholesterol level, urinalysis proteinuria, urinalysis hematuria, and serum creatinine level. Compared with persons who had normal weight (BMI, 18.5 to 24.9 kg/m2), the adjusted relative risk for ESRD was 1.87 (95% CI, 1.64 to 2.14) for those who were overweight (BMI, 25.0 to 29.9 kg/m2), 3.57 (CI, 3.05 to 4.18) for those with class I obesity (BMI, 30.0 to 34.9 kg/m2), 6.12 (CI, 4.97 to 7.54) for those with class II obesity (BMI, 35.0 to 39.9 kg/m2), and 7.07 (CI, 5.37 to 9.31) for those with extreme obesity (BMI > or = 40 kg/m2). Higher baseline BMI remained an independent predictor for ESRD after additional adjustments for baseline blood pressure level and presence or absence of diabetes mellitus.
Similarly, a recent large cohort study of 177570 individuals found obesity to be one of the most potent risk factors for the development of ESRD.

3. How obesity causes kidney disease

Obesity is associated with multiple other conditions that are known to cause compromised renal function, including hypertension, diabetes, hyperuricemia, and the metabolic syndrome that can independently have a detrimental effect on renal function. However, as we can gauge from the evidence quoted in the above section, obesity has been found to cause kidney disease and ESRD even after adjustment for these factors. Hence, the pathogenesis of obesity related kidney disease can be sub-classified in to direct and indirect effects.

3.1 Direct effects of obesity on kidney function

Data from the Framingham Offspring study, the Hypertension Detection and Follow-Up Program, and the Multiphasic Health Testing Services Program suggest that obesity may be independently associated with the risk of developing chronic kidney disease. Obesity seems to cause a change in the renal hemodynamics that promotes progressive kidney disease. These changes begin early in the course of obesity, even before overt renal manifestations of obesity are clinically apparent. This was shown in a landmark study from a center conducting kidney biopsies on obese patients who presented for weight loss/bariatric surgery in Spain. The investigators studied the glomerular architecture in renal biopsies of 95 patients undergoing bariatric surgery for extreme obesity but whose renal function was clinically normal. These subjects had no known prior history of any kidney disease. These patients were then compared with a control group of 40 patients undergoing nephrectomy or donating a kidney, and having protocol biopsies. This second control group had patients who had normal weight and renal function, and were non-diabetic and non-hypertensive. Logistic regression models were then applied to determine associations between the clinical and biochemical variables and glomerular lesions. Focal and segmental glomerulosclerosis (FSGS) was present in only five extremely obese patients but absent in controls. Increased mesangial matrix, podocyte hypertrophy, mesangial cell proliferation, and glomerulomegaly were more frequent in the obese cohort than in the control group. Body mass index was found to be a significant independent risk factor associated with glomerular lesions in all 135 patients and in the 95 extremely obese patients. This was hence an elegant demonstration of the fact that even in patients with no overt clinical renal symptoms, there were a variety of glomerular abnormalities that correlated with body mass, even after adjustment for other factors like high blood pressure, diabetes, metabolic syndrome, and sleep apnea.

3.1.1 The role of adipokines

One of the keys to unravel obesity's effect on the kidneys is understanding the concept of body-fat as an independent endocrine organ, rather than simply a passive storage depot for triglycerides. The overarching factor in this is the dysregulated production of bioactive substances called "adipokines" by adipose cells that cause systemic effects, and directly influence insulin sensitivity and vascular injury.

Adipokines, and other neuro-humoral factors, have already been well studied in the pathogenesis of obesity. Serum levels of adipokines like leptin correlate with the total body fat content. Hence, the levels tend to be higher in the obese. In normal-weight subjects, food intake is reduced by systemic leptin administration, but the response to leptin decreases as the subjects become obese. This leads to a vicious circle of hyperphagia and obesity. Another interesting hormone that plays a role in the pathogenesis of obesity is ghrelin, a peptide produced by the stomach and duodenum. This peptide stimulates growth hormone secretion, and increases food intake in rodents and humans. Serum concentrations are suppressed by food ingestion in normal-weight subjects. However, this suppression is impaired in the obese, leading to increased food intake.

Not surprisingly, dysregulated adipokine production also leads to hemodynamic and structural changes in the kidney, and has been shown to play an important pathophysiologic role in obesity related kidney disease. These adipokines include cytokines like leptin, adiponectin, interleukin-6, tumor necrosis factor-alpha, resistin, and angiotensinogen. Whereas some of these adipokines act in an autocrine or paracrine manner, others act as signaling molecules in remote tissues like liver, skeletal muscle, and endothelium. These cytokines then induce a pro-inflammatory state causing glomerular capillary hypertension, and fibrosis in the renal parenchyma. Of these adipokines, one of the best understood roles is that of angiotensinogen. Angiotensinogen is an α-2-globulin that is produced constitutively, mainly by the liver. However, plasma levels of angiotensin are also positively correlated with body fat mass, indicating increased production of this molecule from adipocytes. In fact, all other components of the renin-angiotensin system (RAS), including renin, angiotensin converting enzyme, angiotensin II, and AT-1 and AT-2 receptors, are expressed as well as secreted from adipocytes. Increased angiotensinogen kick-starts the RAS, and in turn increases the downstream effects of this system, namely, fluid retention and increased vascular tone. Elevated levels of angiotensinogen and angiotensin II then lead to efferent arteriolar constriction in the glomerulus. This increases the intraglomerular pressure, leading to a rise in the GFR. From an evolutionary standpoint, acutely this adaptation served to preserve GFR and prevent low blood pressure in the face of volume depletion. However, over the long term, this effect becomes maladaptive. Raised intraglomerular pressure causes injury to the glomerulus and subsequent hyperfiltration. Eventually, the kidneys start to spill protein in to the urine and begin to undergo permanent irreversible fibrosis.

The relation between RAS and body fat is actually a two-way street. In 1998, Karlsson et al demonstrated that angiotensin-II stimulated preadipocyte differentiation, and hence stimulates adipogenesis. Thus, the RAS itself may also be involved in regulation of body weight and development of obesity. RAS has also been postulated to play an important role in the development of the cardiomyopathy commonly occurring in obesity. The discovery of these mechanisms has had immense clinical implications. Drugs that block the RAS now form the mainstay of treatment to decrease glomerular hyperfiltration and proteinuria, and have found clinical applications in the prevention and treatment of endothelial dysfunction, obesity-related glomerulopathy, diabetic nephropathy, cardiomyopathy etc. Clinical trials of strategies to block the RAS after coronary angioplasty have demonstrated significant decreases in inflammatory markers of systemic inflammation, including IL-6, CRP, and TNF-alpha in response to inhibition of the renin-angiotensin axis.

3.1.2 Other hemodynamic and structural effects

The first large renal-biopsy based clinico-pathologic study on obesity-related kidney disease studied the incidence and structural changes seen in obesity-related glomerulopathy (ORG). This study reviewed 6818 kidney biopsies and reported the presence of structural changes like hyperplasia of the juxta-glomerular apparatus, consistent presence of glomerulomegaly and foot process fusion in patients who were diagnosed to have ORG. Another histologic feature noted in some ORG patients was the presence of focal changes in the form of mild focal mesangial sclerosis or mild focal thickening of glomerular/tubular basement membranes. These changes were not very dissimilar to changes that are more often associated with the presence of diabetic nephropathy.

Obese patients have also been shown to have elevations in both renal plasma flow and GFR. A study investigated differential solute clearances to characterize glomerular function in 12 nondiabetic subjects with severe obesity (body mass index >38). Glomerular filtration rate (GFR) and renal plasma flow (RPF) was found to exceed the control value by 51 and 31%, respectively. Consequently, the filtration fraction was increased as well. The augmented RPF suggests a state of renal vasodilatation involving mainly the afferent arteriole. The analysis suggests that the high GFR in very obese subjects may be the result of an increase in transcapillary hydraulic pressure difference. An abnormal transmission of increased arterial pressure to the glomerular capillaries through a dilated afferent arteriole could account for the augmentation in this transcapillary pressure.

3.2 Indirect effects

Certain co-morbid conditions that come as a "package deal" in patients afflicted with obesity serve as indirect agents of destruction of renal function. The strong association between obesity and the dreaded metabolic syndrome, hypertension, diabetes, hyperuricemia, dyslipidemia, and sleep apnea indirectly has deleterious effects on kidney function.

3.2.1 Effect of hypertension on kidney function

Long standing hypertension causes changes in the kidneys' glomeruli, vasculature, and the tubulointerstitium. These changes are broadly referred to as hypertensive nephrosclerosis.

Intimal thickening and luminal narrowing of the renal arteries and glomerular arterioles is seen. This is thought to be a consequence of a hypertrophic response to chronic hypertension causing medial hypertrophy, followed by deposition of plasma protein constituents such as inactive C3b in to the damaged vessel wall. Abnormal metabolism of nitric oxide is thought to play a major role in this process. This can eventually lead to an ischemic state within the kidney.

The glomeruli may undergo focal global/segmental sclerosis as a consequence of the ensuing ischemic injury. This ischemia also causes alterations in antigen expression on the surface of the tubular cells, inciting an inflammatory response that leads to chronic interstitial nephritis. These alterations cause a decrease in GFR.

3.2.2 Effect of diabetes on kidney function

Glomerular hyperfiltration and hypertension is a well studied phenomenon that develops early in the course of diabetes. However, elevated glucose levels are known to stimulate mesangial cell matrix production. Non-enzymatic glycation of tissue proteins also may contribute to the development of diabetic nephropathy. In this process, excess glucose combines with free amino acids on circulating or tissue proteins eventually leading to the formation of advanced glycation end products (AGEs). These AGEs then crosslink with collagen and cause vascular complications. Glomerular permeability is also thought to increase via activation of protein kinase C that happens in diabetes.

Other molecules that have been postulated to have a role in the development of nephropathy in diabetes include prorenin (which activates protein kinases, and hence mitosis), and other cytokines that cause inflammation and fibrosis. These cytokines include vascular endothelial growth factor (VEGF), transforming growth factor-beta (TGF-beta) etc.

3.2.3 Hyperuricemia and kidney function

Elevated levels of uric acid, or hyperuricemia, that can progress to gout is more prevalent in the obese population. It has been proposed that hyperuricemia may contribute to worsening of renal function by decreasing renal perfusion. This happens because of arteriolosclerosis of the afferent arterioles. It is believed that uric acid stimulates afferent arteriolar vascular smooth muscle cell proliferation. Long standing hyperuricemia and gout can potentially cause chronic urate nephropathy, and uric acid stones to form in the kidneys or the urinary tract.

3.2.4 Hyperlipidemia and renal function

It has been shown in animal models that hyperlipidemia can cause mesangial cell proliferation by activating LDL receptors present on mesangial cells. This also leads to increased production of inflammatory growth factors and reactive oxygen species.

3.2.5 Metabolic syndrome

Metabolic syndrome is the dreaded constellation of clinical signs that include increased waist circumference, insulin resistance, hypertension, and dyslipidemia. These comorbidities act in concert to cause kidney dysfunction through the pathways outlined above.

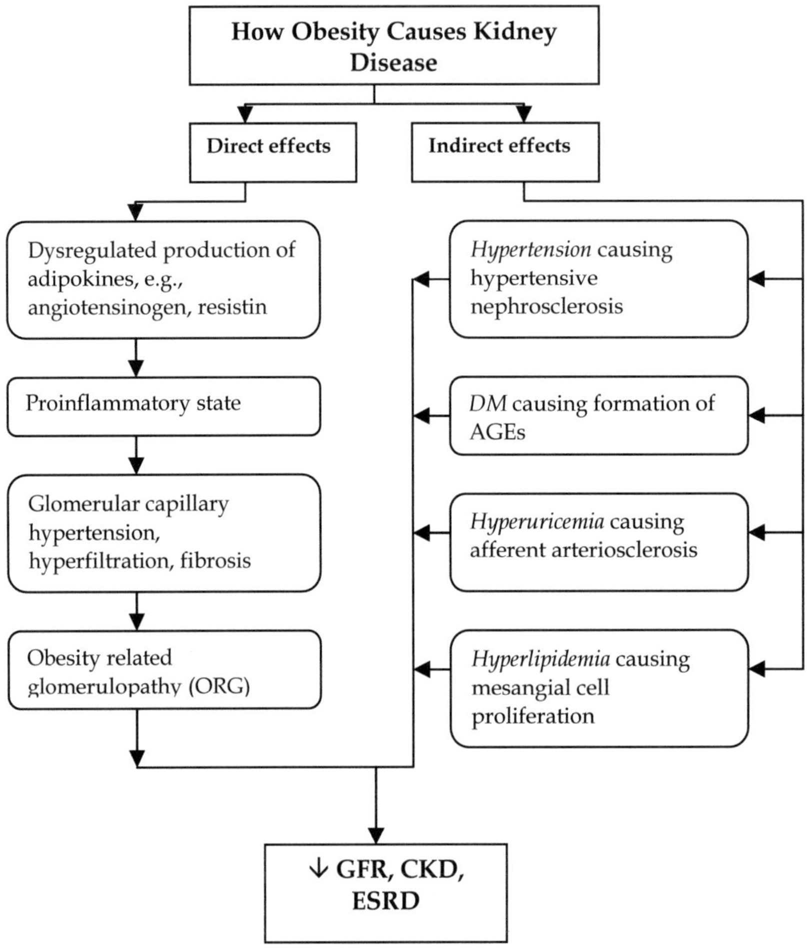

4. Obesity and kidney disease: The clinico-pathologic manifestations

Before clinical kidney disease is apparent in obesity, patients might already have very limited renal disease in a few glomeruli, as discussed in section 3.1. Subclinical disease, with sclerotic lesions in a few glomeruli (with no overt proteinuria) was demonstrated in a series of 95 patients who had renal biopsies while undergoing bariatric surgery for extreme obesity. FSGS was observed in approximately 5 percent of extremely obese patients but not in any of the non-obese patients. Mesangial and podocyte hypertrophy also occurred more frequently in obese patients.

Early markers of glomerular disease like microalbuminuria and albuminuria have been reported in as much as 41% and 4% of the extremely obese patients, respectively. Focal segmental glomerulosclerosis (FSGS) and obesity-related glomerulopathy (ORG), characterized by glomerular enlargement and mesangial expansion have been described in patients with severe obesity, and clinically manifest initially with proteinuria, and in severe states can progress to renal failure. Obesity-related glomerulopathy may be reversible with weight loss.

The term "obesity-related glomerulopathy" is sometime used interchangeably with FSGS associated with obesity. However, multiple studies have shown that these might be different processes pathologically. It is entirely possible that these entities represent a spectrum of kidney disease. In 1985, Wesson et al were one of the first ones to report nephrotic range heavy proteinuria in patients who had no glomerulosclerosis and no epithelial cell injury or foot process fusion on renal biopsy. Later studies reported some of such patients to only have mesangial expansion and glomerular capillary loop enlargement leading to glomerulomegaly. Classically, ORG is considered to be distinct from idiopathic FSGS, with a lower incidence of nephrotic syndrome and a more indolent course. Glomerulomegaly is typically more consistent in ORG, as is milder foot process fusion.

Obese patients with FSGS tend to have elevated glomerular filtration rates and increased glomerular size. Serum levels of an adipokine, adiponectin may be seen in the obese. FSGS in obese subjects presents with proteinuria that may reach the nephrotic range. Both weight loss and ACE inhibitors have been shown to reduce this protein excretion by up to 85 percent. However, just like the other causes of secondary FSGS, nephrotic syndrome is atypical and the presence of edema is uncommon.· Praga et al studied 15 patients with obesity associated FSGS with significant proteinuria (mean of 3.1 g/day), and found that edema and hypoalbuminemia were not observed in any individual.

It has been suggested that the difference between obesity-related glomerulonephropathy or secondary-FSGS from obesity, and idiopathic FSGS is that only some nephrons leak protein in the former, as opposed to global nephron involvement in idiopathic FSGS. This leakage of protein then leads to abnormal renal handling of sodium, which subsequently causes retention of salt and water. Hence ORG and obesity-related secondary FSGS is not associated with edema while the edema in idiopathic FSGS is severe.

Kambham et al reported in their landmark study that the mean age of patients at the time of biopsy diagnosis of ORG was 42.9 years (range 8–71 years). The youngest patients in the study group included an 8-year-old girl [height 4.0 ft (121.9 cm), weight 190 lbs (86.4 kg)]. The patients' weights ranged from 81.8 kg to 186.4 kg. The mean BMI was 41.7 kg/m^2 (range of 30.9 to 62.7); 38 patients had BMI> 40 kg/m^2 and 33 had BMI <40 kg/m^2. Their was a slight male preponderance with a male-to-female ratio of 44:27 (1.6). The majority of patients were Caucasian (75%), followed by African American (21%) and Hispanic (4%). None of these patients had renal biopsy findings of diabetic nephropathy. Forty-four patients had a prior history of hypertension and eight patients carried a diagnosis of obstructive sleep apnea syndrome prior to renal biopsy.

There are other ways in which obesity can affect renal function. Obesity and weight gain during adulthood have been known to increase the risk of kidney stones. In women, obesity is an important risk factor for urinary incontinence.

4.1 Clinical course

As stated above, weight loss, and drugs like ACE inhibitors can stem the progression of kidney disease in obesity and actually reverse the changes (unless most of the glomeruli are already fibrosed). Weight loss may result in remission of proteinuria. This was demonstrated in a study of 63 patients with biopsy-demonstrated ORG. Patients who started the study had a mean protein excretion of 1.48 g/day. These patients were then followed for two years. Protein excretion was reduced from 1.7 to 1 g/24 hours among 29 patients who successfully lowered their BMI but increased among 9 patients whose BMI went up.

In patients in whom this does not happen, the disease can progress relentlessly with a progressive decrease in GFR. Uremic symptoms can ensue below a GFR of 15 ml/min, and eventually, symptoms like failure to thrive, dysgeusia, nausea, vomiting, itching, insomnia, hyperkalemia, fluid overload, or acidosis can mandate the initiation of dialysis.

5. Managing the disease

Obesity associated kidney disease is a ticking time bomb, and the affected patient stands a huge risk of progression to End Stage Renal Disease (ESRD) that mandates dialysis, a treatment that is hugely cumbersome and expensive. It is hence imperative that the disease be diagnosed and managed aggressively from the outset. It goes without saying that weight loss is of utmost importance and can itself cause remission of the disease to a certain extent. However, treatment of associated risk factors like hypertension, diabetes or insulin resistance, sleep apnea, dyslipidemia is also necessary.

Medications that block the renin-angiotensin axis in the kidney like the angiotensin converting enzyme (ACE) inhibitors, or angiotensin receptor blockers (ARBs) have been shown to have a beneficial effect on reducing glomerular hypertension and proteinuria, and preventing disease progression. Praga at al demonstrated this in 17 obese patients with proteinuria>1 g/day. Their age was 34-70 years; 11 were females and 6 males. Renal biopsy was done in five of these patients. This showed focal glomerulosclerosis in 2 cases, minimal changes in 2 and mesangial proliferation in 1. Nine patients (group 1) were then put on hypocaloric diets and followed for one year. There was a significant correlation between body weight loss and decrease in proteinuria. A second group of eight patients were started on captopril, an ACE inhibitor (without any dietary changes). BMI in this group remained stable but proteinuria showed a dramatic decrease, similar to that in group 1. Given the findings of this study, it makes clinical sense to prescribe both body weight loss and ACE inhibitor treatment to patients suspected to have obesity related kidney disease.

6. Conclusion

The World Health Organization considers obesity an international epidemic, stating in 1997 that "obesity's impact is so diverse and extreme that it should now be regarded as one of the greatest neglected public health problems of our time with an impact on health which may well prove to be as great as that of smoking." Despite scientific evidence to the contrary, the effect of obesity on the function of the kidneys is less well-known. There now is a well established risk between obesity and the development of kidney disease. The Framingham Offspring reported obesity as a major risk factor for the development of kidney disease Kidney disease from obesity can progress to End Stage Renal Disease (ESRD), which mandates the use of dialysis to keep the patient alive. It is hence a huge risk factor for morbidity and mortality.

Obesity is associated with multiple other conditions that are known to cause compromised renal function, including hypertension, diabetes, hyperuricemia, and the metabolic syndrome that can independently have a detrimental effect on renal function. However, obesity has been found to cause kidney disease and ESRD even after adjustment for these factors. The pathogenesis of obesity related kidney disease can be sub-classified in to direct and indirect effects.

Obesity seems to cause a change in the renal hemodynamics that promotes progressive kidney disease. These changes begin early in the course of obesity, even before overt renal manifestations of obesity are clinically apparent. One of the keys to unravel obesity's effect on the kidneys is to understand the concept of body fat as an independent endocrine organ rather than simply a passive storage depot for triglycerides. A central factor in this is the dysregulated production by adipose cells of bioactive substances, called "adipokines" that cause systemic effects and directly influence insulin sensitivity and vascular injury. This results in hemodynamic and structural changes in the kidney. These adipokines include cytokines like leptin, adiponectin, interleukin-6, tumor necrosis factor-alpha, resistin, and angiotensinogen. These cytokines then induce a pro-inflammatory state causing glomerular capillary hypertension and fibrosis in the renal parenchyma. Of these adipokines, one of the best understood roles is that of angiotensinogen. Increased angiotensinogen kick-starts the RAS and in turn increases the downstream effects of this system, namely, fluid retention and increased vascular tone. Elevated levels of angiotensinogen and angiotensin II then lead to efferent arteriolar constriction in the glomerulus. This increases the intraglomerular pressure, leading to a rise in the GFR.

Obese patients have been shown to have elevations in both renal plasma flow (RPF) and GFR. The augmented RPF suggests a state of renal vasodilatation involving mainly the afferent arteriole. The analysis suggests that the high GFR in very obese subjects may be the result of an increase in transcapillary hydraulic pressure difference. An abnormal transmission of increased arterial pressure to the glomerular capillaries through a dilated afferent arteriole could account for the augmentation in this transcapillary pressure.

Certain pathognomonic changes are seen in the kidney as a result of long standing obesity. These changes encompass what is referred to as Obesity Related Glomerulopathy (ORG). These include structural changes like hyperplasia of the juxta-glomerular apparatus, consistent presence of glomerulomegaly, and foot process fusion. Another histologic feature noted in some ORG patients is the presence of focal changes in the form of mild focal mesangial sclerosis or mild focal thickening of glomerular/tubular basement membranes. These changes are not very dissimilar to changes that are more often associated with the presence of diabetic nephropathy.

The strong association between obesity and other entities like the dreaded metabolic syndrome, hypertension, diabetes, hyperuricemia, dyslipidemia, and sleep apnea also causes indirect effects on renal structure and function. Long standing hypertension causes changes in the kidneys' glomeruli, vasculature, and the tubulointerstitium. These changes are broadly referred to as hypertensive nephrosclerosis. Intimal thickening and luminal narrowing of the renal arteries and glomerular arterioles is seen. The glomeruli may undergo focal global/segmental sclerosis as a consequence of the ensuing ischemic injury. Glomerular hyperfiltration and hypertension is a well studied phenomenon that develops early in the course of diabetes. Elevated glucose levels are known to stimulate mesangial cell matrix production. Non-enzymatic glycation of tissue proteins also may contribute to the development of diabetic nephropathy. It has been proposed that hyperuricemia may contribute to worsening of renal function by decreasing renal perfusion. This happens because of arteriolosclerosis of the afferent arterioles. It is believed that uric acid stimulates afferent arteriolar vascular smooth muscle cell proliferation. It has been shown in animal models that hyperlipidemia can cause mesangial cell proliferation by activating LDL receptors present on mesangial cells. This leads to increased production of inflammatory growth factors and reactive oxygen species.

Before overt clinical kidney disease becomes clinically apparent in obesity, patients may start to develop limited renal disease in a few glomeruli. Early markers of glomerular disease like microalbuminuria and albuminuria have been reported in as much as 41% and 4% of the extremely obese patients, respectively. Focal segmental glomerulosclerosis (FSGS) and obesity-related glomerulopathy (ORG), as explained above, have been described in patients with severe obesity, and manifest initially with proteinuria. These can, in severe states, progress to renal failure. However, as is the case with other causes of secondary FSGS, nephrotic syndrome is atypical and the presence of edema is uncommon. It has been suggested that the difference between obesity-related glomerulonephropathy or secondary-FSGS from obesity, and idiopathic FSGS is that only some nephrons leak protein in the former, as opposed to global nephron involvement in idiopathic FSGS.

Weight loss, and drugs like ACE inhibitors (eg captopril, lisinopril) or angiotensin receptor blockers (like losartan, irbesartan) can stem the progression of kidney disease in obesity, and are sometimes able to actually reverse the changes induced by obesity related kidney disease. However, this is less likely to happen if most of the glomeruli are already fibrosed. In such cases, the disease can progress relentlessly with a progressive decrease in GFR. Uremic symptoms can ensue below a GFR of 15 ml/min, and eventually, symptoms like failure to thrive, dysgeusia, nausea, vomiting, itching, insomnia, hyperkalemia, fluid overload, or acidosis can mandate the initiation of dialysis. It thus makes clinical sense to prescribe both weight loss and ACE inhibitor/angiotensin receptor blocker treatment to patients suspected of having obesity related kidney disease.

7. Methods

We searched PubMed for English, German, French, and Spanish language references published as of June 2011, using combinations of the following terms: "obesity", "kidney disease", "glomerulopathy", "FSGS", "gastric bypass", "diabetes mellitus", "dyslipidemia", "hypertension", "metabolic syndrome", "metabolic effects", "renal effects", "nutrition", "epidemiology". The bibliographies of the articles thus obtained, as well as those of relevant review articles were also reviewed for inclusion of publications.

8. References

Bellomo G., et al. (2010). Association of uric acid with change in kidney function in healthy normotensive individuals. *Am J Kidney Dis,* Vol. 56, No. 2, (2010 Aug), pp. 264-272

Caballero, B. (2007). The global epidemic of obesity: an overview. *Epidemiol Rev,* Vol. 29, pp 1-5. (Epub 2007 Jun 13)

Chagnac A., et al. (2000). Glomerular hemodynamics in severe obesity. *Am J Physiol Renal Physiol,* Vol. 278, No. 5, (2000 May), pp. 817-822

Choi, H., et al. (2005). Obesity, weight change, hypertension, diuretic use, and risk of gout in men: the health professionals follow-up study. *Arch Intern Med,* Vol. 165, No. 7, (2005 April), pp. 742-748

Flegal, K, et al. (2010). Prevalence and trends in obesity among US adults, 1999-2008. *JAMA,* Vol. 303, No. 3, (2010 Jan), pp. 235-241

Fox, C., et al. (2004). Predictors of new-onset kidney disease in a community-based population. *JAMA,* Vol. 291, No. 7, (2004 Feb), pp. 844-850

Gröne E., & Gröne H. (2008). Does hyperlipidemia injure the kidney? *Nat Clin Pract Nephrol,* Vol. 4, No. 8, (2008 Aug), pp. 424-425

Harris, R., et al. (1991). Global glomerular sclerosis and glomerular arteriolar hyalinosis in insulin dependent diabetes. *Kidney Int,* Vol. 40, No. 1, (1991 July), pp. 107-114

Hsu, C., et al. (2006). Body mass index and risk for end-stage renal disease. *Ann Intern Med,* Vol. 144, No. 1, (2006 Jan), pp. 21-28

Hsu, C., et al. (2009). Risk factors for end-stage renal disease: 25-year follow-up. *Arch Intern Med,* Vol. 169, No. 4, (2009 Feb), pp. 342-350

Hutley, L., Prins, J. (2005). Fat as an endocrine organ: relationship to the metabolic syndrome. *Am J Med Sci,* Vol. 330, No. 6, (2005 Dec), pp. 280-289

Kambham, N., et al. (2001). Obesity-related glomerulopathy: an emerging epidemic. *Kidney Int,* Vol. 59, No. 4, (2001 Apr), pp. 1498-1509

Karlsson, C., et al. (1998) Human adipose tissue expresses angiotensinogen and enzymes required for its conversion to angiotensin II. *J Clin Endocrinol Metab,* Vol. 83, No. 11, (1998 Nov), pp. 3925–3929

Kramer, H., et al. (2005). Obesity and prevalent and incident CKD: the Hypertension Detection and Follow-Up Program. *Am J Kidney Dis,* Vol. 46, No. 4, (2005 Oct), pp. 587-594

Malik, F., et al. (1997). Renin-angiotensin system: genes to bedside. *Am Heart J,* Vol. 134, No. 3, (1997 Sep), pp. 514–526

Morales E., et al. (2003). Beneficial effects of weight loss in overweight patients with chronic proteinuric nephropathies. *Am J Kidney Dis,* Vol. 41, No. 2, (2003 Feb), pp. 319-327

Praga M., et al. (2001). Clinical features and long-term outcome of obesity-associated focal segmental glomerulosclerosis. *Nephrol Dial Transplant,* Vol. 16, No. 9, (2001 Sep), pp. 1790-1798

Praga M., et al. (1995). Effects of body-weight loss and captopril treatment on proteinuria associated with obesity. *Nephron,* Vol. 70, No. 1, (1995), pp. 35-41

Schieffer, B., et al. (2004). Comparative effects of AT1-antagonism and angiotensin-converting enzyme inhibition on markers of inflammation and platelet aggregation in patients with coronary artery disease. *J Am Coll Cardiol,* Vol. 44, No. 2, (2004 July), pp. 362–368

Serra, A., et al. (2008). Renal injury in the extremely obese patients with normal renal function. *Kidney Int,* Vol. 73, No. 8, (2008 Apr), pp. 947-955

Shen W., et al. (2010). Obesity-related glomerulopathy: body mass index and proteinuria. *Clin J Am Soc Nephrol,* Vol. 5, No. 8, (2010 Aug), pp. 1401-1409

Taylor E., et al. (2005). Obesity, weight gain, and the risk of kidney stones. *JAMA,* Vol 293, No. 4, (2005 Jan), pp. 455-462

The world health report 2002 - Reducing Risks, Promoting Healthy Life, Geneva, Switzerland, 2002

Wesson D., et al. (1985). Massive obesity and nephrotic proteinuria with a normal renal biopsy. *Nephron,* Vol. 40, No. 2, (1985), pp. 235-237

5

Uric Acid and Renal Function

Guilherme Ambrosio Albertoni, Fernanda Teixeira Borges and Nestor Schor
Department of Medicine, Nephrology Division, Federal University of São Paulo (UNIFESP)
Brazil

1. Introduction

Since the discovery of hyperuricemia as the cause of gout in the early 1800s, hypertension, cardiovascular disease and kidney disease have also been related to increased serum uric acid (UA) levels in subsequent years (Nakagawa et al., 2006); patients with gout had a much higher prevalence of hypertension (25-50%), mild-to-moderate kidney disease (20-60%) (Kutzing & Firestein, 2008) and cardiovascular disease (90%) compared to the general population. However, conflicting results regarding the role of UA as the causative factor in diseases other than gouty arthritis resulted in a shift of interest away from UA. In recent years, uric acid regained the lost popularity due to new findings in a number of disease states including hypertension, renal disease, metabolic syndrome and many more (Feig et al., 2008).

Hyperuricemia arises from excess dietary purine or ethanol intake, decreased renal excretion of UA, or from tumor lyses in lymphoma, leukaemia, or solid tumours (Kutzing & Firestein, 2008). Finally, several drugs alter UA handling by the kidney, for example drug therapy with candesartan (Li et al., 2008) or both loop- and thiazide diuretics, all of which increase the net urate reabsorption (Suliman et al., 2006). In the majority of individuals, hyperuricemia will be asymptomatic, but as UA tends to precipitate in tissues and in other body fluids, persistent hyperuricemia may eventually lead to the accumulation of urate crystals in many places, resulting in either acute painful conditions, like gout/tophaceous gout/gouty arthritis, urolithiasis, or, in severe cases, like tumor lysis syndrome, in acute UA nephropathy (Riegersperger et al., 2011).

In recent years, increased fructose intake, particularly via sweetened beverages, started to attract more attention from the medical community. During the last two centuries, at least in the western world, dietary fructose intake dramatically increased, with corresponding increases in serum UA levels (Feig et al., 2008). The increase in fructose intake and hyperuricemia is now being associated to the development of metabolic syndrome.

Hyperuricemia is associated with an increased risk for developing CKD (Obermayr et al., 2008) and a risk factor for renal dysfunction in patients with rheumatoid arthritis (Daoussis et al., 2009). Retrospective data suggest an influence of hyperuricemia on graft loss after kidney transplantation (Haririan et al., 2010). A screening among 18,020 individuals with chronic kidney diseases (CKD) found a 20.6% prevalence of hyperuricemia. A cross-sectional study in individuals aged over 40 years found 10.5% prevalence of CKD, and among these, 26% were hyperuricemic (Shan et al., 2010). A multi-center study of 2,145 consecutive patients with essential hypertension found a prevalence of hyperuricemia of 35% in males and 43% in females, and this was associated with elevated serum creatinine levels (Lin et al., 2010). A screening among 5,722 individuals found a 5.4% incidence of chronic kidney disease, and serum UA (sUA) correlated with serum creatinine levels (Chen et al., 2009). A cross-sectional study in 9,375 participants of a health-screening program found 14.5% hyperuricemic individuals (Kuo et al., 2010). A screening study found a higher incidence of end-stage renal disease among hyperuricemic women (Iseki et al., 2004), and a post-hoc analysis in 294 patients initiating renal replacement therapy found that half of these were hyperuricemic with a twofold increase in mortality when UA levels were ≥9.0 mg/dL (≥535 µmol/l) (Suliman et al., 2006).

2. Uric acid metabolism

UA is the end-product of purine nucleotide metabolism in humans. In contrast to many lower vertebrates, human lack UA oxidase (uricase), an enzyme which further catalyses UA to allantoin, more soluble end product (Sautin & Johnson, 2008). Humans have higher serum UA levels when compared to other mammals due to the lack of uricase (Johnson et al., 2003). UA is primarily excreted via the urine. The balance between dietary intake, endogenous metabolism of purines and the urinary excretion rate of UA determines plasma UA levels (Kutzing & Firestein, 2008).

Almost all serum UA is present in the ionized form, monosodium urate, and only about 5% of urate is protein bound at physiological pH. The definition of hyperuricemia is currently arbitrary and varies from >6 mg/dL (360µmol/l) in women and >7 mg/dL (416µmol/l) in men, to ≥6.5 mg/dL (387µmol/l), or to >8.3 mg/dL (494 µmol/l), regardless of gender. UA levels physiologically and gradually rise during the human lifetime; in female individuals, UA levels additionally rise after menopause (Hak et al., 2008).

Renal handling. Kidneys eliminate two-thirds, and the gastrointestinal tract eliminates one-third of the UA load. Urate is filtered completely at the renal glomerulus. However, the normal fractional excretion of UA is only 8% to 12%. Therefore, postglomerular reabsorption and secretion are the ultimate factors regulating the amount of UA excretion (Gutman et al., 1968; Steele et al., 1973). The proximal tubule is the site of UA reabsorption and secretion. Almost complete reabsorption of urate occurs at the S1 segment of the proximal tubule. However, in the S2 segment of the proximal tubule urate is secreted at a range greater than reabsorption via transporters URAT1, OAT1, -2, and -3, -4, and -10, the multi-drug resistance proteins ABCC4 and ABCG2, and the glucose transporters GLUT 9a and b, and others. Finally, post-secretory resorption occurs at a more distal site of the proximal tubule. Approximately 10% of the filtered urate appears in the urine (Shekarriz et al., 2002).

UA Chemistry. UA is a weak acid with 2 dissociation constants. Two factors contribute to UA solubility: UA concentration and solution pH. However, the solubility of UA in urine is primarily determined by urinary pH. The first pKa of UA is at a pH of 5.5, resulting in the loss of 1 proton from UA and the formation of anionic urate (Finlayson, 1974). The second pKa is 10.3, which has no physiological significance in humans. The supersaturation of urine with UA occurs when urinary pH is less than 5.5. In contrast, at a pH of more than 6.5 the majority of UA is in the form of anionic urate. The solubility of urate salts is affected by the relative concentrations of cations present in the urine. Increased urinary sodium concentrations promote formation of the monosodium urate complex, which is more soluble than undissociated UA. Urine is frequently supersaturated with sodium urate but stones of this type are infrequent. However, supersaturation with sodium urate may contribute to calcium oxalate stone formation via heterogeneous nucleation.

UA pool. UA may be derived by endogenous or exogenous routes. The endogenous production of UA from purine synthesis, and tissue catabolism under normal circumstances, is relatively constant at 300 to 400mg per day. However, the exogenous pool varies significantly with diet. A diet rich in animal protein contributes significantly to the purine pool and subsequent UA formation by a series of enzymatic reaction involving xanthine oxidase as the final step.

Excretion. Renal excretion is the primary mode of UA clearance, accounting for two-thirds of its elimination. Intestine, skin, hair and nails account for the remaining one-third of UA excretion. In the intestine bacteria catabolise UA into carbon dioxide and ammonia, which are then eliminated as intestinal air or absorved and excreted in the urine.

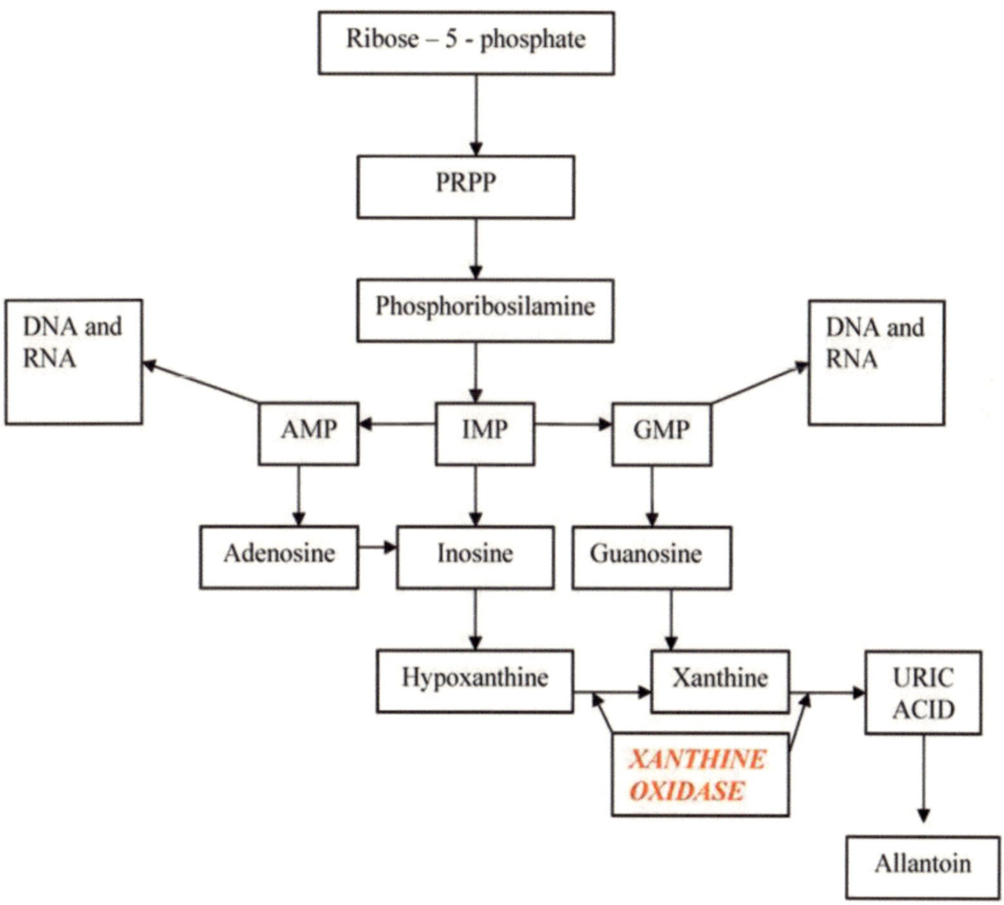

Fig. 1. Schematic representation of the metabolism of Uric Acid

3. Mechanisms of uric acid-induced hypertension

It is well established that when UA is deposited in tissues in the crystalline form, it initiates a proinflammatory state, as seen in gouty arthritis (Sanchez-Lozada et al., 2006). However, the precise pathogenetic role of soluble UA in the serum is somewhat less clear. Moreover, markedly elevated serum UA is clearly associated with gouty arthritis and nephrolithiasis, whereas the importance of subtle elevation in UA levels still remains to be established.

For many years, UA was regarded as a metabolically inert substance. However, several lines of evidence have demonstrated that soluble UA is a strong antioxidant (Ames et al., 1981).

Despite these well-recognized antioxidant effects, UA also behaves as a pro-oxidant and proinflammatory factor. A few points should be emphasized to better understand this apparent paradox. First, UA acts differently inside the cells or in the extracellular milieu, where it is present in soluble form. While being a potent antioxidant in extracellular fluid, UA exerts pro-oxidative effects once inside the cell (Sautin et al., 2007; Corry et al., 2008; Convento et al., 2011).

Second, one isoform of xanthine oxidoreductase - xanthine dehydrogenase - undergoes extensive phenotypic conversion to xanthine oxidase under local ischemic conditions. Unlike xanthine dehydrogenase, xanthine oxidase uses molecular oxygen instead of Nicotinamide Adenine Dinucleotide (NAD) as an electron acceptor (Glantzounis et al., 2005).

In addition to interference with free radical production, UA has some direct effects on endothelial and smooth muscle cells of the vascular wall, which ultimately lead to endothelial dysfunction (Mazzali et al., 2002). In endothelial cells, UA blocks nitric oxide (NO) release, inhibits endothelial proliferation and stimulates C-reactive protein production (Khosla et al., 2005). Several experimental studies also showed that UA can activate smooth muscle cells via activation of specific MAP kinases, nuclear transcription factors, stimulation of ciclooxigenase-2 (Cox-2), and various inflammatory mediators such as the tissue renin-angiotensin system (Corry et al., 2008; Watanabe et al., 2002; Kang et al., 2002). Recent evidence also suggests that hyperuricemia increased cellular proliferation, angiotensin II (AII) and endothelin-1 (ET-1) in human mesangial cells (Albertoni et al., 2010), which could contribute to reduce GFR.

In a landmark study by Mazzali et al., 2001 pharmacologically induced mild-to-moderate hyperuricemia via oxonic acid administration in rats resulted in the development of hypertension. Conversely, when UA elevation was treated with allopurinol or with a uricosuric agent, development of hypertension could be prevented. Other experimental studies show that at a concentration of 10 mg/dL UA significantly decreases the production of ET-1 in mesangial cells after 24h of treatment. This effect was blocked by Losartan (LOS), an AII receptor type 1 antagonist (Albertoni et al, 2010).

It is also possible that genetic polymorphisms of transporters or enzymes involved in UA metabolism affect blood pressure, especially in younger subjects. For example, hypertension has been associated with polymorphisms of xanthine oxidoreductase (Chaves et al., 2007).

4. Uric acid and acute renal failure

Uric acid, as the end-product of purine metabolism in humans, presents a clinical impact since its has a relative insolubility, particularly in the acidic environment of the distal nephron. As a result, states of enhanced purine catabolism increases the urate load on the kidney, leading to intrarenal precipitation. Major causes of increases on purine metabolism are malignancies with rapid cell turnover, such as leukemia and lymphomas, and the added acceleration of cell lyses that occurs with chemotherapy and radiation. Serum urate levels rise rapidly, and acute renal failure occurs as a consequence of tubular deposition and obstruction of urate and uric acid. The keys to the diagnosis of acute uric acid nephropathy are the appropriate clinical settings as cell lyses increases, oliguria, marked hyperuricemia, and hyperuricosuria. A urinary uric acid-to-creatinine ratio greater than 1 helps to distinguish acute uric acid nephropathy from other catabolic forms of acute renal failure in which serum urate is elevated. Preventive treatment involves pharmacologic xanthine oxidase inhibition with allopurinol and alkaline diuresis. Occasionally, acute renal failure occurs despite allopurinol due to tubular precipitation of the metabolites precursors, such as xanthine, which accumulate with xanthine oxidase inhibition. Dialysis therapy may be required both to correct azotemia and to reduce the body burden of urate. Hemodialysis is preferred since it can achieve greater clearance than other dialysis modes. (Conger, 1990).

5. Uric acid and kidney disease

Association of UA with chronic kidney disease dates back to 1890s. Any functional declive which reduces glomerular filtration rates (GFR) and tubular reabsorption secondarily leads to UA elevation, but also the decrease in glomerular filtration rate can increase serum UA (Feig, 2009). To determine which comes first was the principal endeavor of UA researchers in the last two decades.

Experimental studies performed by Mazzali et al., 2002, demonstrated that hyperuricemic rats developed hypertension, afferent arteriolopathy, glomerular hypertrophy, and increased glomerular pressure, tubulointerstitial damage and macrophage infiltration (Mazzali et al., 2002; Sanchez-Lozada et al., 2005; Nakagawa et al., 2003).

Several works analyzed the effects of UA in kidney cells and hyperuricemic animal models. Firstly, hyperuricemia induces endothelial dysfunction and inflammation (Yu et al., 2010, Khosla et al., 2005). UA has the ability to increase monocyte chemoattractant protein (MCP-1) in cultured vascular smooth muscle cells (Kanellis et al., 2003) and human proximal tubular epithelial cells (Cirillo et al., 2006). UA can induce the contraction (Albertoni, et al., 2010) and reactive oxygen species produced in mesangial cells (Convento et al., 2011).

6. Uric acid, metabolic syndrome and diabetes

The relationship between hyperuricemia, hypertension, and the metabolic syndrome has long been debated. Are the conditions different manifestations of a common underlying metabolic disorder? Is hyperuricemia in part responsible for hypertension? Recent evidences from animal studies and epidemiology suggest that hyperuricemia has a primary role in both hypertension and the metabolic syndrome. Rats that were made hyperuricemic rapidly developed hypertension through activation of the renin-angiotensin system, induction of endothelial dysfunction, and vascular smooth muscle proliferation. Lowering UA in these animals prevented this effect (Johnson et al., 2005). In a longitudinal study in children, there was a strong correlation between hyperuricemia and the subsequent development of hypertension (Feig et al., 2006). Recent epidemiological data suggest also that hyperuricemia is an independent risk factor for developing hypertension. In a group of subjects who did not have the metabolic syndrome, normotensive men with baseline hyperuricemia had 80% more risk of develop hypertension compared with those who did not have hyperuricemia (Krishnan et al., 2007). Finally, the degree of hyperuricemia is strongly correlated with the prevalence of the metabolic syndrome (Yoo et al., 2005; Choi et al., 2007; Facchini et al., 1992).

Metabolic syndrome has many components which may independently mediate or lead to kidney damage, including increased inflammation (Calabro & Yeh, 2008), insulin resistance and endothelial dysfunction (Kim et al., 2006). Additionally, diets high in fructose constitute one of the major predisposing factors for the metabolic syndrome epidemia (Cirillo et al., 2006). Fructose is unique among sugars by its ability to rapidly deplete ATP, with resultant purine nucleotide degradation and eventual UA generation.

Experimental studies in rodents have suggested that UA may contribute to the development of the metabolic syndrome, hypertension, and kidney disease (Feig et al., 2008) and recently clinical studies focusing on UA and the development and progression of diabetic kidney disease have been published (Hovind et al., 2011). In the early report of the Modification of Diet in Renal Disease Study (Hunsicker et al., 1997), UA was not found to be an independent predictor for renal disease. Others large epidemiologic studies have revealed conflicting results in this respect. While the majority (Iseki et al., 2001; Domrongkitchaiporn et al., 2005; See et al., 2010; Chang et al., 2010; Obermayr et al., 2008) of these studies suggest an independent predictive role for UA in renal disease, others (Tomita et al., 2000; Sturm et al., 2008; Madero et al., 2009) argue against it.

Historically, the elevated level of UA observed in the metabolic syndrome has been attributed to hyperinsulinemia, since insulin reduces renal excretion of UA (Quinõnes et al., 1995).

Hyperuricemia, however, often precedes the development of hyperinsulinemia (Nakagawa et al., 2005; Carnethon et al., 2003), obesity (Masuo et al., 2003), and diabetes (Nakanishi et al., 2003; Dehghan et al., 2008; Chien et al., 2008). Hyperuricemia may also be present in the metabolic syndrome in people who are not overweight or obese.

The strongest evidence of a role for UA in the development of the metabolic syndrome has been from studies models showing that decreasing UA levels can prevent or reverse features of the metabolic syndrome (Nakagawa et al., 2006; Sanchez-Lozada et al., 2008; Reungjui et al., 2007). Two mechanisms have been suggested to explain how hyperuricemia might induce the metabolic syndrome. The first mechanisms is related to the fact that glucose uptake in skeletal muscle depend in part on increases in blood flow mediated by the insulin-stimulated release of NO from endothelial cells. Features of the metabolic syndrome develop in mice lacking endothelial nitric oxide synthase (iNOs) (Cook et al., 2003). The observations that hyperuricemia can induce endothelial dysfunction in rats (Khosla et al., 2005) and that treatment with allopurinol can improve endothelial function in patients with hyperuricemia (Mercuro et al., 2004) would support this mechanism. The second mechanism concerns the inflammatory and oxidative changes UA induces in adipocytes (Sautin et al., 2007), a process that is key in causing the metabolic syndrome in obese mice (Furukawa et al., 2004).

The prevalence of diabetes, and for that matter the associated complications, has increased dramatically. Presently, diabetes is the leading cause of end-stage renal disease in the western world (United States Renal Data System, 2008). Although the progression of renal disease can be halted partially, diabetic nephropathy is still regarded as an irreversible and progressive disease (Parving et al., 2008).

Therefore, it has become increasingly essential to determine the pathophysiological mechanisms underlying the development and progression of diabetic nephropathy. Evidence is available of a complicated interaction between different contributors to the disease process. It is possible that genetic susceptibility, metabolic abnormalities,

hemodynamic changes, upregulated growth factors, and cytokines may all play a part in the development of diabetic glomerulopathy; however, the complex pathogenesis of development of diabetic nephropathy has not been fully clarified (Hovind et al., 2011).
Recently clinical studies focusing on UA, albuminuria and diabetic kidney disease have been published (Bonakdaran et al., 2011; Kim et al., 2010; Kuo et al., 2010). The new evidence suggests that UA could be a risk factor for the development of diabetic nephropathy; however, the significance of serum UA as pathogenic factor in the development of diabetic nephropathy is not yet fully clarified (Hovind et al., 2011).

7. Uric acid stones

A high concentration of urate and low pH are the determinants of UA stone formation. The prevalence of UA stones in the United States is estimated to be 5% to 10% (Gutman et al., 1968). Interestingly, these data originate from studies performed more than 30 years ago. Therefore, the current incidence of UA stones in the United States may be different. In a more recent study from Veterans Administration hospital stone analyses revealed that 12% of stones contained some UA component and 9.7% comprised pure UA (Mandel et al., 1989). Incidence also may vary with age. The incidence of UA stones was 11% in a geriatric population (Gentle et al., 1997). The frequency of UA stones also varies in different geographical locations within the United States. In southern states the incidence has been reported at 4% compared with 17% in Chicago (Riese et al., 1992). Other industrialized countries have wide variations in UA stone rates, with Germany reporting 17% to 25%, Sweden 4% and Israel up to 40% (Hesse et al., 1975; Scholz et al., 1979; Grenabo et al., 1985; Atsmon et al., 1963). Urate stones have frequently been reported in Iran and Pakistan. However, the majority of these stones are ammonium acid urate (Minon et al., 1983). These apparent geographical variations indicate that genetic, dietary and environmental factors may have an important role in the formation of UA stones.
Composition and different types of UA stones. UA stones can be classified based on crystalline composition as anhydrous uric acid, uric acid dehydrate, sodium acid urate monohydrate or ammonium acid urate (Halabe et al., 1994). The anhydrous form is thermodynamically the most stable crystal. The dehydrate form is unstable and undergoes dehydration to the anhydrous form. Uric acid dehydrate has been identified in 20% of UA calculi and may represent the entire component. Ammonium acid urate precipitation requires high urate and ammonium concentrations and occurs at a higher pH. Recently, a classification of UA stones based on their crystalline growth pattern has been suggested (Grases et al., 2000).
Mechanism of stone formation. UA stone formation requires supersaturation of urinary UA. Three factors contribute to the formation of these calculi: acidic urine, hyperuricemia and decreased urinary volume. One or more of these conditions may coexist in a specific patient and contribute to stone disease severity (Shekarriz et al., 2002).
Hyperuricosuria. Hyperuricosuria is defined as a mean 24-hour urinary UA excretion of more than 600 mg/24 hr in 2 of 3 collected samples (Pak et al., 1980). Hyperuricosuria may be associated with hyperuricemia, such as in primary gout, or may manifest as an isolated abnormality due to various factors such as diet or medications. The degree of hyperuricemia correlates with the incidence of UA stone formation. In patients with gout the incidence of UA stones was 23% in those with urinary UA levels less than 600 mg/24hr compared with

50% in those with UA levels greater than 1,000 mg/24 hr (Yu et al., 1967). In other study 11% of patients with UA excretion less than 300 mg/24 hr had UA stones (Hall et al., 1967; Katz et al., 1970). In patients with gout the rate of stone formation is higher when uricosuric drugs are administered.

Urinary pH. All conditions contributing to acidic urine promote uric acid stone formation. Urinary pH is abnormally low in a significant number of patients with gout and in idiopathic UA stone formers (Gutman et al., 1968; Yu et al., 1967; Zechner et al., 1982; Ito et al., 1995). Urinary alkalization is the cornerstone of medical management of UA stones. The concept of UA stone dissolution is not new. Shekarriz et al., 2002 observed impressive dissolution of large burden UA renal stones with oral alkalization. UA stone dissolution by oral alkalization is generally effective, with a reported success rate of 80% (Shekarriz et al., 2002). Continued alkalization will help prevent future stones, but in the treatment of gout, alkalinization of urine (over pH 6.5) to maintain the solubility may precipitate calcium phosphate crystals (Meyer et al., 1990).

8. Gout

Gout is a disease of ancient origin and its association with UA stones has long been recognized. In 1683 London physician Thomas Sydenham, who suffered from renal stones, described the clinical features of gout. Michelangelo's special interest in anatomy and kidney function has been ascribed to his own urinary stone disease (Eknoyan et al., 2000).

Studies of the composition of urinary calculi were limited before the advent of modern chemistry. Gout is an inflammatory process initiated by tissue deposition of monosodium urate (MSU) crystals. A typical attack is an acute monoarthritis accompanied by classical signs of inflammation. However, inflammation can occur in any tissue in which MSU is deposited, as typified by tophaceous gout and by urate nephropathy due to renal medullary deposition of MSU crystals (So, 2008).

Multiple risk factors may interact and lead to development of gout:

Genetics - Monogenic disorders that result in overproduction of UA via enzyme defects in purine metabolism are extremely rare. Nevertheless, common primary gout in men often shows strong familiar predisposition, although the genetic basis remains unknown. Twin studies have show high heritability for both UA renal clearance (60%) and UA: creatinine ratio (87%) and several susceptibility loci for this have been reported (Roddy et al., 2007).

Gender and age - Men have higher urate levels than women and an increased prevalence of gout at all ages, though less pronounced in older age. Estrogens have a uricosuric effect, making gout very rare in younger women. However, after the menopause, urate levels rise and gout becomes increasingly prevalent. Ageing is an important risk factor in both men and women, possibly due to multiple factors including: an increase in sUA levels (mainly due to reduced renal function); increased use of diuretics and others drugs that raise sUA; age-related changes in connective tissues, which may encourage crystal formation (Roddy et al., 2007).

Diet - Historically, gout has long been linked with a rich lifestyle involving excesses of meat and alcohol, but it is only recently that population studies have been undertaken to determine the risk associated with individual dietary components. Data from the large Health Professionals Follow-up Study (HPFS) have show that the relative risk of gout is higher in people who eat a high red meat diet: the relative risk of a first attack of gout associated with an additional daily portion of meat was 1.21 (95% CI 1.04, 1.41). Higher consumption of seafood was associated with a lesser, but still significant, increase in risk. Diets high in purine-rich vegetables did not increase the risk, while diets high in low-fat dairy products were associated with reduced risk (relative risk with additional daily 0.79; 95% CI 0.71, 0.87) (Choi et al., 2004).

Alcohol - Some alcoholic drinks are rich in purines, notably beer which contains guanosine. Alcohol is though to increase the risk of gout because the metabolism of ethanol to acetyl CoA leads to adenine nucleotide degradation, resulting in increased formation of adenosine monophosphate, a precursor of UA. Alcohol also raises the lactic acid level in blood, which inhibits UA excretion. In the HPFS, overall the higher the daily alcohol intake, the higher the risk of gout (Choi et al., 2004). However, differences in risk were observed with different alcoholic drinks. Beer had the greatest effect, probably because of its high purine content, then alcohol, whereas wine had no increased risk (Choi et al., 2004).

Drugs - Many drugs which either increase sUA levels (e.g. diuretics and pyrazinamide) or reduces sUA levels (e.g.uricosurics such as benzbromarone, sulphinpyrazone and vitamin C) effect these changes via interaction with urate transporters such as URAT1 (Anzai et al., 2005) and GLUT9 (Caulfield et al., 2008).

RENAL DISEASE AND GOUT - Gout frequently associates with kidney disease, each being a risk factor for the other. Primary kidney disease can lead to hyperuricemia and it has been suggested that the increasing prevalence of end-stage renal disease may be one cause of recent increases in gout (Roddy et al., 2007). Kidney damage secondary to gout is associated with urate crystals and microtophi in the interstitium and/or UA crystals within tubules. Evidence from animal studies suggests that hyperuricemia may accelerate chronic kidney disease, and several studies have demonstrated a significant and independent association between sUA levels and the progression of chronic kidney disease (Kang et al., 2002; Kang et al., 2005). A history of gout is an independent risk factor for urolithiasis in men (Kramer et al., 2003). The increased risk is not just for UA stones, but also for more common calcium phosphate stones. High urinary levels of UA increase the risk of stone formation and in gout patients, the higher the excretion of UA, the greater the risk of stone formation (Yu et al., 1967). However, the most important risk factor for UA stone formation is persistently acidic urine, favoring the precipitation of urate (Shekarriz et al., 2002). In patients with UA stones, a high urinary UA: creatinine ratio indicates overproduction of UA, which should prompt a search for an abnormality of purine metabolism.

9. Advances in therapy of hyperuricemia and gout

The treatment of hyperuricemia and gout remains a challenge even though we appear to have a number of effective drugs. Many clinicians recognize that our existing treatment choices are often limited in the routine clinical setting. Allopurinol, the most commonly used drug to treat hyperuricemia, can provoke severe allergic-type reactions and needs to be used with caution in renal failure. Fortunately, the incidence of these rare reactions is low, but skin rashes are frequently reported (Hung et al., 2005). Benzbromarone, a very effective uricosuric drug, was recently withdrawn from general distribution because of a number of cases of hepatic failure associated with its use. Other hypouricemic drugs are therefore needed. Recently, a new xanthine-oxidase inhibitor, febuxostat, underwent clinical trials and was show to be as effective as allopurinol in reducing hyperuricemia (Becker et al., 2005). Febuxostat, unlike allopurinol, is not a purine analog and does not cross-react with allopurinol. In clinical trials, when administered at a daily dose of either 80 or 120 mg, it was more effective than a 300 mg daily dose of allopurinol in achieving the target value of uricemia (less than 6 mg/dL or less than 360 µmol/L), a target that has been recommended in treatment guidelines for gout and hyperuricemia (Zhang et al., 2006).

10. Conclusion

It is becoming clear that the role of UA is no longer confined solely to gout and nephrolithiasis. Increasing evidence now points to a significant relation of UA to hypertension and renal disease. Moreover, recent studies have started to unveil the causal nature of this relationship in both hypertension and renal disease. Despite considerable progress, given the numerous confounders, more compelling evidence is needed before ultimately labelling UA as a causative factor in hypertension and renal disease. Persistently acidic urine resulting in supersaturation of UA is the only metabolic abnormality found in many patients with UA stones. Although the mechanism responsible for acidic urine in many patients remains unclear, urinary alkalization is the cornerstone of medical management and should be the primary mode of treatment in the absence of absolute indications for surgical intervention. Furthermore, prophylaxis with urinary alkalization using oral alkali prevents stone recurrence and associated morbidity. Hyperuricemia is the central risk factor for gout and is a key component of the metabolic syndrome, is also an independent risk factor for cardiovascular disease, although at present there is no evidence to support urate-lowering therapy for asymptomatic hyperuricemia. More studies in this exciting and provocative area of research are being conducted and published (Kanbay et al., 2007; 2010; Turgut et al., 2009).

11. References

Albertoni G, Maquigussa E, Pessoa E, Barreto JA, Borges F, Schor N. (2010). Soluble uric acid increases intracellular calcium through an angiotensin II-dependent mechanism in immortalized human mesangial cells. *Experimetal Biological Medicine,* Vol. 235, No.7, (July 2010), pp.825-832, ISSN 1535-3702.

Ames BN, Cathcart R, Schwiers E, Hochstein P. (1981). Uric acid provides an antioxidant defense in humans against oxidant- and radical-caused aging and cancer: a hypothesis. *Proccedings of the National Academy of Science USA,* Vol. 78, No.11, (November 1981), pp.6858-6862, ISSN 0027-8424.

Anzai N, Enomoto A, Endou H. (2005). Renal urate handling: clinical relevance of recent advances. *Curr Rheumatol Rep,* Vol. 7, No 3, (June 2005), pp.227-35, ISSN 1534-6307.

Atsmon A, de Vries A, Frank M. (1963). Uric acid lithiasis. New York: Elsevier Publishing Co.

Becker MA, Schumacher HR Jr., Wortmann RL, MacDonald PA, Eustace D, Palo WA, Streit J, Joseph-Ridge N. (2005). Febuxostat compared with allopurinol in patients with hyperuricemia and gout. *N Engl J Med,* Vol. 353, No 23, (December 2005), pp.2450-61, ISSN 1533-4406.

Bonakdaran S, Hami M, Shakeri MT.. (2011). Hyperuricemia and albuminuria in patients with type 2 diabetes mellitus. *Iranian Journal of Kidney Dieases,*Vol. 5, No.1, (January 2011), pp. 21-24, ISSN 1735-8582.

Calabro P. Yeh ET. (2008). Intra-abdominal adiposity, inflammation, and cardiovascular risk: new insight into global cardiometabolic risk. *Current Hypertension Report,* Vol. 10, No.1, (February 2008), pp.32-38, ISSN 1522-6417.

Carnethon MR, Fortmann SP, Palaniappan L, Duncan BB, Schmidt MI, Chambless LE. (2003). Risk factors for progression to incident hyperurinsulinemia: the atherosclerosis risk in communities study. *American Journal of Epidemiology,* Vol. 158, No.11, (December 2003), pp.1058-1067, ISSN 1476-6256.

Caulfield MJ, Munroe PB, O'Neill D, Witkowska K, Charchar FJ, Doblado M, Evans S, Eyheramendy S, Onipinla A, Howard P, Shaw-Hawkins S, Dobson RJ, Wallace C, Newhouse SJ, Brown M, Connell JM, Dominiczak A, Farrall M, Lathrop GM, Samani NJ, Kumari M, Marmot M, Brunner E, Chambers J, Elliott P, Kooner J, Laan M, Org E, Veldre G, Viigimaa M, Cappuccio FP, Ji C, Iacone R, Strazzullo P, Moley KH, Cheeseman C. (2008). SLC2A9 is a high-capacity urate transporter in humans. *PLoS Med,* Vol. 5, No 10, (October 2008), pp.197, ISSN 1549-1676.

Chang HY, Tung CW, Lee PH, Lei CC, Hsu YC, Chang HH, Yang HF, Lu LC, Jong MC, Chen CY, Fang KY, Chao YS, Shih YH, Lin CL. (2010). Hyperuricemia as an independent risk factor of chronic kidney disease in middle-aged and elderly population. *American Journal of the Medical Science,* Vol. 339, No.6, (June 2010), pp. 509-515, ISSN 0002-9629.

Chaves FJ, Corella D, Blesa S, Mansego ML, Marín P, Portoles O, Sorlí JV, González-Albert V, Tormos MC, García-García AB, Sáez G, Redon J. (2007). Xanthine oxidoreductase polymorphisms: influence in blood pressure and oxidative stress levels. *Pharmacogenetics and Genomics* Vol. 17, No.8, (August 2007), pp.589-596, ISSN 1744-6872.

Chen YC, Su CT, Wang ST, Lee HD, Lin SY. (2009). A preliminary investigation of the association between serum uric acid and impaired renal function. *Chang Gung Med J,* Vol. 32, No 1, (Jan-Feb 2009), pp.66-71, ISSN 2072-0939.

Chien KL, Chen MF, Hsu HC, Chang WT, Su TC, Lee YT, Hu FB. (2008). Plasma uric acid and the risk of type 2 diabetes in a Chinese community. *Clinical chemistry* Vol. 54, No.2, (February 2008), pp.310-316, ISSN 0009-9147.

Choi HK, Atkinson K, Karlson EW, Willett W, Curhan G. (2004). Purine-rich foods, dairy and protein intake, and the risk of gout in men. *N Engl J Med,* Vol. 350, No 11, (March 2004), pp. 1093-103, ISSN 1533-4406.

Choi HK, Willett W, Curhan G. (2007). Coffee consumption and risk of incident gout in men: a prospective study. *Arthritis Rheum,* Vol. 56, No 6, (June 2007), pp.2049-55, ISSN 1529-0131.

Cirillo P, Sato W, Reungjui S, Heinig M, Gersch M, Sautin Y, Nakagawa T, Johnson RJ. (2006). Uric acid, the metabolic syndrome, and renal disease. *Journal of the American Society Nephrology,* Vol. 17, No. 12 Suppl, (December 2006), pp. S165-S168, ISSN 1046-6673.

Conger JD. (1990). Acute uric acid nephropathy. *Med Clin North Am,* Vol. 74, No 4, (July 1990), pp.859-71, ISSN 1557-9859.

Convento MS, Pessoa E, Dalboni MA, Borges FT, Schor N. (2011). Pro-inflammatory and oxidative effects of noncrystalline uric acid in human mesangial cells: contribution to hyperuricemic glomerular damage. *Urological Research,* Vol. 39, No.1, (June 2010), pp.21-27, ISSN 0300-5623.

Cook S, Hugli O, Egli M, Vollenweider P, Burcelin R, Nicod P, Thorens B, Scherrer U. (2003). Clustering of cardiovascular risk factors mimicking the human metabolic syndrome X in eNOs null mice. *Swiss Med Weekly* Vol. 136, No.24-26, (June 2003), pp.360-363, ISSN 1424-3997.

Corry DB, Eslami P, Yamamoto K, Nyby MD, Makino H, Tuck ML. (2008). Uric acid stimulates vascular smooth muscle cell proliferation and oxidative stress via the vascular renin-angiotensin system. *Journal of Hypertension*, Vol. 26, No.2, (February 2008), pp.269-275, ISSN 0263-6352.

Daoussis D, Panoulas V, Toms T, John H, Antonopoulos I, Nightingale P, Douglas KM, Klocke R, Kitas GD. (2009). Uric acid is a strong independent predictor of renal dysfunction in patients with rheumatoid arthritis. *Arthritis Res Ther*, Vol.11, No 4, (July 2009), PP.116, ISSN 1478-6362..

Dehghan A, van Hoek M, Sijbrands EJ, Hofman A, Witteman JC. (2008). High serum uric acid as a novel risk factor for type 2 diabetes. *Diabetes Care*, Vol. 31, No.2, (February 2008), pp. 361-2, ISSN 0149-5992.

Domrongkitchaiporn S, Sritara P, Kitiyakara C, Stitchantrakul W, Krittaphol V, Lolekha P, Cheepudomwit S, Yipintsoi T. (2005). Risk factors for development of decreased kidney function in a southeast Asian population: a 12-year cohort study. *Journal of the American Society Nephrology*, Vol.16, No.3, (March 2005), pp.791-9, ISSN 1046-6673.

Eknoyan G. (2000). Michelangelo: art, anatomy, and the kidney. *Kidney Int*, Vol.57, No 3, (March 2000), pp.1190-201, ISSN 1523-1755.

Facchini F, Chen YD, Hollenbeck CB, Reaven GM. (1991). Relationship between resistance to insulin-mediated glucose uptake, urinary uric acid clearance, and plasma uric acid concentration. *The Journal of the American Medical Association*, Vol. 266, No.21, (December 1991), pp.3008-3011, ISSN 0098-7484.

Feig DI, Kang DH, Johnson RJ. (2008). Uric acid and cardiovascular risk. *New England Journal of Medicine*, Vol.359, No.17, (October 2008), pp.1811-1821, ISSN 0028-4793.

Feig DI, Kang DH, Nakagawa T, Mazzali M, Johnson RJ. (2006). Uric acid and hypertension. *Curr Hypertens Rep*, Vol. 8, No 2, (May 2006), pp.111-5, ISSN 1534-3111.

Feig DI. (2009). Uric acid: a novel mediator and marker of risk in chronic kidney disease? *Current Opinion in Nephrology and Hypertension*, Vol.18, No.6, (November 2009), pp.526-530, ISSN 1062-4821.

Finlayson B. (1974). Symposium on renal lithiasis. Renal lithiasis in review. *Urol Clin North Am*, Vol. 01, No 2, (June 1974), pp.181-212, ISSN 1558-318X.

Furukawa S, Fujita T, Shimabukuro M, Iwaki M, Yamada Y, Nakajima Y, Nakayama O, Makishima M, Matsuda M, Shimomura I. (2004). Increased oxidative stress in obesity and its impact on metabolic syndrome. The *Journal of Clinical Investigation*, Vol.114, No.12, (December 2004), pp.1752-1761, ISSN 0021-9738.

Gentle DL, Stoller ML, Bruce JE, Leslie SW. (1997). Geriatric urolithiasis. *J Urol*, Vol.158, No 6, (December 1997), pp.2221-4, ISSN 1527-3792.

Glantzounis GK, Tsimoyiannis EC, Kappas AM, Galaris DA. (2005). Uric acid and oxidative stress. *Current Pharmaceutical Design*, Vol.11, No.32, pp.4145-4151, ISSN 1381-6128.

Grases F, Villacampa AI, Costa-Bauza A, Sohnel O. (2000). Uric acid calculi: types, etiology and mechanisms of formation. *Clin Chim Acta*, Vol. 302, No 1-2, (September 2000), pp.89-104, ISSN 1873-3492.

Grenabo L, Hedelin H, Petterson S. (1985). The severity of infection stones compared to other stones in the upper urinary tract. *Scand J Urol Nephrol,* Vol. 19, No 4, pp.285-9, ISSN 1651-2065.

Gutman AB, Yu TF. (1968). Uric acid nephrolithiasis. *Am J Med,* Vol. 45, No 5, (November 1968), pp.756-79, ISSN 1555-7162.

Hak AE, Choi HK. (2008). Menopause, postmenopausal hormone use and serum uric acid levels in US women - the third national health and nutrition examination survey. *Arthritis Res Ther,* Vol. 10, No 5, (September 2008), pp.116, ISSN 1478-6362.

Halabe A, Sperling O. (1994). Uric acid nephrolithiasis. *Electrolyte Metab,* Vol. 20, No 6, (1994), pp.424-31, ISSN 0378-0392.

Hall AP, Barry PE, Dawber TR, McNamara PM. (1967). Epidemiology of gout and hyperuricemia. A long-term population study. *Am J Med,* Vol. 42, No 1, (January 1967), pp.27-37. ISSN 1555-7162.

Haririan A, Noguiera JM, Zandi-Nejad K, Aiyer R, Hurley H, Cooper M, Klassen DK, Weir MR. (2010). The independent association between serum uric acid and graft outcomes after kidney transplantation. *Transplantation,* Vol. 89, No 5, (March 2010), pp.573-9, ISSN 1534-6080.

Hesse A, Schneider HJ, Berg W, Hienzsch E. (1975). Uric acid dehydrate as urinary calculus component. *Invest Urol,* Vol. 12, No 5, (March 1975), pp.405-9, ISSN 0021-0005.

Hovind P, Rossing P, Johnson RJ, Parving HH. (2011). Serum uric acid as a new player in the development of diabetic nephropathy. *Journal of Renal Nutrition,* Vol.21, No.1, (January 2011), pp.124-127, ISSN 1051-2276.

Hung HY, Appel LJ, Choi MJ Gelber AC, Charleston J, Norkus EP, Miller ER 3rd. (2005). The effects of vitamin C supplementation on serum concentrations of uric acid: results of a controlled trial. *Arthritis Rheum,* Vol. 52, No 6, (June 2005), pp.1843-7, ISSN 1529-0131.

Hunsicker LG, Adler S, Caggiula A, England BK, Greene T, Kusek JW, Rogers NL, Teschan PE. (1997). Predictors of the progression of renal disease in the Modification of Diet in Renal Disease Study. *Kidney International,* Vol.51, No.6, (June 1997), pp.1908-1919, ISSN 0098-6577.

Iseki K, Ikemiya Y, Inoue T , Iseki C, Kinjo K, Takishita S. (2004). Significance of hyperuricemia as a risk factor for developing ESRD in a screened cohort. *Am J Kidney Dis,* Vol. 44, No 4, (October 2004), pp642-50, ISSN 1523-6838.

Iseki K, Oshiro S, Tozawa M, Iseki C, Ikemiya Y, Takishita S. (2001). Significance of hyperuricemia on the early detection of renal failure in a cohort of screened subjects. *Hypertension Research,* Vol. 24, No 6, (November 2001), pp.691-697, ISSN 0916-9636.

Ito H, Kotake T, Nomura K, Masai M. (1995). Clinical and biochemical features of uric acid nephrolithiasis. *Eur Urol,* Vol. 27, No 4, pp.324-8, ISSN 1873-7560.

Johnson RJ, Kang DH, Feig D, Kivlighn S, Kanellis J, Watanabe S, Tuttle KR, Rodriguez-Iturbe B, Herrera-Acosta J, Mazzali M. (2003). Is there a pathogenetic role for uric acid in hypertension and cardiovascular and renal disease? *Hypertens*ion, Vol. 41, No 6, (April 2003), pp.1183-1190, ISSN 0194911X.

Johnson RJ, Segal MS, Srinivas T, Ejaz A, Mu W, Roncal C, Sánchez-Lozada LG, Gersch M, Rodriguez-Iturbe B, Kang DH, Acosta JH. (2005). *J Am Soc Nephrol,* Vol. 16, No 7, (July 2005), pp.1909-19, ISSN 1533-3450.

Kanbay M, Ozkara A, Selcoki Y, Isik B, Turgut F, Bavbek N, Uz E, Akcay A, Yigitoglu R, Covic A. (2007). Effect of treatment of hyperuricemia with allopurinol on blood pressure, creatinine clearance, and proteinuria in patients with normal renal function. *Int Urol Nephrol,* Vol. 39, No 4, (August 2007), pp.1227-33, ISSN 1573-2584.

Kanbay M, Sanchez-Lozada LG, Franco M (2010). Microvascular disease and its role in the brain and cardiovascular system: a potential role for uric acid as a cardiorenal toxin. *Nephrol Dial Transpalnt,* Vol. 26, No 2, (February 2010), pp. 430-7, ISSN 1460-2385.

Kanellis J, Watanabe S, Li JH, Kang DH, Li P, Nakagawa T, Wamsley A, Sheikh-Hamad D, Lan HY, Feng L, Johnson RJ. (2003). Uric acid stimulates monocyte chemoattractant protein-1 production in vascular smooth muscle cells via mitogen-activated protein kinase and cyclooxygenase-2. *Hypertension,* Vol. 41, No 6, (May 2003), pp.1287-1293, ISSN 0194911X.

Kang DH, Nakagawa T, Feng L, Watanabe S, Han L, Mazzali M, Truong L, Harris R, Johnson RJ. (2002). A role for uric acid in the progression of renal disease. *Journal of the American Society Nephrology,* Vol. 13, No 12, (December 2002), pp.2888-2897, ISSN 1046-6673.

Kang DH, Nakagawa T. (2005). Uric acid and chronic renal disease: possible implication of hyperuricemia on progression of renal disease. *Sem Nephrol.* Vol.25, No 01, (January 2005), pp.43-9, ISSN 1558-4488.

Katz WA, Schubert M. (1970). The interaction of monosodium urate with connective tissue components. *J Clin Invest,* Vol. 49, No 10, (October 1970), pp.1783-9, ISSN 1365-2362.

Khosla UM, Zharikov S, Finch JL, Nakagawa T, Roncal C, Mu W, Krotova K, Block ER, Prabhakar S, Johnson RJ. (2005). Hyperuricemia induces endothelial dysfunction. *Kidney International,* Vol. 67, No 5, (May 2005), pp.1739-1742, ISSN 0098-6577.

Kim ES, Kwon HS, Ahn CW, Lim DJ, Shin JA, Lee SH, Cho JH, Yoon KH, Kang MI, Cha BY, Son HY. (2010). Serum uric acid level is associated with metabolic syndrome and microalbuminuria in Korean patients with type 2 diabetes mellitus. *Journal of Diabetes and itsComplications,* [epub ahead of print], (December 2010), ISSN 1056-8727.

Kim JA, Montagnani M, Koh KK, Quon MJ. (2006). Reciprocal relationships between insulin resistance and endothelial dysfunction: molecular and pathophysiological mechanisms. *Circulation,* Vol. 113, No 15, (April 2006), pp.1888-1904, ISSN 0009-7322.

Krishnan E, Kwoh CK, Schumacher HR, Kuller L. (2007). *Hypertension,* Vol. 49, No 2, (February 2007), pp.298-303, ISSN 1524-4563.

Kuo CF, Luo SF, See LC, Ko YS, Chen YM, Hwang JS, Chou IJ, Chang HC, Chen HW, Yu KH. (2010). Hyperuricaemia and accelerated reduction in renal function. (2006). *Scandinavian Journal of Rheumatology,* [Epub ahead of print], (September 2010), ISSN 0301-3847.

Kutzing, MK & Firestein, BL. (2008). Altered uric acid levels and disease states. *Journal of Pharmacology and Experimental Therapeutics,* Vol. 324, No 1, (September 2008), pp.1-7, ISSN 0022-3565.

Li Y, Sato M, Yanagisawa Y Mamada H, Fukushi A, Mikami K, Shirasaka Y, Tamai I. (2008). Effects of angiotensin II receptor blockers on renal handling of uric acid in rats. *Drug Metab Pharmacokinet,* Vol. 23, No 4, (2008), pp.263-70, ISSN 1880-0920.

Lin CS, Hung YL, Chen GY, Tzeng TF, Lee DY, Chen CY, Huang WP, Huang CH. (2010). A multicenter study of the association of serum uric acid, serum creatinine, and diuretic use in hypertensive patients. *Int J Cardiol,* Vol. 148, No 3, (May 2010), pp.325-30, ISSN 1874-1754.

Madero M, Sarnak MJ, Wang X, Greene T, Beck GJ, Kusek JW, Collins AJ, Levey AS, Menon V. (2009). Uric acid and long-term outcomes in CKD. *Am J Kidney Dis,* Vol. 53, No 5, (May 2009), pp.796-802. ISSN 1523-6838.

Mandel NS, Mandel GS. (1989). Urinary tract stone disease in the United States veteran population. II. Geographical analysis of variations in composition. *J Urol,* Vol. 142, No 6, (December 1989), pp.1516-21, ISSN 1527-3792.

Masuo K, Kawaguchi H, Mikami H, Ogihara T, Tuck ML. (2003). Serum uric acid and plasma norepinephrine concentrations predicts subsequent weight gain and blood pressure elevation. *Hypertension,* Vol. 42, (October 2003), pp.474-80, ISSN 0194911X.

Mazzali M, Hughes J, Kim YG, Jefferson JA, Kang DH, Gordon KL, Lan HY, Kivlighn S, Johnson RJ. (2001). Elevated uric acid increases blood pressure in the rat by a novel crystal-independent mechanism. *Hypertension,* Vol. 38, No 5, (November 2001), pp. 1101-1106, ISSN 0194911X.

Mazzali M, Kanellis J, Han L, Feng L, Xia YY, Chen Q, Kang DH, Gordon KL, Watanabe S, Nakagawa T, Lan HY, Johnson RJ. (2002). Hyperuricemia induces a primary renal arteriolopathy in rats by a blood pressure-independent mechanism. *American Journal of Physiology. Renal Physiology,* Vol. 282, No 6, (June 2002), pp.F991-F997, ISSN 0363-6127.

Mercuro G, Vitale C, Cerquetani E, Zoncu S, Deidda M, Fini M, Rosano GM.. (2004). Effect of hyperuricemia upon endothelial function in patients at increased cardiovascular risk. *American Journal of Cardiology,* Vol. 94 7, (October 2004), pp. 932-935, ISSN 0002-9149.

Meyer JL. (1990). Physicochemistry of stone formation. *Urolithiasis a Medical Surgical Reference,* WB Saunders, Philadelphia, pp.11-34.

Minon Cifuentes J, Pourmand G. (1983). Mineral composition of 103 stones from Iran. *Br J Urol,*Vol. 55, No 5, (October 1983), pp.468-8, ISSN 0007-1331.

Nakagawa T, Hu H, Zharikov S, Tuttle KR, Short RA, Glushakova O, Ouyang X, Feig DI, Block ER, Herrera-Acosta J, Patel JM, Johnson RJ. (2006). A causal role for uric acid in fructose-induced metabolic syndrome. *American Journal of Physiology. Renal Physiology,* Vol. 290, No 3, (March 2006), pp. F625-F631, ISSN 0002-9149.

Nakagawa T, Mazzali M, Kang DH, Kanellis J, Watanabe S, Sanchez-Lozada LG, Rodriguez-Iturbe B, Herrera-Acosta J, Johnson RJ. (2003). Hyperuricemia causes glomerular hypertrophy in the rat. *American Journal of Nephrology,* Vol. 23, No 2, pp. 2-7, ISSN 0250-8095.

Nakagawa T, Tuttle KR, Short RA, Johnson RJ. (2005). Fructose-induced hyperuricemia as a causal mechanism for the epidemic of the metabolic syndrome. *Nature Clinical Practice. Nephrology,* Vol. 1, No 2, (December 2005), pp. 80-86, ISSN 1745-8323.

Nakanishi N, Okamoto M, Yoshida H, Matsuo Y, Suzuki K, Tatara K. (2003). Serum uric acid and risk for development of hypertension and impaired fasting glucose or type II diabetes in Japanese male office workers. *European Journal of Epidemiology,* Vol. 18, No 6, pp. 523-30, ISSN 0393- 2990.

Obermayr RP, Temml C, Gutjahr G, Knechtelsdorfer M, Oberbauer R, Klauser-Braun R. (2008). Elevated uric acid increases the risk for kidney disease. *Journal of the American Society of Nephrology,* Vol. 19, No 12, (December 2008), pp. 2407-2413 ISSN 1046-6673.

Pak CYC, Britton F, Peterson R, Ward D, Northcutt C, Breslau N, McGuire J, Sakhaee K, Bush S, Nicar M, Norman DA, Peters P. (1980). Ambulatory evaluation of nephrolithiasis. Classification, clinical presentation and diagnostic criteria. *Am J Med,* Vol. 69, No 1, (July 1980), pp.19-30, ISSN1555-7162.

Parving, H-H. Mauer, M. Ritz E. (2008). Diabetic nephropathy, In: *Brenner BM,* (ed.) Brenner & Rector's The Kidney, 8th pp. 1265-1298, Boston

Quiñones Galvan A, Natali A, Baldi S, Frascerra S, Sanna G, Ciociaro D, Ferrannini E. (1995). Effect of insulin on uric acid excretion in humans. *American Journal of Physiology. Endocrinology and Metabolism,* Vol. 268, No 1, (January 1995), pp. E1-E5, ISSN 0193-1849.

Reungjui S, Roncal CA, Mu W, Srinivas TR, Sirivongs D, Johnson RJ, Nakagawa T. (2007). Thiazide diuretics exacerbate fructose-induced metabolic syndrome. *Journal of the American Society of Nephrology,* Vol. 18, No 10, (October 2007), pp. 2724-2731, ISSN 1046-6673.

Riegersperger M, Covic A, Goldsmith D. (2011). Allopurinol, uric acid, and oxidative stress in cardiorenal disease. *Int Urol Nephrol,* Vol. 43, No 2, (June 2011), pp.441-9, ISSN 1573-2584 .

Riese RL, Sakhaee K. (1992). Uric acid nephrolithiasis: pathogenesis and treatment. *J Urol,* Vol. 148, No 3, (September 1992), pp.765-71, ISSN 1527-3792.

Roddy E, Zhang W, Doherty M. (2007). The changing epidemiology of gout. *Nat Clin Pract Rheumatol,* Vol. 3, No 8, (August 2007), pp. 443-9, ISSN 1745-8390.

Sánchez-Lozada LG, Nakagawa T, Kang DH, Feig DI, Franco M, Johnson RJ, Herrera-Acosta J. (2006). Hormonal and cytokine effects of uric acid. *Current Opinion in Nephrology and Hypertension,* Vol. 15, No 1, (January 2006), pp. 30-33, ISSN 1062-4821.

Sánchez-Lozada LG, Tapia E, Bautista-García P, Soto V, Avila-Casado C, Vega-Campos IP, Nakagawa T, Zhao L, Franco M, Johnson RJ. (2008). Effects of febuxostat on metabolic and renal alterations in rats with fructose-induced metabolic syndrome. *American Journal of Physiology. Renal Physiology,* Vol. 294, No 4, (April 2008), pp.F710-F718, ISSN 0002-9149.

Sánchez-Lozada LG, Tapia E, Santamaría J, Avila-Casado C, Soto V, Nepomuceno T, Rodríguez-Iturbe B, Johnson RJ, Herrera-Acosta J. (2005). Mild hyperuricemia induces vasoconstriction and maintains glomerular hypertension in normal and remnant kidney rats. *Kidney International,* Vol. 67, No 1, (January 2005), pp. 237-247, ISSN 0098-6577.

Sautin YY & Johnson RJ. (2008). Uric acid: the oxidant-antioxidant paradox. *Nucleosides Nucleotides Nucleic Acids,* Vol. 27, No 6, (June 2008), pp.608-19, ISSN 1525-7770.

Sautin YY, Nakagawa T, Zharikov S, Johnson RJ. (2007). Adverse effects of the classic antioxidant uric acid in adipocytes: NADPH oxidase-mediated oxidative/nitrosative stress. *American Journal of Physiology. Cell Physiology,* Vol. 293, No 2, (April 2007), pp. C584-C596, ISSN 0363-6143.

Scholz D, Schwille PO, Ullbrich D, Bausch WM, Sigel A. (1979). Composition of renal stones and their frequency in a stone clinic: relationship to parameters of mineral metabolism in serum and urine. *Urol Res,* Vol. 7, No 3, (September 1979), pp.161-70, ISSN 1434-0879.

See LC, Kuo CF, Chuang FH, Shen YM, Ko YS, Chen YM, Yu KH. (2010). Hyperuricemia and metabolic syndrome: associations with chronic kidney disease. *Clinical Rheumatology,* [Epub ahead of print], (April 2010), ISSN 0770-3198.

Shan Y, Zhang Q, Liu Z, Hu X, Liu D. (2010). Prevalence and risk factors associated with chronic kidney disease in adults over 40 years: a population study from Central China. *Nephrology,* Vol. 15, No 3, (April 2010), pp.354-61, ISSN 1440-1797.

Shekarriz B, Stoller ML. (2002). Uric acid nephrolithiasis: current concepts and controversies. *J Urol,* Vol. 168, No 4, (October 2002), pp.1307-14, ISSN 1527-3792.

So A. (2008). Developments in the scientific and clinical understanding of gout. *Arthritis Res Ther,* Vol. 10, No 5, (October 2008), PP.221-27, ISSN 1478-6362.

Steele TH. (1973). Urate secretion in man: the pyrazinamide suppression test. *Ann Int Med,* Vol. 79, No 5, (November 1973), pp.734-7, ISSN 1539-3704.

Sturm G, Kollerits B, Neyer U, Ritz E, Kronenberg F; MMKD Study Group. (2008). Uric acid as a risk factor for progression of non-diabetic chronic kidney disease? The Mild to Moderate Kidney Disease (MMKD) Study. *Experimental Gerontology,* Vol. 43, No 4, (April 2008), pp. 347-52, ISSN 0531-5565.

Suliman ME, Johnson RJ, Garcia-Lopez, Qureshi AR, Molinaei H, Carrero JJ, Heimbürger O, Bárány P, Axelsson J, Lindholm B, Stenvinkel P. (2006). J-shaped mortality relationship for uric acid in CKD. *Am J Kidney Dis,* Vol. 48, No 5, (November 2006), pp.761-71, ISSN 1523-6838.

Tomita M, Mizuno S, Yamanaka H, Hosoda Y, Sakuma K, Matuoka Y, Odaka M, Yamaguchi M, Yosida H, Morisawa H, Murayama T. (2000). Does hyperuricemia affect mortality? A prospective cohort study of Japanese male workers. *Journal of Epidemiology,* Vol. 10, No 6, (November 2000), pp. 403-9, ISSN 0917-5040.

Turgut F, Kasopoglu B, Kanbay M. (2009). Uric acid, cardiovascular mortality, long-term outcomes in CKD. *Am J Kidney,* Vol. 54, No 3, (September 2009), pp.582-3, ISSN 1523-6838.

United states renal data system, available at: www.usrds.org, 2008.

Watanabe S, Kang DH, Feng L, Nakagawa T, Kanellis J, Lan H, Mazzali M, Johnson RJ. (2002). Uric acid, hominoid evolution, and the pathogenesis of salt-sensitivity. *Hypertension,*Vol. 40, No 3, (September 2002), pp. 355-360, ISSN 0194911X.

Yoo TW, Sung KC, Shin HS, Kim BJ, Kim BS, Kang JH, Lee MH, Park JR, Kim H, Rhee EJ, Lee WY, Kim SW, Ryu SH, Keum DG. (2005). Relationship between serum uric acid concentration and insulin resistence and metabolic syndrome. *Circ J,* Vol. 69, No 8, (August 2005), pp.928-33, ISSN 1347-4820.

Yu MA, Sánchez-Lozada LG, Johnson RJ, Kang DH. (2010). Oxidative stress with an activation of the renin-angiotensin system in human vascular endothelial cells as a novel mechanism of uric acid-induced endothelial dysfunction. *Journal of Hypertension,* Vol. 28, No 6, (June 2010), pp. 1234-1242, ISSN 0263-6352.

Yu T, Gutman AB. (1967). Uric acid nephrolithiasis in gout. Predisposing factors. *Ann Intern Med,* Vol. 67, No 6, (December 1967), pp.1133-48, ISSN 1539-3704.

Yu TF, Gutman AB. (1967). Uric acid nephrolithiasis in gout: predisposing factors. *Ann Intern Med,* Vol. 67, No 6, (December 1967), pp.1133-48, ISSN 1539-3704.

Zechner O, Pfluger H, Scheiber V. (1982). Idiopathic uric acid lithiasis: epidemiologic and metabolic aspects. *J Urol,* Vol. 128, No 6, (December 1982), pp.1219-23, ISSN 1527-3792.

Zhang W, Doherty M, Pacual E, Bardin T, Barskova V, Conaghan P, Gerster J, Jacobs J, Leeb B, Lioté F, McCarthy G, Netter P, Nuki G, Perez-Ruiz F, Pignone A, Pimentão J, Punzi L, Roddy E, Uhlig T, Zimmermann-Gòrska I. (2006). EULAR evidence based recommendations for gout. Part I: Diagnosis. Report of a task force of the Standing Committee for International Clinical Studies Including Therapeutics (ESCISIT).*Ann Rheum Dis,* Vol. 65, No 10, (October 2006), pp.1301-11, ISSN 1468-2060.

6

Renal Disease and Pregnancy

Marius Craina, Elena Bernad, Răzvan Nițu, Paul Stanciu, Cosmin Cîtu, Zoran Popa, Corina Şerban and Rodica Mihăescu
University of Medicine and Pharmacy
"Victor Babeş" Timişoara
Romania

1. Introduction

Pregnancy in women with different renal diseases has important consequences for the developing fetus and maternal health. Kidneys and the urinary tract have to adapt to the pregnancy status and therefore suffer significant anatomical, hemodynamic and endocrine changes. Failure to adapt can aggravate the preexisting maternal disease and can also create suboptimal environment for fetal development and increase the risk of obstetric complications. Knowledge and correct interpretation of the renal functional tests is necessary for the modern obstetrician, avoiding an incorrect diagnosis for renal disease where only specific renal changes during pregnancy are present, but meanwhile a correct evaluation of the renal function and changes can detect a pathology that can aggravate both the mother's and the baby's condition. Improvement and better understanding of the renal pathophysiology in pregnancy made possible that pregnant woman look forward for a good outcome, including here also the women with renal transplant. Nowadays is underlined the concept of multidisciplinary teamwork, a very important concept of modern medicine. The obstetrician should consider nephrologists as key players in the team and in our opinion should refer to them the pregnant women for a routine check-up of the renal status in the 2nd or beginning of 3rd trimester by ultrasound, beside the usual blood and urine analysis. The nephrologists and urologists should be involved in the management of severe medical conditions, such as preeclampsia, acute and chronic renal failure and never the less in the complex management of dialysis or renal transplant patients. In pregnancy it can be encountered several renal diseases, some of them preexisting the pregnancy and other developed or being direct influenced by pregnancy. This chapter will discuss briefly the basic evaluation of renal status in order to present and better understand the acute and chronic renal disorders in pregnancy. The chapter will focus on the most common preexisting diseases in pregnancy such as: chronic glomerulonephritis, secondary glomerular nephropathies, interstitial nephropathies (chronic pyelonephritis, renal tuberculosis), diabetes nephropathy, unique surgical kidney, chronic renal failure. From the renal diseases directly influenced by pregnancy it will be discussed: asymptomatic bacteriuria, symptomatic urinary infection, urolithiasis and acute renal failure in pregnancy.

It will be presented also the management of dialysis in pregnancy and pregnant women with renal transplant.

2. Evaluation of the renal function in pregnancy

Evaluation of the renal function is very important in pregnant women. *Serum uric acid, blood urea nitrogen (BUN),* and *serum creatinine levels* are important indices of renal function in pregnancy. *Urinalysis* is a useful tool for screening, further testing being necessary if changes in renal status are detected. Another useful method is the *24 hour urine sample,* used especially for total protein analysis. Most investigators consider the value of up to 260 mg/day of total urinary protein normal in pregnancy. Usually higher values indicate a decline of renal function due to preeclampsia. It should be noted that when serial 24-hour urine samples are performed in order to evaluate the change of renal status, it is crucial that the collection be standardized [Airoldi, 2007]. The total amount of creatinine excreted in 24 hour is considered to be the best method to compare two urine samples, as the cleared creatinine in a day should remain constant through pregnancy. The significance of dipstick or microscopic hematuria in pregnancy is uncertain, but some studies suggested it is associated with a greater risk for preeclampsia [Brown, 2005]. A study of McNair and collaborators compared urinalysis with uroculture for screening of asymptomatic bacteriuria [McNair, 2000]. They found that urinalysis has a sensitivity of 80.6% and specificity of 71.5% in their population. Given the 19.4% of false negative rate and the morbidity of the undiagnosed bacteriuria it is recommended that urine culture should be used as the primary method for screening in pregnant women. Although baseline creatinine clearance is decreased in patients with chronic renal insufficiency, it should still be elevated in pregnancy. Pregnancy may lead to permanent worsening of renal function in more than 40% women with serum creatinine (SCr) of 250 μmol/l or greater or creatinine clearance < 50 ml/minute and therefore it should serve as a contraindication to pregnancy. However, at that level of impaired renal function fertility is reduced and pregnancy is rare. The treatment of microalbuminuria with ACE-inhibitors should be interrupted in women that want to become pregnant. A moderate decrease of creatinine clearance is often observed during late gestation in women with renal disease. Typically this decrease is more severe in women with diffuse glomerular disease and it usually reverses after delivery. The long-term effect of pregnancy on renal disease remains controversial. Pregnant women with renal disease that have normal or near normal renal function at conception and a SCr < 120 μmol/L carry only a slightly increased risk of a long-term damage to their kidneys from pregnancy compared with never pregnant women with mild renal disease. In a larger multicenter study, 40% of women with moderate renal impairment (SCr 124-168 μmol/L; 1.49-1.90 mg/dL) had pregnancy related deterioration in renal function that persisted after delivery in almost 50% of cases [Williams, 2004]. One of the series from this study showed that only 2% of the pregnancies in women with initial SCr below 2.00 mg/dL rapidly decline to ESRF [Jungers, 1995; Jones, 1996; Epstein, 1996; Sibai, 2002]. Two-thirds of women with SCr > 2.0 mg/dL have a gestational deterioration in renal function that nearly always persists in the post-partum period. The recovery of the renal function after the delivery is rare. One third of women will develop ESRF during or following pregnancy. If renal function significantly worsens during pregnancy, studies showed that the termination of pregnancy will not improve the maternal outcome, therefore abortion cannot be routinely recommended for pregnant women with SCr over 1.5 mg/dL. Ideally before conception counseling should be provided for women with renal chronic disease. Severe hypertension is considered to be the greatest threat to pregnant woman with chronic renal disease, as uncontrolled hypertension can lead to intracerebral hemorrhage, or worse renal status. Diastolic blood pressure > 110 mmHg or greater will develop in ~ 20% of the patient with hypertension, a bigger chance of eclampsia being present in these cases. Proteinuria usually increases in chronic renal disease during pregnancy often reaching nephrotic ranges. A study remarked a correlation between low serum albumin and low birth weight [Studd, 1969].

Estimated glomerular filtration rate is another useful marker of renal function that depends on the value of serum creatinine and variables like patient age and gender. In the United Kingdom, estimated glomerular filtration rate is usually calculated using the four-variable Modification of Diet in Renal Disease (MDRD) formula although importantly this is not validated for use in pregnancy and it is inaccurate at values greater than 60 ml/min [Hall, 2010].

3. Pregnancy and underlying chronic renal disease

Historically, pregnancy has been commonly regarded as very high risk in women with chronic renal disease. Attempts have been made to clarify these risks in the settings of chronic renal insufficiency, dialysis, and transplanted kidneys. Chronic renal disease can be silent until advanced stages. As obstetricians routinely examine the patient's urine for presence of protein, glucose and ketones, they may be the first to detect chronic renal disease. The effect of pregnancy-related changes in women with preexisting renal disease depends on the type of renal impairment and complications such as hypertension, proteinuria and infection. Advice to women with renal impairment regarding pregnancy must take into account all these parameters in an effort to answer the two most important questions:

- What effect will the pregnancy have on the mother's kidney disease?
- What effect will the mother's kidney disease have on the pregnancy?

The features that are detrimental to long-term maternal renal function and pregnancy outcome are:

- The impaired renal function (preconception SCr > 177 µmol/L (2.00 mg/dL) or glomerular filtration rate (GRF) < 25 mL/min) will lead in 2/3 of mothers to have an accelerated decline in renal function and one third to develop End-Stage Renal Failure (ESRF) in association with pregnancy. There is also considerable risk for preterm labor, intrauterine growth restriction (IUGR) and preeclampsia
- Hypertension increases risk of preeclampsia, IUGR, preterm labor and can accelerate the decline of maternal renal function
- Proteinuria in nephritic levels is associated with maternal thromboembolism, IUGR, preterm labor and poorer long-term maternal renal prognosis
- Reduced plasma volume with IUGR
- Hyperglycemia leads to large-for-gestational-age babies, but when associated with microvascular disease there is increased risk of IUGR

Although fertility is diminished in chronic kidney disease (CKD), even women on dialysis may in rare instances become pregnant. Most women will experience an increase of blood pressure and proteinuria and decrease of GRF, which can be irreversible. Affected women are at increased risk of fetal loss, intrauterine growth retardation, and early labor, especially if they experience an acute onset of kidney disease, nephritic syndrome, or hypertension. Additionally, high maternal blood urea nitrogen levels can act as an osmotic diuretic in the fetal kidney and can cause early labor and fetal loss. Progression of the underlying maternal disease depends less on the specific disease than on its severity.

One third of women with moderate kidney disease (GFR < 70 mL/min or serum creatinine > 1.4 mg/dL) are at risk for more rapid declines of renal function than are patients with less severe CKD. Dilated afferent arterioles associated with hypertension in pregnancy can further increase the already elevated intraglomerular pressures. If kidney function deteriorates quickly in early pregnancy, especially with no apparent diagnosis, renal biopsy should be considered and can be performed safely. According to Katz, 85% of women with chronic renal disease will have a surviving infant if renal function is well preserved, earlier reports being more pessimistic [Katz, 1980]. Many studies underlined that if there isn't a good control of the blood pressure there is a high likelihood of pregnancy loss. Developing of the antepartum fetal surveillance and advances in neonatal care have improved the perinatal outcome. Hou and collaborators reported a 13.8% of fetal loss rate, including miscarriage, stillbirths and neonatal deaths, this percent being close to the general population's one [Hou, 1999]. Holley and collaborators appreciated that early pregnancies losses are more common in patients with preexisting renal disease [Holley, 1996]. Higher rates of preterm delivery and IUGR were observed in women with normal or near normal renal function and mild to moderate renal impairment. Preexisting severe renal impairment (SCr > 220 umol/L) is associated with more preterm deliveries and lower birth weights than a lower SCr. A higher rate of cesarean section is seen in these women and older studies, before 1995, the perinatal outcome was good. Most authors agreed that it is difficult to assess the independent contribution to poor fetal outcome of maternal hypertension, proteinuria and renal impairment. The balance of evidence suggested that each parameter is individually and cumulative detrimental to fetal outcome. A blood pressure higher than 140/90 mmHg in the context of chronic renal disease leads to a fetal mortality of ~23%, 6 times higher than in normal population. Treatment of maternal hypertension in pregnancy is also challenging because only few classes of antihypertensive drugs are permitted in pregnancy: methyldopa, labetolol, nifedipine, or alpha antagonists. A study showed that increased proteinuria in pregnancy is associated with decreased infant weight. The risk of thromboembolism is also higher in pregnant women with nephrotic syndrome. The authors still have controversy on administration of prophylactic low-dose aspirin during pregnancy in attempt to prevent glomerular capillary thrombi, preserve maternal renal function and reduce the risk of preeclampsia [Katz, 1980; Barcello, 1986; Coomarasamy, 2003].

4. Specific renal diseases in pregnancy

Glomerular diseases such as membrane-proliferative glomerulonephritis, focal glomerulosclerosis, and reflux nephropathy were associated with poorer renal outcomes. In addition, pregnant women with autosomal dominant polycystic kidney disease that are hypertensive have a high risk for fetal and maternal complications, but women who are normotensive with mild kidney disease usually have uncomplicated pregnancies. In women with systemic lupus erythematosus, the best outcomes occur in stables inactive lupus for 6 months or longer before conception. Usually renal flares in pregnancy associated with proteinuria, hypertension, and decreased GFR, makes the distinction from preeclampsia very difficult. However, low complement levels may be helpful in distinguishing between women with preeclampsia and those with active lupus nephritis. All these women should be screened for anti-SSA (Ro) antibodies, due to the risk of congenital heart block. Treatment is difficult because usually used drugs in lupus therapy like cyclophosphamide and mycophenolate mofetil are potentially teratogenic in early pregnancy. Pregnant women with diabetic nephropathy may also develop proteinuria and hypertension.

4.1 Preeclampsia

Preeclampsia rarely causes acute renal failure severe enough to require dialysis. Acute renal failure (ARF) has become a rare complication of pregnancy in developed countries [Prakash, 2006]. Studies show that temporary dialysis was needed in hemorrhage due to placental abruption or HELLP syndrome. Women with preexisting renal disease as presented before are more vulnerable to preeclampsia, a higher risk population being that with chronic hypertension. A meta-analysis of trials investigating the effectiveness of low-dose aspirin administration (50-150 mg/day) in pregnant women with moderate to severe renal disease revealed significant reduction in the risk of preeclampsia and perinatal death [Drakely, 2002]. Delivery of the baby and placenta is the cure of severe preeclampsia. This will halt the general progression of preeclampsia, but postpartum maternal renal function usually deteriorates before improving [Rosenne-Montella, 2008]. Dialysis is limited to few cases, HELLP syndrome or placental abruption and SCr doubled in 24-48 hours, being such cases. Fluid balance is essential in the management of ARF in pregnancy, as well as the control of hypertension.

4.2 Primary glomerulonephritis

Acute primary glomerular disease rarely coincides with pregnancy. Barnes, from all available records observed a fetal salvage of only 43 600 and a maternal mortality of 20-25% during pregnancy but made it clear that such statistics would be improved with modern treatment [Barnes, 1970]. Self-limited glomerular disease preceding pregnancy has, however, no adverse effects [Tillman, 1951; Felding, 1968]. Chronic glomerular diseases, mainly on account of their diverse pathogenesis, have a less clear-cut relationship to pregnancy. Some are more progressive than others, their courses often punctuated by remissions and relapses. An established proteinuria before pregnancy may worse during it, considering increased GRF. Augmented by salt and water retention, it may produce a full nephrotic syndrome. However, assuming the edema is adequately controlled by diuretics and that neither hypertension nor renal failures supervene, the outlook for both mother and fetus is good. Several studies sustained this idea. In 1963, Johnston and collaborators studied 29 pregnancies in 10 patients with nephrosis (uncomplicated in five cases and complicated in five cases). In 1969, Studd and Blainey recorded only two infant deaths in 31 nephrotic pregnant women. In uncomplicated group were registered 11 live births from 12 pregnancies and in complicated group were 2 miscarriages, six abortion and only nine successful deliveries. In a 10-year follow up of 23 nephrotic patients involving 35 pregnancies were recorded 33 normal deliveries although infant weights were reduced relative to their maturities [Blainey, 1971]. Only two mothers with severe proliferative glomerulonephritis showed serious deterioration of renal function requiring dialysis or transplantation. In another study of 41 pregnancies in 25 patients whose renal diseases had been defined by renal biopsy were obtained favourable results [Strauch, 1974].

4.3 Lupus nephritis in pregnancy

Glomerulopathies form an important aspect of several systemic diseases of which systemic lupus erythematosus (SLE) is one of the more important. About 50% of women with this disease experience renal involvement in a wide variety of forms which may range from a focal proliferative glomerulonephritis to a more indolent and diffuse thickening of glomerular basement membranes. This variety of glomerular involvement, together with changing treatment over the years, accounted for some of the controversy which surrounds its relationship to pregnancy. 20 years ago, women with systemic lupus erythematosus (SLE) were advised against pregnancy due to fear of irreversible consequences for the mother. Today the advent of combined teams of obstetricians and 'lupus doctors' offering coordinated care for both, the mother and the baby improved significantly these terms [Ruiz-Irastorza, 2009]. The fertility rate in women with SLE is relatively normal compared to the general population; however, fetuses born to mothers with SLE may face major complications [Mok, 2001]. Multiple adverse pregnancies such as fetal loss, preterm birth, and pre-eclampsia are associated with SLE. The risk is caused by the ability of maternal autoantibodies to cross the placenta and initiate pathogenesis of the fetus. One of the most severe SLE-associated conditions is the formation of congenital heart block and can develop as a result of the passage of maternal autoantibodies. A lot of researchers studied the interrelationship of pregnancy and SLE and concluded that a great number of complications are possible in pregnant women with SLE. The presence of proteinuria, thrombocytopenia and arterial hypertension in the first semester in pregnant mother with SLE are major risks factors for pregnancy loss. The women with such risk factors have a probability of pregnancy loss of 30-40% [Clowse, 2006]. A study performed in United States from 2000-2003, compared maternal and pregnancy complications for all pregnancy-related admissions for women with and without systemic lupus erythematosus. Of more than 16.7 million admissions for childbirth over the 4 years, 13,555 were to women with systemic lupus erythematosus. The study related a maternal mortality of 20-fold higher among women with systemic lupus erythematous [Clowse, 2008]. Different signs and symptoms of pregnancy may easily be confused with signs of active lupus. Symptoms such as fatigue, melasma, palmar erythema and facial hair in the postpartum dyspnea, arthralgia, and headache are frequent in a normal pregnancy. Arthralgias are common among pregnant women due to increased weight as well as the effect of relaxin on the joints [Clowse, 2007]. A complete set of auto-antibodies should be done in every pregnant women with SLE, especially anti-phospholipid antibodies (aPL), both anti-cardiolipin antibodies (aCL) and lupus anticoagulant (LA) and anti-Ro and anti-La antibodies, given their close link with specific pregnancy complications (thrombosis, embryo/fetal loss, pre-eclampsia and congenital heart block) [Ruiz-Irastorza, 2009]. During pregnancy, C_3 and C_4 may be elevated, though a flare may occur despite apparently normal levels. However, a decrease of C_3 or C_4 levels by more than 25% may be considered an indicator of disease activity [Buyon 1999]. Lymphopenia, but not leucopenia, should be considered an indicator of SLE activity in pregnancy, because a neutrophil leucocytosis can occur in the third trimester [Motha, 2009]. Elevated uric acid levels indicates toxemia, while the presences of hematuria and/or cellular casts, extrarenale activity, elevated anti-DNA antibody levels, and decreased complement levels indicate lupus nephritis [Mackillop, 2007]. The treatment in pregnant with SLE is based on hydroxychloroquine, low-dose steroids, azathioprine and in patients with anti-phospholipid antibodies, low-dose aspirin ± low molecular weight heparin. It is recommended a close surveillance, with monitoring of blood pressure, proteinuria and placental blood flow by Doppler studies [Ruiz-Irastorza, 2009]. Maintenance of the autoantibody levels in the mother's blood is essential and a key method in sustaining the health of the fetus by preventing the likelihood of maternal-fetal exchange of SLE-associated autoantibodies. Another major contributor to adverse SLE pregnancy outcomes is antiphospholipid syndrome (APS), defined as the presence of an antiphospholipid antibody (APL) in association with clinic features of venous/arterial thrombosis or specific pregnancy complications [Smith, 2009]. Optimal management is not over with the birth of a healthy baby. Postnatal maternal monitoring by a nephrologist is indicated for optimization of hypertension and lupus nephritis treatment, without concerns for medication-related fetal adverse effects. A close surveillance in the first 4 weeks after delivery is warranted, especially in women with recent activity or previous severe disease. However, no specific prophylactic therapy (such as increasing the dose of steroids) is recommended [Ruiz-Irastorza, 2009].

4.4 Urinary tract infections and pyelonephritis in pregnancy

Urinary tract infections (UTIs) are one of the most common medical complications of pregnancy [Berard, 2011]. It is estimated that one in three women of childbearing age will have a UTI [Duarte, 2008]. The incidence of asymptomatic bacteriuria is 2% to 10%, which is the same during pregnancy as it is in sexually active nonpregnant women [Hooton, 2000]. However, the structural and immune changes the urothelium of the renal tract in pregnancy make it more likely that a lower UTI will ascend to cause acute pyelonephritis. Studies mention that between 12.5% and 30% of patients with untreated asymptomatic bacteriuria will develop acute pyelonephritis, causing significant morbidity to both mother and fetus [Little, 1966; Nowicki, 2000]. The most common uropathogens are: Escherichia Coli (70-80%), Klebsiella, Proteus, Enterobacter and Staphylococcus saphrophyticus. Asymptomatic bacteriuria beside its risk to progress to acute pyelonephritis as mentioned has a high recurrence risk, and is also associated with increased risk for preterm delivery and low birth weight [Tincello, 1998]. Although controversial modern literature doesn't advice for asymptomatic bacteriuria screening unless the population has a prevalence of more than 5% (usually the prevalence is ~2.5%), or in particular cases with history of frequent urinary infection, or other subsequent risk factors for urinary infection. Treatment of asymptomatic bacteriuria should take into account that the most frequent agent causing it is Escherichia Coli. Patients can therefore be safely treated with nitrofurantoin, ampicilin, cephalosporins and short-acting sulfa drugs. Therapy should be for 3-7 days and the patient should repeat the urine culture 1 to 2 weeks after finishing the treatment. Aprox 15% will experience reinfection and/or will not respond to the initial therapy [Romero, 1989; Davison, 1989].

Although pyelonephritis affects only 1–2% of pregnant women, it is accompanied by significant maternal morbidity and fetal morbidity and mortality [Gilstrap, 2001]. In 20–30% of pregnant women with pyelonephritis can result premature labor and the babies at high risk of neonatal death [Steer, 2005]. It is the most common non-obstetric cause for hospitalization during pregnancy. It is caused by the same uropathogens that cause asymptomatic bacteriuria. Studies reflect that the screen for asymptomatic bacteriuria in high risk population (history of asymptomatic bacteriuria, previous recurrent UTIs, preexisting renal disease- especially scared kidneys due to reflux nephropathy, structural and neurophatic abnormalities of the renal tract, renal calculi, preexisting diabetes mellitus- but not gestational diabetes, sickle cell disease, low socioeconomic group and less than 12 years higher education)decreases the risk for acute pyelonephritis to less than 1% [Plattner, 1994]. Most women will present pyelonephritis in the second or third trimester of pregnancy and will accuse in over 80% of cases: backache, fever, rigors, and costovertebral angle tenderness, and about half have lower urinary tract symptoms, nausea and vomiting. Bacteremia is present in 15% to 20% and only very few will develop septic shock or more severe complications. High risk cases will present: highest fever (> 39.4 degrees C), tachycardia (>110 bpm) [Cunningham, 1987]. Acute pyelonephritis can trigger uterine contractions and preterm labour, so the tocolytic therapy should be used carefully if there are cervical changes. Pregnant women suspected of acute pyelonephritis should be admitted in hospital for treatment. Those presenting in shock need to be referred to the intensive care unit. The treatment is empiric first, with intravenous antibiotic until sensibilities of blood and urine cultures are known. Usually these patients associate a degree of renal impairment, thrombocytopenia, and hemolysis, suggesting that alveolar capillary endothelium is damaged by endotoxin [Winf, 2001]. As the Gram-Negative bacteria usually causing pyelonephritis are often resistant to ampicilin the first choice of antibiotics should be intravenous cephalosporins, such as cefuroxime 750 mg to 1.5 g every 8 hours, until cultures results are known. Gentamicin can also be used. Intravenous antibiotics should be used until the patient is afebrile for 24 hours, and then the treatment should be followed by oral antibiotics for 7-10 days, as if for lower urinary infections. Following one episode of acute pyelonephritis, the pregnant woman should have monthly urine cultures for the recurrence screen [Dunlow, 1990].

4.5 Acute renal failure and renal cortical necrosis in pregnancy

Acute renal failure in pregnancy is largely a preventable problem usually resulting from obstetric complications and not intrinsic renal disease. With this in mind, pregnancy related acute renal failure (AFR) can be viewed more as a public health problem than a nephrologic problem [Hou, 1998]. Acute renal failure (ARF) represents a plurietiological syndrome characterized by the kidney incapacity to clear the metabolism products of the organisms. It is a very severe condition, fortunately rare in nowadays. Acute renal failure (ARF) and septic abortion is the most frequent form of ARF in early pregnancy especially in developing countries, where pronatality policies forbidden abortion. Such a case was also in Romania during the communist regime (in the seventies and eighties) when the maternal mortality got to ~ 500-600/100000 women. ARF appears due to the severe toxico- infectious syndrome (usually caused by anaerob bacteria- Clostridium velchii) after an abortive maneuver. Renal injuries are represented by acute tubular necrosis, and in very severe cases cortical bilateral necrosis. Evolution is characterized by initial oligoanuria followed by septicemic signs. Treatment addresses the primary septicemic reservoir (hysterectomy, massive antibiotherapy), dialysis. Global mortality I this pathology remain at high levels ~15-20%.

Around the time of delivery, ARF is commonly caused by gestational syndromes such as preeclampsia/hemolysis, elevated liver enzymes and low platelets (HELLP syndrome) and abruption placentae [Spargo, 1959; Redman, 1999; Poston, 2002]. ARF multiple etiologies recognize common causes such as: urinary tract infections (especially acute pyelonephritis), intoxications with drugs or nephrotoxic substances, septicemic states, shock, major hidro-electrolitic disequilibrium, posttransfusion accidents, urological causes (lithiasis, tuberculosis, ureteral obstructions). Specific etiological factors connected to the pregnancy status are: placental abruption, severe preeclampsia/HELLP syndrome, septic abortion, hyperemesis gravidarum, ovarian hyperstimulation syndrome, amniotic fluid embolus, hemolytic uremic syndrome/ thrombotic thrombocytopenic purpura, acute fatty liver of pregnancy and acute obstruction of real tracts. The most common renal lesion is acute tubular necrosis and cortical necrosis usually appears in non pregnant patients. Positive diagnosis of ARF is based on oligoanury (less than 100 ml urine/24 hours) and association of uremic retention, hypercalcemia, hypermagnesemia, metabolic acidosis. ARF is a severe complication that triggers other complications: infectious (pneumopathy, thromboembolism, parotiditis), hidroelectrolitical (edema, hypertension, congestive cardiac failure), hemorragical. Treatment of ARF concentrates on finding the cause and treat it dialysis has more indications nowadays. The obstetric management of the patient has to take into account the gestational age and the fact that pregnancy related acute renal failure has a more severe evolution and prognosis than other causes.

Acute renal cortical necrosis is a rare complication of pregnancy nowadays. In western countries, the frequency of renal cortical necrosis range from 1.9% to 2% [Schreiner, 1979]. Obstetric complications such as abruptio placentae, septic abortion, eclamptic toxemia, post-partum hemorrhage, intrauterine fetal demise, amniotic fluid embolism and puerperal sepsis can cause renal cortical necrosis [Ali, 2003]. By all, the most common obstetric cause is abruptio placentae, responsible for 50-60% of cases [Jeong, 2002]. Acute renal cortical necrosis should be suspected if anuria persists. Definitive diagnosis can be made only by renal biopsy. Incidence of maternal and fetal mortality is still increased [Chugh, 1994].

Hemolytic uremic syndrome (HUS) and thrombotic thrombocytopenic purpura (TTP) are very similar syndromes characterized by microangiopathic hemolytic anemia and thrombocytopenia. They appear more likely in the third trimester of pregnancy and determine a multiorgan disorder, women with these pathology present gastrointestinal or neurological abnormalities. Maternal survival from HUS/TTP has greatly improved since treatment with plasmapheresis [Greer, 2007]. Steroids are often added to the plasma exchange, but there are no randomized controlled trials of their use [Rosene-Montella, 2008]. Antiplatelet regimen with aspirin may also be beneficial [McMinn, 2001].

4.6 Diabetic nephropathy in pregnancy

In the last 10 years an increased number of people with type 2 diabetes mellitus appeared. Diabetes mellitus (DM) is the most common medical complication of pregnancy and it carries a significant risk to the fetus and the mother [Abourawi, 2006]. Gestational DM represents approximately 90% of these cases and affects 2-5% of all pregnancies and varies in direct proportion to type 2 diabetes mellitus in the background population [Ben-Haroush, 2004]. There is a clear association between obesity and adverse pregnancy outcomes (cesarean section, gestational diabetes, hypertensive disorders, birth defects and prematurity) [McIntyre, 2009]. Pregnant women with diabetes are at risk of progression to microvascular diabetic complications, early pregnancy loss, pre-eclampsia, polyhydramnios and premature labour. Glycemic control before and during pregnancy is critical and the benefit may result in a viable, healthy off spring [Hertzel, 2001]. The risk of neonatal macrosomia and hypoglycemia can be reduced by proper management of gestational DM. Appropriate counseling in women with gestational DM and post-partum evaluation of glucose tolerance may help decrease the high risk of subsequent type 2 diabetes in the long-term [Kitzmiller, 2007]. Metabolic changes occur in normal pregnancy in response to the increase in nutrient needs of the fetus and the mother. There are two main changes which are seen during pregnancy, progressive insulin resistance that begins near mid-pregnancy and progresses through the third trimester to the level that approximates the insulin resistance seen in individuals with type 2 diabetes mellitus [Abourawi, 2006]. The insulin resistance appears to result from a combination of increased maternal adiposity and the placental secretion of hormones (progesterone, cortisol, placental lactogen, prolactin and growth hormone). The fact that insulin resistance rapidly abates following delivery suggests that the major contributors to this state of resistance are placental hormones. The second change is the compensatory increase in insulin secretion by the pancreatic beta-cells to overcome the insulin resistance of pregnancy [Ben-Ziv, 2008]. Circulating glucose levels are maintained normal. If there is maternal defect in insulin secretion and in glucose utilization, then GDM will occur as the diabetogenic hormones rise to their peak levels. Maternal diabetes complications are frequent in women with both type 1 and type 2 diabetes [Abourawi, 2006]. Diabetic retinopathy and diabetic nephropathy may progress or start de novo during the pregnancy.

Diabetic pregnant woman can have maternal complications such as: diabetic ketoacidosis, hypoglycemia, and retinopathy, deterioration of nephropathy, vomiting (gastric neuropathy), miscarriages, preeclampsia, polyhydramnios, and premature delivery. In order that diabetic pregnant women have a healthy baby and avoid maternal morbidity it is recommended a multidisciplinary pre-pregnancy consult. Ideally this is carried out by a team, which includes an obstetrician, a nephrologist and a diabetologist for optimum care. Clinical trials of pre-conception care to achieve stringent blood glucose control in the pre-conception period and during the first trimester of pregnancy have demonstrated striking reductions in rates of malformation compared with infants of diabetic women who did not participate in pre-conception care [Ray, 2001]. In approximately two thirds of women with diabetes, may appear pregnancy, without an adequate pre-conception care and a lot of malformations in their infants. Oral hypoglycemic agents should be interrupted before pregnancy and insulin started if needed, and also statins and ACE-inhibitors should be discontinued. Safer drugs like Methyldopa, Nifedipine or Labetalol should be administered for arterial hypertension. It is necessary be evaluated and treated all the diabetic complications. Regular self-monitoring should be encouraged to optimize control. At least at four weeks pre-conception it should be administered Folic acid. Glycemic control should be optimized with the aim of pre-prandial blood glucose < 5.5 mmol/l (< 95 mg/dl) and HbA1c < 7%. Home blood glucose monitoring is an essential part of maintaining euglycemic state and its goal is to detect glucose concentration to allow fine-tuning of insulin adjustment, pre-prandial glucose level < 5.5 mmol/l (< 95mg/dl), and postprandial level glucose < 7.8 mmol/ l (<140 mg/dl). Post-prandial glucose levels have been shown to correlate more with macrosomia than do fasting levels. Diabetes in early pregnancy studies found that third trimester post-prandial glucose levels were the strongest predictors of percentile birth weight [Setji, 2005]. Diet in pregnancy should provide an adequate nutrition for both mother and fetus, with sufficient calories for appropriate maternal weight gain, for maintaining normal glycemia and avoiding ketosis. It is recommended that pregnant women with diabetes to eat three small to moderate size meals and three snacks per day. Monitoring with a pre-breakfast ketone measurement is recommended for patients who are on a hypo-caloric or carbohydrate restricted diet [Franz, 2002]. Before conception, a baseline assessment of renal function by serum creatinine and some measure of urinary protein excretion (urine albumin/creatinine ratio or 24-hour albumin excretion) should be done. Women with microalbuminuria may experience transient worsening during pregnancy; however, those with established nephropathy with overt proteinuria are at increased risk of pre-eclampsia and intra-uterine growth retardation and premature delivery [Abourawi, 2006]. A frequent associated pathology of diabetes is arterial hypertension. Patients with type 1 diabetes frequently develop hypertension in association with diabetic nephropathy, as manifested by the presence of overt proteinuria. Patients with type 2 diabetes more commonly have hypertension as a concomitant disease. In addition, pregnancy induced hypertension is a potential problem for the women with diabetes. In pregnancy, arterial hypertension may worse diabetic nephropathy and retinopathy. ACE-inhibitors, beta-blockers and diuretics should be avoided in women contemplating pregnancy if are used for hypertension. Methyl-Dopa or Labetalol should be substituted. Considering the earlier studies in this domain [Purdy, 1996; Reece, 1998; Ekbom, 2001; Rossing, 2002], the management of diabetic nephropathy should follow:

- Prepregnancy: advise that pregnancy with diabetic nephropathy and SCr > 124 μmol/L is associated with 40% risk of gestational decline in renal function; advise that increase risk of adverse pregnancy outcome; try and achieve euglycemia
- Prenatal: every 4-6 week monitor blood pressure, blood urea nitrogen, glucose, midstream urinalysis until 24 week of gestation, then every 2 week until 32 weeks of pregnancy and after that weekly; try and achieve euglycemia; give aspirin 75 mg once daily to reduce the risk of preeclampsia, control hypertension to < 140/90 mmHg; screen for preeclampsia; fetal surveillance; give LMW heparin when > 1-3 g proteinuria/24 hour and hipoalbuminemia; a diuretic may be necessary for symptomatic relief of gross edema with nephrotic syndrome
- Postnatal: reassess the renal function (GFR) postpartum

Treatment with medical nutrition therapy, close monitoring of glucose levels, and insulin therapy if glucose levels are above goal can help to reduce these complications [Setji, 2005].

4.7 Unique surgical kidney and pregnancy

Women undergoing nephrectomy (despite the cause of the surgical procedure) will have a pregnancy evolution in normal parameters if the remaining kidney has its morph functional integrity. Multidrug resistant urinary infection can be an indication for ending the pregnancy in order to preserve the renal function. Authors consider that pregnancy won't influence the renal function and evolution of the renal disease if the blood pressure can be controlled and urinary infection treated promptly if they appear.

4.8 Renal calculi and pregnancy

Renal calculi, congenital renal tract abnormalities or a gestational overdistension syndrome can produce renal obstruction in pregnancy [Rosene-Montella, 2008]. The incidence of renal calculi in pregnant women appears to be no greater than in the nonpregnant population. Their presence and especially their migration in the urinary tract are associated with renal colic, UTI. Treatment and management of renal colic is similar as for nonpregnant women. Women born with congenital obstructive urophaties are at increased risk for urine outflow obstruction in second trimester of pregnancy and also for recurrent UTI [Meyers, 1985]. Overdistension of urinary tracts isn't very frequent in pregnancy. The patients will present severe loin pain, most commonly on the right part and radiating to the lower abdomen. Spontaneous rupture of the kidney is uncommon, and in severe cases ureteric stent or nephrostomy is performed.

4.9 Acute fatty liver of pregnancy

Acute fatty liver of pregnancy was first described in 1940 by H. L. Sheehan as an "acute yellow atrophy" of the liver. Acute renal failure due to acute fatty liver of pregnancy is a rare life-threatening complication, specific to pregnancy. If unrecognized or untreated, the disorder may progress to fulminant hepatic failure with jaundice, encephalopathy, disseminated intravascular coagulation, uncontrollable gastrointestinal and uterine bleeding, and death [Kaplan, 1994]. Although the exact pathogenesis is unknown, it seems to be caused by a disordered metabolism of fatty acids by mitochondria in the mother, caused by deficiency in long-chain 3-hydroxyacyl-coenzyme A dehydrogenase enzyme [Bellig, 2004]. Acute fatty liver of pregnancy may be confused with acute hepatitis or toxemia on both clinical and histological grounds [Burroughs, 1982]. The diagnosis of acute fatty liver of pregnancy is suggested by jaundice with a lesser elevation of liver enzymes, elevated white blood cell count, disseminated intravascular coagulation, and a clinically unwell patient [Riely, 1999]. Usually such patients will present with nausea, vomiting, and abdominal cramps. First appear an impaired renal function and reduced plasma antithrombin levels, liver dysfunction following this [Castro, 1999]. Maternal renal impairment is aggravated by hypotension secondary to hemorrhage, which it is most likely to follow an emergency cesarean section. Renal dysfunction, hemorrhage, and disseminated intravascular coagulation secondary to liver failure require a complex intensive therapy in a multidisciplinary team. Treatment includes supportive care in order to maintain adequate fluid balance for renal perfusion, replacing blood, correcting the coagulopathy. Temporary dialysis might be necessary [Pereira, 1997].

4.10 Pregnancy in women on dialysis

End-stage renal disease requiring dialysis is associated with a marked decrease in fertility. Pregnancy occurs in approximately 1% of women, usually within the first few years of starting dialysis. The cause of infertility is not entirely clear, but it is probably multifactorial. An estimated 42% of women receiving dialysis who are of childbearing age have regular menses, but many more are likely anovulatory. Anemia probably also plays a role. In fact, some investigators suggest that the regular use of erythropoietin improves the pregnancy rate. Generally pregnancy is a contraindication in women on dialysis. The fetal outcome is quite poor. Only 23-55% of pregnancies result in surviving infants, and a large number of second-trimester spontaneous abortions occur. In addition, surviving infants have significant morbidities. Approximately 85% of surviving infants are born premature, and 28% are born small for gestational age. Maternal complications occur as well, including reports of several maternal deaths. Hypertension worsens in more than 80% of pregnant females on dialysis and is a major concern. The diagnosis of pregnancy in these patients is also difficult, because levels of beta-human chorionic gonadotropin (beta-hCG) are normally elevated in patients receiving dialysis. If pregnancy is considered likely and the beta-hCG level is high, obtain an ultrasonogram to aid in diagnosis. Some general recommendations apply to patients who become pregnant while receiving dialysis. Place the patient on a transplant list (if not on already), because outcomes with allograft transplant patients are markedly better. During hemodialysis, pursue uterine and fetal monitoring and make every attempt to avoid dialysis-induced hypotension. Some evidence indicates that judicious use of erythropoietin may improve fetal survival; however, no findings from randomized studies support this. Erythropoietin can also increase hypertension and must be used cautiously. An increased frequency of dialysis may improve mortality and morbidity. Aggressive dialysis to keep blood urea nitrogen levels less than 50 mg/dL may be pursued with daily dialysis. Controlling uremia in this fashion may avoid polyhydramnios, control hypertension, and improve the mother's nutritional status [Hou, 1998; Holley, 2003].

4.11 Pregnancy after renal transplantation

The first reported successful pregnancy occurred in a recipient of a kidney transplant from an identical twin sister performed in 1958 [Murray, 1963]. Fertility is usually restored in women with renal transplants. Pregnancy is then common, occurring in 12% of women at childbearing age in one series [Sturgiss, 1992]. Pregnancy success rates are also quite good, with more than 90% fetal survival rates after the first trimester. Pregnancy can be anticipated, planned, and even encouraged. In patients with chronic renal insufficiency, factors such as uncontrolled or worsening hypertension, worsening proteinuria, and poor prepregnancy renal function are important prognostic indicators for the risk of renal function deterioration. Whether pregnancy itself induces a significant risk to the transplanted kidney's function is unclear. Obstruction of the transplant ureter by the pregnant uterus is quite rare but has been reported. Further long-term studies are indicated. Current opinion holds that the graft function is not adversely affected by pregnancy in the setting of women with a creatinine level of less than 1.4 mg/dL who are treated with prednisone and/or azathioprine. An elevated prepregnancy creatinine level (> 1.4 mg/dL) is associated with a higher risk of renal decline but also with a decreased fetal survival rate. The fetal survival rate is approximately 74% in patients with a creatinine level of more than 1.4 mg/dL, whereas it increases to about 96% in patients with a creatinine level of less than 1.4 mg/dL [EBPG Expert Group on Renal Transplantation, 2002; Davison, 1995].

5. Conclusion

In pregnancy associated with different renal diseases, laboratory tests play an important role Pregnant women with any renal disease must be prepregnancy counseled, prenatal monitored, and receive a skilled obstetric management in a multidisciplinary manner, since the most common cause of mortality and morbidity in these cases is preterm labor.

6. References

Abe S. (1991). An overview of pregnancy in women with underlying renal disease, *American Journal of Kidney Disease,* Vol. 17, pp. 112-115

Abourawi FI. (2006). Diabetes mellitus and pregnancy, *Libyan Journal of Medicine,* Vol. 1, No. 1, (July, 2006), pp. 28–41.

Airoldi J, Weinstein L. (2007). Clinical significance of proteinuria in pregnancy. *Obstetrics and Gynecology Survey,* Vol. 62, pp. 117–24.

Ali SS, Rizvi SZH, Muzaffar S et al. (2003). Renal cortical necrosis: A case series of nine patients and review of literature. *Journal of Ayub Medical College Abbottabad,* Vol. 15, pp. 41–44.

Bérard, A.; Santos, F.; Ferreira E.; Perreault, S. (2011). Urinary tract infections during pregnancy, Urinary Tract Infections, Peter Tenke (Ed.), ISBN: 978-953-307-757-4, InTech.

Barnes, C. G. (1970). Medical Disorders in Obstetric Practice, 3rd ed. Blackwell, Oxford.

Ben-Haroush A, Yogev Y, Hod M. (2004). epidemiology of gestational diabetes and its association with type 2 diabetes mellitus. *Diabetic Medicine,* Vol. 21, No.2, pp.103-113.

Ben-Ziv, R. G., & Hod, M. (2008). Gestational diabetes mellitus. *Fetal and Maternal Medicine Review,* Vol. 19, No.3, pp. 245-269.

Blainey, J. D., and Studd, J. W. (1971). Nephritis and pregnancy, *Quart Journal of medicine* 40, pp. 566-567.

Brown MA, Holt JL, Mangos GJ, Murray N, Curtis J, Homer C. (2005). Microscopic hematuria in pregnancy: Relevance to pregnancy outcome. *American Journal of Kidney Disease,* Vol. 45, pp. 667–673.

Buyon JP, Kalunian KC, Ramsey-Goldman R, Petri MA, Lockshin MD, Ruiz-Irastorza G, et al. (1999). Assessing disease activity in SLE patients during pregnancy. *Lupus,* Vol. 8, pp. 677–684.

Castro MA, Fassett Mj, et al. (1999). Reversible peripartum liver failure: A new perspective on the diagnosis, treatment, and cause of acute fatty liver of pregnancy, based on 29 consecutive cases. *American Journal of Obstetrics and Gynecology,* Vol. 181, pp. 389- 395.

Chugh KS, et al. (1994). Acute renal cortical necrosis- a study of 113 patients. *Renal Failure* Vol. 16, pp. 37-47.

Clowse M. (2007). Lupus activity in pregnancy. Rheum Dis Clin North Am, Vol.33, pp. 237–52.

Clowse ME, Magder LS, Witter F, Petri M. (2006). Early risk factors for pregnancy loss in lupus. *Obstetrics and Gynecology,* Vol. 107, No.2, pp. 293-299.

Clowse ME, Jamison M, Myers E, James AH. (2008). A national study of the complications of lupus in pregnancy. *American Journal of Obstetrics and Gynecology,* Vol. 199;127. e1-6.

Coomarasamy A, et al. (2003). Aspirin for prevention of preeclampsia in women with historical risk factors: A systematic review. *Obstetrics and Gynecology,* Vol.101, pp. 1319-1332.

Cunningham FG, et al. (1987). Pulmonary injury complicating antepartum pyelonephritis. *American Journal of Obstetrics and Gynecology,* Vol. 156, pp. 797-807.

Cunningham FG, Cox SM, Harstad TW, Mason RA, Pritchard JA. (1990). Chronic renal disease and pregnancy outcome. *American Journal of Obstetrics and Gynecology.* Vol. 163, No.2, (August, 1990), pp.453-459.

Cunningham FG, Gant NF, Leveno KJ. (2001). Renal and urinary tract disorders. In: Cunningham FG, Gilstrap LC, Gant NF, Leveno KJ, Hauth JC, Wenstrom KD, eds. Williams Obstetrics. ed. New York, NY: McGraw-Hill.

Cunningham, Leveno, Bloom, Hauth, Rouse, Spong. (2010). Williams Obstetrics, 23rd edition, The McGraw-Hill Companies, Vol. c48, pp. 1033-1048.

Davison JM, et al. (1989). The effect of covert bateriuria in schoolgirls on renal function at 18 years and during pregnancy. *Lancet,* No.2, pp. 651.

Davison JM. (1995). Towards long-term graft survival in renal transplantation: Pregnancy. *Nephrology, Dialysis and Transplantation,* Vol. 10, pp.85-89.

Drakely AJ, et al. (2002). Acute renal failure complicating severe preeclampsia requiring admission to a obstetric intensive care unit. *American Journal of Obstetrics and Gynecology,* Vol. 186, pp. 253-256.

Duarte G, Marcolin AC, Quintana SM, Cavalli RC. (2008). Urinary tract infection in pregnancy. *Revista Brasileira de Ginecologia e Obstetricia,* Vol. 30, No. 2, (February, 2008), pp.93-100.

Dunlow SG, et al. (1990). Prevalence of antibiotic-resistant uropathogens in obstetric patients with acute pylonepritis. *Obstetrics and Gynecology,* Vol. 76, pp. 241-245.

EBPG Expert Group on Renal Transplantation. (2002). European Best practice guidelines for renal transplantation. Section IV: Long-term management of the transplant recipient. *Nephrology, Dialysis and Transplantation,* Vol. 17, No. 4, pp. 50-55.

Ekbom P, e al. (2001). Pregnancy outcome in type I diabetic patients with microalbuminuria; *Diabetes Care,* Vol. 24, pp. 1739-1744.

Epstein FH. (1996). Pregnancy and renal disease *New England Journal of Medicine,* Vol. 335, pp. 277-278.

Franz MJ, Bantle JP, Beebe CA, Brunzell JD, Chiasson JL, Garg A, et al. (2002). Evidence-based nutrition principles and recommendations for the treatment and prevention of diabetes and related complications (Technical Review). *Diabetes Care,* Vol. 25, pp. 148-198.

Gilstrap III LC, Ramin SM. (2001). Urinary tract infections during pregnancy. *Obstetrics and Gynecology of Clinical North America,* Vol. 28, pp. 581- 591.

Greer IA, Nelson-Piercy C, Walters B. (2007). Maternal Medicine, Medical Problems in Pregnancy Churchill Livingstone, Edinburgh.

Hall M, Brunskill N. (2010). Renal disease and Pregnancy. *Obstetrics, Gynecology, and Reproductive Medicine* 2010; doi:10.1016/j.ogrm.2010.02.006.

Holley JL, Reddy SS. (2003). Pregnancy in dialysis patients: A review of outcomes, complications and management. *Seminars in Dialysis,* Vol. 16, pp. 384-387.

Hooton, T.M., Scholes, D., Stapleton, A.E., Roberts, P.L., Winter, C., Gupta, K., (2000). A prospective study of asymptomatic bacteriuria in sexually active young women. *New England Journal of Medicine,* Vol. 343, pp. 992-997.

Hou S, Firanek C. (1998). Management of the pregnant dialysis patient. Adv Ren Replace Ther, Vol. 5, pp.24-30.

Hou S, Peano C. (1998). Acute Renal Failure in Pregnancy. *Saudi Journal of Kidney Disease and Transplantation,* Vol. 9, pp. 261-6.

Hou S. (1999). Pregnancy in chronic renal insufficiency and end-stage renal disease. *American Journal of Kidney Disease,* 33(2), (February, 1999), pp. 235-252.

Hou S. (1998). The kidney in pregnancy. In: Primer on Kidney Diseases. 2nd ed. Greenberg A: Academic Press; pp.388-394.

James DK, Steer PJ, Weiner, CP.; Gonik., B. (2005). High risk pregnancy: management options - 3rd edition, Elsevier Saunders, 2005, ISBN: 13: 978-0-7216-0132-8; chapter 50, pp. pag 1098-1124.

Jones Dc, et al. (1996). Outcome of pregnancy in women with moderate or severe renal insufficiency. *New England Journal of Medicine,* Vol. 335, pp. 226-232.

Jungers, Houillier, Forget et al. (1995). Influence of pregnancy on the course of primary glomerulonephritis. *Lancet,* Vol. 346, pp. 1122-1124.

Katz AI, Davison JM, Hayslett JP, Singson E, Lindheimer MD. (1980). Pregnancy in women with kidney disease. *Kidney International.* Vol. 18, No. 2, (Aug 1980), pp.192-206.

Kaplan MM. (1985). Acute fatty liver of pregnancy. *New England Journal of Medicine,* Vol. 313, pp. 367-70.

Kitzmiller J, Dang-Kilduff L, Taslimi M. (2007). Gestational diabetes after delivery: short-term management and long-term risks. *Diabetes Care,* Vol. 30, pp. S225–S235.

Ko H, Yoshida EM. (2006). Acute fatty liver of pregnancy. *Canadian Journal of Gastroenterology,* Vol. 20, pp. 25–30.

Landau L, et al. (1999). Perinatal vasoconstrictive renal insufficiency associated with maternal nimesulide use. *American Journal of Perinatology,* Vol.26, pp. 2163-2166.

Li DK, Liu L, Odouli R. (2003). Exposure to non-steroidal anti-inflammatory drugs during pregnancy and risk of miscarriage: population based cohort study. *British Medical Journal,* Vol. 327, pp. 368-371.

Little PJ. (1966). The incidence of urinary infection in 5000 pregnant women. *Lancet,* Vol. 2, pp. 925-928.

Mackillop LH, Germain SJ, Nelson-Piercy C. (2007). Systemic lupus erythematosus. *British Medical Journal,* Vol. 335, pp.933–936.

McIntyre HD, Thomae MK, Wong SF, Idris N, Callaway LK. (2009). Pregnancy in type 2 diabetes mellitus–problems & promises. *Current Diabetes Reviews,* Vol. 5, No.3, pp.190-200.

McMinn JR, George JN. (2001). Evaluation of women with clinically suspected TTP/HUS during pregnancy. *Journal of Clinical Apheresis,* Vol. 16, No.4, pp. 202-209.

McNair, MacDonald, Dooley, Peterson. (2000). Evaluation of the centrifuged and Gram-stained smear, urinalysis, and reagent strip testing to detect asymptomatic bacteriuria in obstetric patients, *American Journal of Obstetrics and Gynecology,* Vol. 182, No.5, (May, 2000), pp. 1076-1079.

Meyers SJ, Lee RV, Munschauer. (1985). Dilatation and nontraumatic rupture of the urinary tract during pregnancy: a review. *Obstetrics and Gynecology,* Vol. 66, pp.809-815.

Mok, C. C. and R. W. Wong (2001). Pregnancy in systemic lupus erythematosus. Postgrad Med J 77(905): 157-165.

Motha MBC, Wijesinghe PS, Systemic lupus erythematosus and pregnancy - a challenge to the clinician, *Ceylon Medical Journal,* Vol.54(4) 2009: 107-109.

Murray JE, Reid DE, Harrison JH et al. (1963). Successful pregnancies after human renal transplantation. *New England Journal of Medicine,* Vol. 269, pp. 346.

Nowicki B. (2000). Urinary tract infection in pregnant women: Old dogmas and current concepts regarding pathogenesis. *Current Infectious Disease Reports,* Vol. 4, pp. 529-535.

Pereira SP,et al. (1997). Maternal and perinatal outcome in severe pregnancy-related liver disease. *Hepatology,* Vol. 26, pp. 1258-1262.

Plattner MS. (1994). Pyelonephritis in pregnancy. Journal of Perinatology and Neonatal Nursing, Vol. 8, pp. 20.

Poston L, et al. (2002). Vascular function in normal pregnancy and preeclampsia. Cambridge University Press, pp. 398-425.

Prakash J, H. Kumar and D.K. Sinha, et al. (2006). Acute renal failure in pregnancy in a developing country: twenty years of experience. *Renal Failure,* Vol. 28, pp. 309-313.

Purdy LP, et al. (1996). Effect of pregnancy on renal function in patients with moderate to severe diabetic renal insufficiency. *Diabetes Care,* Vol. 19, pp.1067-1074.

Ray JG, O'Brien TE, Chan WS. (2001). Preconception care and the risk of congenital anomalies in the offspring of women with diabetes mellitus: a meta-analysis. *QJM.* Vol. 94, No. 8, pp.435–444.

Redman CW, et al. (1999). Preeclampsia: an excessive maternal inflammatory response to pregnancy. *American Journal of Obstetrics and Gynecology,* Vol. 180, pp. 499-506.

Reece EA et al. (1998). Pregnancy performance and outcomes associated with diabetic nephropathy, *American Journal of Perinatology,* Vol. 15, pp. 413-421.

Riely CA (1999). Liver disease in the pregnant patient. American College of Gastroenterology. *American Journal of Gastroenterology,* Vol. 94, No.77, pp. 1728–1732.

Romero R, et al. (1989). Meta-analysis of relationship between asymptomatic bacteriuria and preterm delivery/low birth weight babies. *Obstetrics and Gynecology,* Vol. 73, pp. 576.

Rosene-Montella K, Keely K, Barbour L, Lee R. (2008). Medical care of the pregnant patient. 2a Ed. ACP Press, American College of Physicians, Philadelphia.

Rossing K, et al. (2002). Pregnancy and progression of diabetic nephropathy, *Diabetologia,* Vol.45, pp. 36-41.

Ruiz-Irastorza G, Khamashta MA. (2009). Managing lupus patients during pregnancy. *Best Practice Research in Clinical Rheumatology,* Vol. 23, pp. 575-582.

Sarris, Bewley, Agnihotri. (2009). Training in Obstetrics and Gynecology- the essential curriculum, Oxford University Press, c6: 112-113; c 7: 144-145; 166-167; 176-179.

Schreiner GE. (1979). Bilateral cortical necrosis. In: Hamburger J, Crosnier J, Grunfeld JP (Eds): Nephrology. New York, Wiley, pp 411-30.

Setji T, Brown A, Feinglos M. (2005). Gestational diabetes mellitus. *Clinical Diabetes.* Vol. 23, pp. 17-22.

Sibai BM. (2002). Chronic hypertension in pregnancy. *Obstetrics and Gynecology,* Vol. 100, pp. 369–377.

Sheehan HL (1940). The pathology of acute yellow atrophy and delayed chloroform poisoning. *Journal of Obstetrics and Gynecology Br. Emp.* Vol. 47, pp. 49–62.

Spargo B, et al. (1959). Glomerular capillary endotheliosis in toxaemia of pregnancy. *Archives of Pathology,* Vol. 63, pp. 593-599.

Steer P. (2005). The epidemiology of preterm labor—a global perspective. *Journal of Perinatal Medicine,* Vol. 33, pp. 273 - 276.

Tincello DG, Richmond DH. (1998). Evaluation of reagent strips in detecting asymptomatic bacteriuria in early pregnancy: prospective case series. *British Medical Journal,* Vol. 316, pp. 435-437.

Winf DA: Pyelonephritis in pregnancy. Treatment options for optimal outcomes. Drugs 2001; 61:2087-2096.

Williams D. Renal disease in pregnancy. Curr Opin Obstetr Gynecol 2004; 14: 166–174.

7

Arterial Hypertension and Renal Disease

Corina Şerban, Rodica Mihăescu, Lavinia Noveanu,
Ioana Mozoş, Ruxandra Christodorescu and Simona Drăgan
University of Medicine and Pharmacy „Victor Babeş" Timişoara
Romania

1. Introduction

The past decade has witnessed enormous advances in understanding the association between arterial hypertension and renal disease. This chapter aims to provide a comprehensive review about new insights generated from recent experimental and clinical studies that should shed light on the role of the kidney in causing hypertension but also the role of hypertension in causing renal disease. It will focus on pathogenic mechanisms that connect arterial hypertension with target renal damage and new markers able to identify subclinical target-renal damage.

Nowadays, the most important causes of renal failure and dialysis in the world arterial are hypertension and diabetes mellitus. The kidneys have a central role in the control of sodium homeostasis through the important mechanism of regulation of blood pressure. Arterial hypertension is also a well known consequence of chronic kidney disease (CKD), and at the same time one of the main factors causing diabetic and/or non-diabetic chronic renal failure progression (Ljutić, 2003).

Kidneys can be damaged by arterial hypertension by several mechanisms. Because autoregulation of glomerular pressure is impaired in CKD, elevations in systemic blood pressure are associated with increased glomerular capillary pressure. Glomerular hypertension results in increased protein filtration and endothelial damage, causing increased release of cytokines and other soluble mediators, promoting replacement of normal kidney tissue by fibrosis. An important factor contributing to progressive renal disease is activation of the renin-angiotensin system, which tends to increase blood pressure and also promotes cell proliferation, inflammation, and matrix accumulation (Dworkin, 1999). An important part of the standard of care in clinics is the evaluation of microalbuminuria in order to detect renal organ damage that may influence the occurrence of future cardiovascular events. Screening for renal organ damage is part of classification schemes and clinical assessment process and influences the therapy to prevent disease progression and delay or prevent future cardiovascular events. The presence of target organ damage defines a high-risk population that develops complications due to suboptimal disease control or accelerated development and progression of the atherosclerotic process (Lockhart, 2009).

The renin-angiotensin system (RAS) is the most important mechanism for blood pressure regulation and electrolyte homeostasis. It was suggested that the major fraction of angiotensin II present in renal tissues is locally generated from angiotensinogen delivered to the kidney as well as from angiotensinogen locally produced by the proximal tubule cells (Kobori, 2007). Renin is produced by the cells of the juxtaglomerular apparatus cells and then delivered in the renal interstitium and vascular compartment resulting local generation of angiotensin. Angiotensin-converting enzyme is abundant in the kidney and is present in the proximal tubules, distal tubules, and collecting ducts (Kobori, 2010). Angiotensin I delivered to the kidney can also be converted to angiotensin II (Komlosi, 2003). All of the components necessary to generate intrarenal angiotensin II are present along the nephron (Navar, 2002; Kobori, 2007). Recently, in the Bogalusa Heart Study was proved that urinary level of angiotensinogen can be a new and potential marker of intrarenal RAS status in kidney disease due to arterial hypertension (Kobori, 2010). An important role in progression of inflammation and fibrosis seems to involve the renin-angiotensin system, and specifically the angiotensin-converting enzyme (ACE)-angiotensin (Ang) II-AT_1 receptor axis. ACE_2, a new component of the renin-angiotensin system, has emerged as a key enzyme that selectively degrades Ang II and generates Ang-(1-7), a bioactive peptide with anti-inflammatory and anti-fibrotic actions (Chappell, 2010). The deficiency of angiotensin-converting enzyme 2 is associated with elevated tissue and circulating levels of angiotensin II, reduced levels of angiotensin and progressive glomerulosclerosis in the kidneys (Tikellis, 2011). Definitely, the overexpression of angiotensin-converting enzyme 2 may produce adverse cardiac effects, and angiotensin-converting enzyme 2 and its metabolic products may promote epithelial-to-mesenchymal transition (Tikellis, 2011).

Increased activity of the intrarenal RAS is another concept considered responsible for initiating and maintaining an elevated blood pressure in patients with hypertension and it is sustained by a lot of studies (Mitchell, 1992; Navar, 1999; Navar, 2002; Guyenet, 2006; Kobori, 2007).

Since current European guidelines on hypertension (Mancia, 2007), stratify individuals based on both known risk factors and early markers of subclinical target-organ damage, the chapter focuses further on new and old available biomarkers that can detect renal damage in arterial hypertension. Blood urea nitrogen and creatinine clearance are well-established biomarkers of renal function that can be measured cheaply and easily. Reduced glomerular filtration rate (GFR) and increased urinary albumin excretion are manifestations of target organ damage in hypertension. New renal biomarkers include: urinary level of angiotensinogen, plasma aldosterone concentration, hyperhomocysteinemia and cystatin C.

Antihypertensive agents like diuretics, angiotensin converting enzyme (ACE) inhibitors, angiotensin II (Ang II) receptor antagonists, ß-blockers, or calcium channel blockers (CCBs) can improve end organ damage and effectively reduce hypertension (Cohuet, 2006).

2. From arterial hypertension to renal organ damage

The increasing prevalence of arterial hypertension in general population is caused by a sum of factors involved in renal disease progression like atherogenic dyslipidemia, metabolic syndrome, type II diabetes, anemia, and disorders of mineral metabolism.

The first form of hypertension most commonly observed in early or borderline hypertension is characterized by salt-resistance, normal or only slightly decreased GFR, relatively normal or mild renal arteriolosclerosis, and normal renal autoregulation. The patients affected by this form of hypertension are at minimal risk for renal progression.

The second form of hypertension, characterized by salt-sensitivity, renal arteriolar disease, and blunted renal autoregulation, defines a group at highest risk for the development of microalbuminuria, albuminuria, and progressive renal disease. This second form is more likely to be observed in blacks, in subjects with gout or hyperuricemia, with low level lead intoxication, or with severe obesity/metabolic syndrome (Johnson, 2005).

Essential hypertension is frequently associated with arteriolar thickening, fibrinoid deposition in the glomeruli, and proteinuria (Cohuet, 2006). The deleterious effects of systemic hypertension on renal vascular bed depend on the degree to which the microcirculation is exposed to elevated pressures. Renal injury occurs when the preglomerular autoregulatory mechanism is insufficient to maintain flow and pressure in the kidney (Griffin, 2003).

Chronic hypertension can lead to nephrosclerosis, a common cause of CKD (Porth, 2011). Clinicians use different terms to identify renal damage caused by hypertension like nephrosclerosis, benign nephrosclerosis, hypertensive kidney disease, or nephroangiosclerosis. Two clinicopathologic patterns have been described until now. The first form is *benign nephrosclerosis* or simply nephrosclerosis, characterised by microvascular changes with hyalinosis of the preglomerular vessel walls and thickening of the intima and reduplication of the internal elastic lamina of the arcuate and interlobar arteries. These modifications can lead to glomerular damage, glomerulosclerosis, patchy tubular atrophy, and interstitial fibrosis. The second form is *malignant nephrosclerosis*, associated with accelerated or malignant hypertension, characterized by fibrinoid necrosis and myointimal hyperplasia and left untreated can cause progressive renal insufficiency. It becomes a rare entity today due to improvements of antihypertensive management (Marin, 2005). Brenner established the central role for nephron injury and loss in glomerular hypertension. The remaining nephrons develop glomerular capillary hypertension accompanied with hyperfiltration (Brenner, 1982). Nephrosclerosis has actually been seen as a form of intrarenal renovascular disease (Marín, 2005). Beside benign and malignant nephrosclerosis, the spectrum of hypertension-induced renal damage is larger. The pathogenetic mechanisms involved in hypertensive renal damage seems to be the systemic blood pressure "load", the degree to which such load is transmitted to the renal vascular bed and the local tissue susceptibility to any given degree of barotrauma (Bidani, 2004).

In 2009 was proposed a new theory about nephrosclerosis induced by hypertension that involves the genetic *MYH9* polymorphisms. The presence of *MYH9* polymorphisms in individuals leads to products that disrupt normal podocyte function, causing podocyte injury, which ultimately leads to glomerulosclerosis (Freedman, 2009). The presence of genetic polymorphisms leading to intrinsic kidney injury suggest that the failure of strict blood-pressure control to prevent CKD progression does not relate to blood pressure alone, but rather relates to factors intrinsic to the kidney that are yet to be defined. In African American Study of Kidney Disease (AASK) could be observed that blood-pressure control alone cannot reverse existing kidney damage or stop progressive kidney damage (AASK) (Appel, 2008).

Tubulointerstitial injury seems to be one of the main histological determinants of hypertension-related kidney damage. This fact is of particular importance because the pathology correlates with the degree and progression of renal impairment, regardless of the type and origin of kidney injury. Long time it was supposed that interstitial and tubular damage is secondary to glomerular and vascular injury and occurs in the final stages of hypertensive nephropathy. However, experimental studies have demonstrated that this type of kidney damage can be present in hypertensive patients before any changes in glomerular vessels (Mai, 1993). Considering the results of these studies, it may be hypothesized that the tubulointerstitium may be an initial site of renal injury in primary hypertension. This hypothesis is based only on animal studies, however, and has not been finally confirmed in clinical research (Tylicki, 2003).

Endothelium seems to be at the crossroads of the risk for renal impairment and cardiovascular complications in individuals with essential hypertension, therefore, combined effects of low-grade inflammation, oxidative stress and hyperuricemia may be the link between arterial hypertension and renal organ damage. Different studies showed that endothelial dysfunction is associated with renal function decline in hypertensive patients with normal or only mildly impaired baseline renal function (Perticone, 2010). It is possible that a reduction of GFR could induce endothelial dysfunction, establishing a vicious circle which, if not interrupted, promotes the progression of both renal and vascular damage. Therefore, systemic endothelial dysfunction represents an important physiopathological mechanism for the appearance and progression of mild renal dysfunction in hypertensive status. Interstitial inflammation together with oxidative stress participates to the development and maintenance of hypertension by reducing the number of nephrons, limiting therefore the sodium filtration (Brenner, 1988). Ultimately, these effects lead to end stage renal disease. In hypertension, the permeability of the glomeruli is altered which leads to an excess of protein infiltration. The toxicity of this protein load generates tubular damage, inflammation and scarring (Cohuet, 2006).

Novel biomarkers of renal damage are currently investigated and could be used to identify the first signs of hypertension-associated renal injury. There are a number of definitions of the term "biomarker". In general, they have in common three components:

1. They are objectively measured indicators of specific anatomic, physiologic, biochemical, or molecular events;
2. They are associated with normal biological processes or accompany the onset, progression and/or severity of specific pathological or toxic conditions;
3. They are useful to assess the progress of injury, disease or the effects of therapeutic intervention.

2.1 Low grade inflammation

The degree of inflammation and fibrosis of the tubulointerstitial compartment are considered strong predictors of the renal function loss and the risk of progression to end-stage renal disease (Leemans, 2009). Tissue fibrosis and chronic inflammation are common causes of progressive renal damage, leading to loss of physiological functions. Renal fibrosis can be defined by the accumulation of interstitial leukocytes and fibroblasts, contributing to abnormal accumulation of extracellular matrix (ECM) and, eventual, tubular atrophy and loss of renal function (Iwano, 2004). Interestingly, the concept of renal inflammation in progressive kidney disease is intertwined with the concept of hemodynamically induced renal injury (Stuveling, 2005). In the last years, low-grade inflammation has acquired progressive recognition as a mechanism facilitating the occurrence of both glomerular and tubulo-interstitial renal damage. Recently, it was shown that Toll-like receptor 2 (TLR2) is expressed in the kidney and activated by endogenous danger signals (Leemans, 2009). The renal fibrosis is considered to be the common final pathway by which kidney diseases with variable etiology progresses to end-stage renal failure. It is therefore important to identify factors that participate in the initiation of tubulointerstitial inflammation and subsequent interstitial fibrosis during progressive renal injury. Toll-like receptor 2 (TLR2) and 4 plays a crucial role in the induction of acute inflammation and early tubular injury in the kidney in a reversible model of acute renal injury (Leemans, 2009).

Among inflammatory markers, high-sensitive C-reactive protein levels has been recently associated with early kidney damage and seems to best identify the subgroup of hypertensive patients at risk for renal involvement (Zoccali, 2006). Subtle elevations in plasma concentration of high-sensitive C-reactive protein, a reliable marker of inflammation, were associated with similarly subtle reductions in creatinine clearance in the Prevention of Renal and Vascular Endstage Disease (PREVEND) study (Stuveling, 2003).

2.2 Oxidative stress

The role of reactive oxygen species (ROS) has been documented in both experimental and human hypertension (Romero, 1999). It was observed that ROS can have direct and indirect effects on the vascular reactivity (Cohuet, 2006). Indeed, by inactivating endothelial nitric oxide, ROS impair vasodilation and can also have direct effects on vascular tone in function of the quantity of ROS produced and the involved vascular bed. The major ROS is the superoxide anion $\cdot O^{2-}$ and the most common response to its stimulus is vasoconstriction directly or potentiation of the constriction due to angiotensin II (Ang II), thromboxane A_2, endothelin-1 (ET-1), and norepinephrine by increasing intracellular calcium in smooth muscle and endothelial cells. In addition, tubulointerstitial inflammation (infiltration and accumulation of lymphocytes and macrophages) appears to be responsible for the mediation of sodium retention in salt-sensitive models of hypertension. Moreover, oxidative stress may have an influence on sodium retention through tubulointerstitial accumulation of Ang II-positive cells. These 2 mechanisms for hypertension pathogenesis are related by their effects on sodium retention via intrarenal Ang II activity. In the kidney, Ang II decreases glomerular filtration rate, increases tubular sodium reabsorption, and impairs pressure-natriuresis contributing to renal insufficiency. Additionally, oxidative stress has proinflammatory effects: firstly, it activates NF-κB, a transcription factor for proinflammatory genes, which promotes leucocytes infiltration by increasing the expression of adhesion molecules and secondly, it induces the expression of heat shock proteins, resulting in cell death and apoptosis in an inflammatory environment.

2.3 Hyperuricemia

Uric acid may mediate aspects of the relationship between hypertension and kidney disease via renal vasoconstriction and systemic hypertension (Weiner, 2008). Hyperuricemia is present in 25–40% of untreated hypertensive individuals, in 50% of those treated with diuretics, and in over 80% of those with malignant hypertension and is associated with cardiovascular disease, but is not clear if it is an independent risk factor or just a marker associated with cardiovascular risk factors like insulin resistance, obesity and arterial hypertension (Feig, 2008). The high serum uric acid levels in hypertension have been attributed to several mechanisms:

1. The reduced renal blood flow that often accompanies the hypertensive state stimulates urate reabsorption in the proximal tubule;
2. The hypertensive microvascular disease leads to local tissue ischemia, the release of lactate that blocks urate secretion in the proximal tubule and increases uric acid synthesis. Tissue ischemia leads to ATP degradation to adenosine and xanthine oxidase. Both increased xanthine and xanthine oxidase result in increased generation of uric acid and oxidant (O^{2-}) formation;

3. Additional factors can contribute to hyperuricemia in hypertension such as alcohol abuse, lead intoxication, and diuretic use.

Animal model studies have shown that hyperuricemia activates the renin-angiotensin system, induces oxidative stress and reduces renal function. In experimental rat models of hypertension it was shown that hyperuricemia is associated with renal vasoconstriction and is positively correlated with plasma renin activity, these data suggest that uric acid may have adverse effects that are mediated by activated RAS (Lee, 2006). Few studies demonstrated an association between hyperuricemia and microalbuminuria in hypertensive patients (Viazzi, 2007). Recent studies proved that hyperuricemia predicts the development of new-onset kidney disease (Obermayr, 2008) and is considered a risk factor for the development and progression of renal disease (Kang, 2002; Johnson, 2005; Nagakawa, 2006; Feig, 2009).

3. From chronic kidney disease to arterial hypertension

Although the relationship between hypertension and CKD has been recognized for several hundred years, the prevalence of CKD among patients with normal blood pressure has not been assessed in randomly sampled populations. Crews et al reported recently that 13.4% of people who have normal blood pressure have CKD (Agarwal, 2010).

From a clinical point of view, kidney diseases can be classified into two categories according to the onset of the renal pathology (but irrespective of the etiology of injury): (i) Acute kidney injury (AKI) and (ii) Chronic kidney disease (CKD).

AKI, also known as acute renal failure or acute kidney failure, is a rapid loss of renal function, with variable evolution (full, partial or no recovery of a normal renal function), resulting in failure of urinary elimination of nitrogenous waste products (urea nitrogen and creatinine). This impairment of renal function results in elevations of blood urea nitrogen and serum creatinine concentrations. While there is no disagreement about the general definition of ARF, there are substantial differences in diagnosis criteria of ARF (eg, magnitude of rise of serum creatinine concentration). From a clinical perspective, for persons with normal renal function and serum creatinine concentration, GFR must be dramatically reduced to result in even modest increments (eg, 0.1 to 0.3 mg/dL) in serum creatinine concentration (Dwinnell, 1999).

AKI and CKD affect patients worldwide and both are associated with a high morbidity and mortality rate (Prunotto, 2011). AKI community-based incidence has increased by 60% in the past few years, affecting up to 15.3% of all hospitalized patients. CKD is a major public health problem throughout the world. CKD affects more than 13% of the population in the USA and in Europe (Prunotto, 2011). The worldwide impact of CKD is significant, yet underestimated. According to the World Health Report 2002 and the global burden of disease project, kidney and urinary tract diseases contribute to 850,000 deaths per year and 15,010,167 in disability-adjusted life years (Staples, 2010).

Chronic kidney failure, also known as chronic renal failure, chronic renal disease, or chronic kidney disease, is a slow progressive loss of kidney function over a period of several years. The definition of CKD is kidney damage or a GFR below 60 mL per minute per 1.73 m^2 for three months or more (National Kidney Foundation, 2004). It has been appreciated for several decades that once GFR has decreased below a critical level, CKD tends to progress relentlessly toward ESRD (Taal, 2006). Earlier recognition of CKD could slow progression, prevent complications, and reduce cardiovascular-related outcomes (Plantinga, 2010). Due to the asymptomatic nature of this disease, CKD is not frequently detected until its later progress, resulting in loss of prevention opportunities. Progress to kidney failure or other adverse outcomes could be prevented or delayed through early detection and treatment of CKD (Locatelli, 2002).

Until now the available literature exploring the epidemiology of CKD overall has not classified individuals according to the underlying etiology. Rather, the available population cohort data gathered via NHANES and the national Kidney Foundation's KEEP have provided information on comorbid conditions associated with CKD, including hypertension, as opposed to providing accurate estimates of CKD resulting from hypertension; as a result, only estimates of CKD associated with hypertension can be provided. The 2010 USRDS report summarizes the NHANES data on CKD and comorbid conditions. Compared to individuals without CKD, individuals with any stage of CKD (stages 1-5) have higher rates of hypertension (Udani, 2011). The strong association of hypertension with CKD was confirmed by data from KEEP. However, the KEEP data suggest that hypertension is more prevalent at early stages of CKD and that individuals with CKD have even higher rates of hypertension than NHANES data suggest. The KEEP investigators found that the overall prevalence of hypertension exceeded 50% in all individuals with CKD, regardless of GFR, and in those with 'normal' renal function (GFR >100 ml/min/1.73 m^2) the prevalence of hypertension was 57%. The two databases, however, included different methods of sampling individuals and, overall, have different demographical data (Udani, 2011).

The attention paid globally to CKD is attributable to five factors: the rapid increase in its prevalence, the enormous cost of treatment, recent data indicating that overt disease is the tip of an iceberg of covert disease, an appreciation of its major role in increasing the risk of cardiovascular disease, and the discovery of effective measures to prevent its progression (Barsoum, 2006). Furthermore, a gender-different prevalence of CKD was revealed in most included studies. Females had a higher prevalence of CKD than males. Females have less muscle mass as compared to males and the muscle mass is a major determinant of serum creatinine concentration (Heimsfiled, 1983).

Hypertension is present in more than 80% of patients with CKD and contributes to progression of kidney disease toward end stage (ESRD) as well as to cardiovascular events such as heart attack and stroke (Toto, 2005). In fact the risk for cardiovascular death in this patient population is greater than the risk for progression to ESRD. Proteinuria is an important co-morbidity in hypertensive patients with CKD and increases the risk of disease progression and cardiovascular events.

3.1 Pathogenesis

Hypertension has long been recognized as a consequence of renal impairment and an important factor in the progression of CKD. The RAS together with genetic background, renal anemia, altered mineral homeostasis, atherogenic dyslipidemia, chronic inflammation, and oxidative stress and others cardiovascular risk factors such as diabetes, smoking, and obesity are the main contributors in the pathogenesis (Wühl, 2008). CKD pathogenesis is characterized by a progressive loss of renal function, and an excessive deposition of extracellular matrix in the glomeruli and tubular interstitium (López-Novoa, 2011). Chronic glomerulonephritis and interstitial nephritis are currently the principal causes of CKD in developing countries, reflecting the high prevalence of bacterial, viral, and parasitic infections affecting the kidneys (Barsoum, 2006).

3.2 Hyperuricemia

Hyperuricemia is highly prevalent in patients with CKD, reflecting reduced efficiency in renal excretion of uric acid associated with hypouricosuria. Evaluating the role of uric acid in the development or progression of CKD is difficult due to the number of confounders to any study (Feig, 2009). A decline in GFR is associated with increased values of serum uric acid because uric acid is predominantly cleared by the kidneys (Marangella, 2005). The role of uric acid in the initiation and progression of CKD remains controversial. Recent epidemiological and experimental evidence suggested that uric acid might be involved in the development of CKD. In animal studies, experimental hyperuricemia is associated with increasing proteinuria, impaired renal function, glomerulosclerosis, renal interstitial fibrosis and preglomerular vasculopathy (Kang, 2002). Increased renal renin expression appears to be involved in these adverse effects of uric acid on renal function. In humans, hyperuricemia also appears to be associated with activation of the intrarenal RAS (Kobori, 2007). In the Cardiovascular Health Study, SUA levels did not predict incident CKD but were independently associated with the progression of pre-existing CKD (Tziomalos, 2010).

3.3 Assessment of kidney function

Blood urea nitrogen and creatinine clearance are well-established biomarkers of kidney function that can be measured cheaply and easily (Tesch, 2010). Increases levels of serum creatinine are the main manifestations of hypertension-associated renal dysfunction. Persistent increases of serum creatinine levels reflect an important renal parenchymal damage and some degree of irreversible kidney dysfunction (Udani, 2011). CKD from glomerular disease associated with arterial hypertension can be detected by markers of renal parenchymal disease, like proteinuria. The evidence of early kidney injury is elusive without overt glomerular disease that can be found in hypertensive nephrosclerosis or early diabetic nephropathy. The diagnosis and staging of CKD is nowadays based upon the presence of signs of kidney damage together with the estimation of the GFR (Montañés, 2011).

3.3.1 Albuminuria

Albumin is the most abundant protein in the circulation and during normal kidney function very little intact albumin is excreted by the kidney (<30 mg/day in humans) (Tesch, 2010). It is known that a slight increase of urinary albumin excretion (microalbuminuria) is a predictor of renal and cardiovascular events in hypertensive patients (Hillege, 2002). Albuminuria is frequently used as an early marker of renal injury because it often precedes a decline in renal function (Tesch, 2010). In arterial hypertension, an increased transglomerular passage of albumin may result from several mechanisms—hyperfiltration, glomerular basal membrane abnormalities, endothelial dysfunction, and nephrosclerosis (Redon, 2002). Microalbuminuria can also be considered a marker of underlying generalized endothelial or vascular dysfunction. The presence of a single measurement microalbuminuria does not confirm the presence of glomerular disease or parenchymal kidney injury (Udani, 2011). A 2010 debate questioned the relevance of microalbuminuria measurements in the diagnosis of kidney disease and controversies regarding its use as a marker of CKD still exist. The results of the Avoiding Cardiovascular events through Combination therapy in Patients living with systolic Hypertension (ACCOMPLISH) study highlights the limits of microalbuminuria as a marker of kidney disease and predictor of CKD progression (Jamerson, 2004).

3.3.2 Serum creatinine and estimated glomerular filtration rate

In clinical practice, serum creatinine became the almost universal biomarker of choice for GFR (Dalton, 2010). Now it appears to be a rather unreliable marker of GRF because creatinine serum concentrations are affected by tubular secretion, age, sex, muscle mass, physical activity, and diet, and therefore creatinine does not have a direct relationship with the GFR (Hsu, 2002). The Cockcroft-Gault and the Modification of Diet in Renal Disease (MDRD) equations, both based on serum creatinine, are being used increasingly because they overcome, at least in part, some of the limitations of creatinine measurements (Cockcroft, 1976; Levey, 1999). Both equations are currently recommended for the estimation of GFR, which is an established method for detection and classification of CKD in clinical practice (National Kidney Foundation, 2002). The development of formula for estimating GFR and disease staging based on serum creatinine reiterate the continuing importance of this biomarker (Dalton, 2010).

3.3.3 Urinalysis

Urinalysis is considered the major noninvasive diagnostic tool available to the clinician. Although examination of the urine can also provide some information about disease severity, such a direct relationship between the urinalysis and disease severity is not always present (Post, 2006). A normalization of the urinalysis in patients with acute glomerulonephritis can be considered the resolution of the active inflammatory process, a recovery or healing with irreversible glomerular scarring and nephron loss. In this setting, repeated renal biopsy may be required to accurately estimate the status of the renal disease. Despite potential limitations, a complete urinalysis should be performed in all patients with renal disease (Post, 2003).

3.3.4 Aldosterone

Aldosterone, the main mineralocorticoid synthesized by the adrenal gland, has an essential function in sodium and water homeostasis and urinary excretion of potassium (Roldán, 2010). It is an important mediator of collagen turnover, stimulating the expression of various profibrotic molecules and inhibiting other antifibrotic molecules, thereby assuming a decisive role in the development of renal fibrosis. Aldosterone also has an important pathogenic role in hypertension and vascular remodeling, in left ventricular hypertrophy, and in renal disease, specifically proteinuria and glomerulosclerosis in patients with hypertension (Roldán, 2010). A lot of experimental studies analysed the damage caused by aldosterone in the mesangium, basement membrane, and renal tubule and indicated an important pathologic role of the hormone in renal function impairment. The contribution of aldosterone to the development of arterial hypertension in the general population has been shown recently by the Framingham Offspring Study in which serum plasma aldosterone levels in normotensive subjects predicted subsequent increases in blood pressure and in the development of incident hypertension (Vasan, 2004). Plasma aldosterone concentration can be used as a marker of impaired renal function in the initial phases of arterial hypertension (Roldán, 2010).

3.3.5 Hyperhomocysteinemia

Another marker of renal damage is hyperhomocysteinemia. Serum homocysteine concentrations are significantly elevated in patients with albuminuria and low GFR

(Ikeyaga, 2005). In the Horn study, high plasma homocysteine was associated with microalbuminuria independently of other risk factors (Hoogeveen, 1998). Several biochemical mechanisms have been proposed to explain the presumed vasculotoxic effects of homocysteine. The main theory is that high homocysteine levels lead to endothelial dysfunction. Impaired endothelial vasomotor responses have been ascribed to a reduced bioavailability of nitric oxide due to auto-oxidation of homocysteine in plasma which leads to oxidative inactivation of nitric oxide (Welch, 1998). Alternatively, homocysteine may lead to the accumulation of asymmetric dimethylarginine by inhibiting its catabolizing enzyme dimethylarginine dimethylaminohydrolase (van Guldener, 2006). Hyperhomocysteinemia could cause subclinical renal interstitial injury, and reduced renal function promotes further rise in plasma homocysteine (Ikegaya, 2005). Both hyperhomocysteinemia and renal injury are associated as pathogenic processes, creating a vicious cycle that results in further impairment of renal function.

3.3.6 Cystatin-C

Recently, Cystatin-C, a protein member of the family of cysteine proteinase inhibitors, was proposed as a new reliable marker of renal function. Because of its small size, cystatin C is freely filtered by the glomerulus. It is not secreted but reabsorbed by tubular epithelial cells and subsequently catabolized so that it does not return to the blood flow (Abrahamson, 1990). It is the product of a gene expressed in all nucleated cells and is produced at a constant rate, therefore permitted calculation of a cystatin C clearance using urine concentrations. Serum levels of cystatin C is a promising early marker of hypertension-associated kidney dysfunction and may accurately reflect eGFR in various populations (Udani, 2011). The use of serum cystatin C to approximate eGFR is based on the same logic as the use of blood urea nitrogen and creatinine, but because it does not return to the bloodstream and is not secreted, the eGFR obtained may be more reflective of actual renal filtration function (McMurray, 2009). The cystatin C concentration is converted and reported in milliliters per minute giving a direct estimation of the GFR. Unlike serum creatinine, it is not influenced by age, sex, muscle mass, exercise or diet. A study from the Prevention of Renal and Vascular End-Stage Renal Disease (PREVEND) cohort found that cystatin C was significantly associated with C-reactive protein (CRP), smoking and body mass index, even after adjustment for creatinine clearance levels (Knight, 2004). The authors concluded that cystatin C levels were influenced by these factors in addition to kidney function. Other longitudinal studies have shown that cystatin C has a stronger and more linear association with cardiovascular disease and mortality outcomes compared to creatinine-based measures. These findings led to the hypothesis that cystatin C`s link to inflammation could explain its advantage over creatinine as a prognostic marker (Singh, 2007).

3.3.7 Advanced Glycation End Products (AGE)

Advanced glycation end products (AGEs) are a heterogeneous group of proteins and lipids covalently bound to sugar residues. It appears that activation of the RAS may contribute to AGE formation through various mechanisms (Bohlender, 2005). Although AGEs could nonspecifically bind to basement membranes and modify their properties, they also induce specific cellular responses including the release of profibrogenic and proinflammatory cytokines by interacting with the receptor for AGE (Bohlender, 2005). AGE levels are grossly elevated in CKD and hemodialysis as a result of decreased clearance, resulting in an increased tissue accumulation. The accumulation of AGE in renal failure is even greater than in diabetes (Noordzij, 2008).

3.3.8 Resistin

Resistin, a newly discovered low molecular weight plasma protein, promotes endothelial dysfunction and proinflammatory activation, contributing to subclinical atherosclerosis (Dimitriadis, 2009). Although classified as an adipokine, resistin in humans is mainly produced by blood-derived leukocytes and mononuclear cells, both within and outside the adipose tissue (Ellington, 2007). Resistin directly induces endothelin-1 production, upregulates adhesion molecules and chemokines, and downregulates TNF receptor-associated factor-3 (Verma, 2003). Resistin-induced mitochondrial dysfunction and imbalance in cellular redox enzymes may be the underlying mechanisms of oxidative stress (Chen, 2010). The humoral factors induced by resistin and their downstream effectors could potentiate mesangial proliferation and interstitial fibrosis, thereby affecting both glomerular and tubular processes. Recently, elevated levels of resistin were proposed to be a risk factor for kidney disease or may even represent overt kidney damage in asymptomatic adults with essential hypertension (Ellington, 2007).

3.3.9 Kidney injury molecule-1 (KIM-1)

The kidney injury molecule-1 (designated as Kim-1 in rodents, KIM-1 in humans) mRNA was identified using techniques of representational difference analysis, a PCR-based technique (Hubank, 1994; Bonventre, 2009). KIM-1 is a type 1 transmembrane protein that is not detectable in normal kidney tissue but is expressed at high levels in human and rodent kidneys with dedifferentiated proximal tubule epithelial cells after ischemic or toxic injury (Han, 2005). KIM-1 is strongly up-regulated in dedifferentiated proximal tubule kidney epithelial cells after an ischemic or toxic injury. It may also play a role in epithelial adhesion, growth, and differentiation (Malyszko, 2010). KIM-1 not only functions as a biomarker but also has predictive value for acute renal injury, but was predictive for adverse clinical outcome in a cohort of 201 hospitalized patients with acute renal failure (Lock, 2010). Urinary Kim-1 levels may serve as a noninvasive, rapid, sensitive, reproducible, and potentially high-throughput method to detect early kidney injury in pathophysiological studies and in preclinical drug development studies for risk-benefit profiling of pharmaceutical agents (Vaidya, 2006).

3.3.10 Asymmetric dimethylarginine

Asymmetric dimethylarginine (ADMA) is a naturally occurring L-arginine analogue, found in plasma and various types of tissues, acting as an endogenous NO synthase inhibitor *in vivo* (Ueda, 2007). Further, plasma level of ADMA is elevated in patients with CKD and found to be a strong biomarker or predictor for future cardiovascular events (Ueda, 2007). In addition, plasma level of ADMA could predict the progression of renal injury in these patients, as well. These findings suggest that elevation of ADMA may be a missing link between CVD and CKD. ADMA levels are markedly elevated in renal impairment, together with the experimental evidence showing ADMA to be a CKD progression factor in animals; four prospective studies have found an association between ADMA level and CKD progression in humans (Kronenberg, 2009).

3.3.11 Interleukin-18 (IL-18)

Interleukin-18 (IL-18) is a proinflammatory cytokine which is induced in PCT and is detected in urine following AKI. It was found to be an early predictor of AKI in patients with adult respiratory distress syndrome with an area under the curve (AUC) of 0.73 (Soni, 2009). It was also found to be an independent predictor of mortality in this study. In another study on patients undergoing cardiac surgery, urinary IL-18 levels increased 6 h after cardiopulmonary bypass (CPB) and peaked at 12 h in patients who were diagnosed to have AKI 2 days later by creatinine criteria (Han, 2009). Elevated urinary IL-18 is more specific for ischemic AKI and its levels are not deranged in CKD, urinary tract infections or nephrotoxic AKI. However, a study by Haase et al. did not find IL-18 to be a useful early predictor of AKI in a group of 100 adult patients undergoing cardiac surgery (Soni, 2009).

3.3.12 Urinary Netrin-1 (Ntn-1)

Netrin-1 (Ntn-1), a laminin-related axon guidance molecule, is highly induced and excreted in the urine after acute kidney injury (AKI) in animals (Ramesh, 2010). Previous studies proved that Ntn-1 is involved in the orchestration of inflammatory responses in vitro or in vivo (Ly, 2005; Rosenberger, 2009). The kidney has one of the highest levels of netrin-1 expression, and administration of recombinant netrin-1 before ischemia reperfusion reduces kidney injury and inflammation (Wang, 2008).

3.3.13 Urinary neutrophil gelatinase-associated lipocalin (NGAL)

Urinary neutrophil gelatinase-associated lipocalin (NGAL) is a small (25 kDa) protein, expressed in renal tubular cells and released into the blood and urine after exposure to ischemia or toxicity (Devarajan, 2010) and represent a promising new renal biomarker able to diagnose acute kidney injury (AKI). It is rapidly induced and released from the injured renal distal nephrons in experimental studies and various human diseases. The changes of body water content could, thus, influence the urinary concentration, like for other urinary biomarkers, too. The release of NGAL occurs within hours after the stimulus and long before an increase in serum creatinine level. Urinary and plasma concentrations of NGAL increase proportionally to severity and duration of renal injury and rapidly decrease with its attenuation. However, NGAL release is not specific to the kidney. Measurements may be readily and easily performed in urine and plasma using clinical laboratory platforms or point of care devices (Haase, 2011). Therefore, the NGAL level was proposed to be a real-time indicator of active kidney damage, whereas creatinine level and GFR are markers of functional nephron number (Kronenberg, 2009).

3.3.14 Liver-type fatty acid binding protein (L-FABP)

Clinical data on associations between liver-type fatty acid binding protein (L-FaBP) and kidney disease are sparse (Kronenberg, 2009). This protein is expressed in proximal tubular cells and increased expression and higher levels are seen in the urine of patients with kidney disease and is considered a promising indicator of tubular but not glomerular damage (Kamijo-Ikemori, 2011). A large health screening program in more than 900 individuals revealed that average urinary levels of L-FaBP were approximately 50% higher in patients with diabetes mellitus, hypertension or chronic hepatitis than in controls. A study investigating L-FaBP levels in patients with type 2 diabetes and different stages of nephropathy showed that urinary L-FaBP was associated with the severity of diabetic nephropathy (Nakamura, 2005). Small studies in patients with mild kidney dysfunction suggest that urinary L-FaBP concentrations are increased in patients whose renal function deteriorates further (Kamijo, 2004).

3.4 Lifestyle modifications

In the general population, the strategies that lower blood pressure include dietary and lifestyle modifications in order to prevent and treat arterial hypertension. Blood pressure and CKD management rely heavily upon the patient's ability to self-manage and willingness to change or maintain health-promoting behaviors. The prevalence of hypertension may be also reduced also by measures like eight loss, sodium restriction, fluid restriction, exercise, and limitation of alcohol intake (Miller, 2003).

The Intersalt Cooperative Research Study, which measured urinary sodium in over 10,000 individuals from 32 countries, found that consumption of more than 100 mmol/day sodium was associated with significantly higher blood pressures (Miller, 2003). Sodium restriction is also a crucial component to dietary intake for patients with CKD. In CKD, extracellular volume expansion as a result of impaired natriuresis is thought to play an important role in the pathogenesis of hypertension. It is therefore recommended that dietary sodium intake should be less than 100 mmol/day. Exercise and weight loss (if body mass index is more than 25 kg/m^2) are also recommended (Thuraisingham, 2011).

The Dietary Approaches to Stop Hypertension (DASH) diet has been shown to produce most benefits in blood pressure reduction through sodium restriction and weight loss, and can also decrease LDL cholesterol. The DASH diet is a result of a feeding study of 459 adults (49% women, 60% African American) with high normal or elevated blood pressure (Sacks, 2001).

3.5 Pharmacologic intervention

The discussed pathophysiology of hypertensive renal damage suggests three broad targets for therapeutic interventions: (1) reduction of BP load; (2) reduction of pressure transmission to the renal microvasculature; and (3) interruption and/or modification of the local cellular/molecular pathways that mediate eventual tissue injury and fibrosis (Bidani, 2004).

Antihypertensive therapy significantly decreases the vascular damage in the kidneys of hypertensive patients. Therapy of hypertension is therefore imperative. The National Kidney Foundation clinical practice guidelines recommend a blood pressure goal of <130 mmHg systolic and <80 mmHg diastolic for all CKD patients. Post-hoc analyses of the Modification of Diet in Renal Disease study indicate that lower blood pressure may provide long-term kidney protection in patients with nondiabetic kidney disease. Specifically a mean arterial pressure < 92 mmHg (e.g. 120/80 mmHg) compared to 102-107 mmHg (e.g. 140/90 mmHg) is associated with a reduced risk for ESRD (Toto, 2005). Citing KDOQI, the seventh report from the Joint National Committee on Prevention, Detection, Evaluation, and Treatment of High Blood Pressure (JNC 7) also recommends a target BP of < 130/80 mmHg for all patients with CKD defined as an GFR<60 ml/min per 1.73m ^{2} or protein-to-creatinine ratio ≥ 200 mg/g.1 A target BP < 130/80 mmHg is also recommended by the American Diabetes Association (ADA) and by JNC 7 for all patients with diabetes (O'Hare, 2009).

The inhibition of the effects of angiotensin II is necessary to ensure the best degree of renal protection by the simultaneous control of blood pressure (BP) and the achievement of the maximal antiproteinuric capacity. The inhibition can be attained through the administration of either an angiotensin-converting enzyme (ACE) inhibitor or an angiotensin II receptor blocker (ARB). Uptitration of antihypertensive therapy is frequently required to achieve the desired BP goal in patients presenting with renal disease, with or without proteinuria. Control of BP is good for both cardiovascular and renal protection (Segura, 2003).

RAS inhibitors have been shown to reduce proteinuria and the rate of loss of renal function in patients with CKD (Ito, 2010). However, the benefits of RAS inhibition seem to depend on the degree of proteinuria at baseline. Namely, RAS inhibition has been shown to be beneficial in patients with at least 0.5 g per day proteinuria, whereas no convincing evidence exists to demonstrate the benefits extended to patients with a lower level of proteinuria (Jafal, 2001). An "adequate" BP control with standard antihypertensive therapy, the kidney is well protected and very few hypertensive patients, less than 2%, will develop renal damage as a consequence of arterial hypertension (Ruilope, 2002). Interestingly, data from the ACCOMPLISH trial demonstrated that use of an ACE inhibitor in combination with a calcium antagonist was associated with a reduced requirement for dialysis than use of an ACE inhibitor and a diuretic in individuals > 65 years of age (Backris, 2010).

Identifying individuals with early signs of CKD might help the targeting of therapies to more effectively prevent disease progression and associated complications. Identifying an appropriate marker of early renal dysfunction, however, remains challenging and depends on the underlying etiology of kidney disease. Early diagnosis on the basis of presence of proteinuria or reduced estimated GFR could permit early intervention to reduce the risks of cardiovascular events, kidney failure, and death that are associated with chronic kidney disease. In developed countries, screening for the disorder is most effective when targeted at high-risk groups including elderly people and those with concomitant illness (such as diabetes, hypertension, or cardiovascular disease) or a family history of chronic kidney disease, although the role of screening in developing countries is not yet clear. Different strategies available now aimed to slow the progression of CKD and to reduce cardiovascular risk (James, 2010). Treatment of high blood pressure is recommended for all individuals with, or at risk of, chronic kidney disease. Use of angiotensin-converting-enzyme inhibitors or angiotensin-receptor blockers is preferred for patients with diabetic CKD or those with the proteinuric non-diabetic disorder (Matthew, 2010).

4. Conclusion

In conclusion, hypertension-associated renal damage would paradoxically originate from subtle, focal renovascular damage, where hypertension would be another mere consequence acting as a magnifying amplifier in the vicious circle of malignancy. The therapeutic strategy aims, at targeting the pathophysiological processes mentioned in this chapter, to prevent, reduce or reverse the renal organ damage due to arterial hypertension.

5. References

Abrahamson, M.; Olafsson, I.; Palsdottir, A.; Ulvsback, M.; Lundwall, A. et al. (1990). Structure and expression of the human cystatin C gene. *Biochemical Journal*, Vol. 268, (June, 1990), pp. 287–294.

Agarwal. R. (2010). Epidemiology of chronic kidney disease among normotensives. But what is chronic kidney disease? *Hypertension*, Vol. 55. (May, 2010), pp. 1097-1099.

Appel, L. J. et al. (2008). Long-term effects of renin-angiotensin system-blocking therapy and a low blood pressure goal on progression of hypertensive chronic kidney disease in African Americans. *Archives of Internal Medicine,* Vol. 168, (April, 2008), pp. 832-839.

Bakris, G. L. et al. (2010). Renal outcomes with different fixed-dose combination therapies in patients with hypertension at high-risk for cardiovascular events (ACCOMPLISH): a prespecified secondary analysis of a randomized clinical trial. *Lancet,* Vol. 375, (April, 2010), pp.1173–1181.

Barsoum, R.S. (2006). Chronic kidney disease in the developing world. *New England Journal of Medicine,* Vol. 354, (March, 2006), pp. 997-999.

Bohlender JM, Franke S, Stein G, Wolf G. (2005). Advanced glycation end products and the kidney. *American Journal of Physiology Renal Physiology,* Vol. 289, Vol.4, (October, 2005), pp. F645–F659.

Bonventre, J. V. (2009). Kidney injury molecule-1 (KIM-1): a urinary biomarker and much more. *Nephrology, Dialisis, Transplantation,* Vol. 24, No.11, (November, 2011), pp. 3265-3268.

Chappell, M.C. (2010). Angiotensin-converting enzyme 2 autoantibodies: further evidence for a role of the renin-angiotensin system in inflammation, *Arthritis research and therapy,* Vol.12, No.3, (June, 2010), pp.128.

Chen C, Jiang J, Lü JM, Chai H, Wang X, Lin PH, Yao Q. (2010). Resistin decreases expression of endothelial nitric oxide synthase through oxidative stress in human coronary artery endothelial cells. *American Journal of Physiology Heart and Circulation Physiology,* Vol. 299, No.1, (July, 2010), pp. H193-H201.

Cockcroft, D.W.; Gault, M.H. (1976). Prediction of creatinine clearance from serum creatinine. *Nephron,* Vol. 16, No.1. pp. 31–41.

Cohuet, G.; Struijker-Boudier, H. (2006). Mechanisms of target organ damage caused by hypertension: therapeutic potential. *Pharmacology and Therapeutics,* Vol. 111, (July, 2006), pp. 81–98.

Dalton, R.N., (2010). Serum creatinine and glomerular filtration rate: perception and reality. *Clinical Chemistry,* Vol. 56, (May, 2010), pp. 687-689.

Devarajan, P., (2010). Neutrophil gelatinase-associated lipocalin: a promising biomarker for human acute kidney injury. Biomarkers in Medicine, Vol. 4, No.2 (Aprilie, 2010), pp. 265–280.

Dimitriadis K, Tsioufis C, Selima M, Tsiachris D, Miliou A, Kasiakogias A et al. (2009). Independent association of circulating resistin with glomeular filtration rate in the early stages of essential hypertension. *Journal of Human Hypertension,* Vol.23, (May, 2009), pp. 668–673.

Dworkin, L.D; Shemin, D.G. (1999). The role of hypertension in progression of chronic renal disease. In: R.W. Schrier, Editor, *Atlas of diseases of the kidneys,* Current Medicine, Inc., Philadelphia (Pa) (1999), pp. 6.1–6.18.

Dwinnell, B.G.; Anderson, R.J. (1999). Diagnostic evaluation of the patient with acute renal failure, in *Atlas of Diseases of Kidney,* edited by Schrier RW, Philadelphia, Current Medicine Inc., 1999, pp 12.1-12.12.

Ellington, A.A.; Malik, A.R.; Klee, G.G.; Turner, S.T.; Rule, A.D.; Mosley TH Jr, Kullo IJ: (2007). Association of plasma resistin with glomerular filtration rate and albuminuria in hypertensive adults. *Hypertension,* Vol. 50, (October, 2007), pp. 708– 714.

Feig, D.I., Rang, D.H., Johnson, R.J. (2008). Uric acid and cardiovascular risk. *New England Journal of Medicine,* Vol. 359, (October, 2008), pp. 1811–1821.

Freedman, B.I. et al. (2009). Polymorphisms in the non-muscle myosin heavy chain 9 gene (MYH9) are strongly associated with end-stage renal disease historically attributed to hypertension in African Americans. *Kidney International,* Vol. 75, (April, 2009), pp. 736-745.

Gomez Campdera FJ, Luno J, Garcia de Vinuesa S, Valderrabano F. (1998). Renal vascular disease in the elderly. *Kidney International,* Vol. 68, (December, 1998), pp.S73-S77.

Griffin, K.A.; Abu-Amarah, I.; Picken, M.; Bidani, A.K. (2003), Renoprotection by ACE inhibition or aldosterone blockade is blood pressure-dependent. *Hypertension,* Vol. 41, (February, 2003), pp. 201–206.

Guyenet PG. (2006). The sympathetic control of blood pressure. *Nature Review Neuroscience,* Vol.7 ,(May, 2006), pp. 335-346.

Haase, M. (2011). NGAL—From discovery to a new era of "Acute Renal Disease" diagnosis? *Clinical Biochemistry,* Vol. 44, No. 7. (May 2011), pp. 499-500.

Han, WK et al. (2005). Human Kidney Injury Molecule-1 is a Tissue and Urinary Tumor Marker of Renal Cell Carcinoma, *Journal of the American Society of Nephrology,* Vol. 16, no. 4, (April, 2005), pp. 1126-1134.

Heymsfield, S.B.; Arteaga, C.; McManus, C.; Smith, J.; Moffitt, S. (1983). Measurement of muscle mass in humans: validity of the 24-hour urinary creatinine method. *American Journal of Clinical Nutrition,* Vol. 37, (March, 1983), pp. 478-494.

Hillege HL, Fidler V, Diercks GF, et al. (2002). Urinary albumin excretion predicts cardiovascular and noncardiovascular mortality in general population, *Circulation,* Vol. 106, (September, 2002), pp. 1777–1782.

Hoogeveen EK, Kostense PJ, Jager A et al. (1998). Serum homocysteine level and protein intake are related to risk of microalbuminuria: the Hoorn Study. *Kidney International,* Vol. 54, pp. 203–209.

Hsu CY, Chertow GM, Curhan GC. (2002). Methodological issues in studying the epidemiology of mild to moderate chronic renal insufficiency. *Kidney International,* Vol. 61, pp. 1567-1576.

Hubank M, Schatz DG. (1994). Identifying differences in mRNA expression by representational difference analysis of cDNA. *Nucleic Acids Research,* Vol. 22, No.25, (December, 1994), pp. 5640–5648.

Ikegaya N, Yanagisawa C, Kumagai H. (2005). Relationship between plasma homocysteine concentration and urinary markers of tubulointerstitial injury. *Kidney International,* Vol. 67, No.1, (January, 2005), pp. 375.

Iwano, M.; Neilson, E.G. (2004). Mechanisms of tubulointerstitial fibrosis. *Current Opinion in Nephrology and Hypertension,* Vol. 13, (May, 2004), pp. 279–284.

Ito S. (2010). Usefulness of RAS inhibition depends on baseline albuminuria. *Nature Review Nephrology,* Vol. 6, (January, 2010), pp. 10–11.

Jafar, T.H. *et al.* (2001). Angiotensin-converting enzyme inhibitors and progression of nondiabetic renal disease. A meta-analysis of patient-level data. *Annals of Internal Medicine,* Vol. 135, (July, 2001), pp. 73–87.

Jamerson KA, Bakris GL, Wun C-C, et al. (2004). Rationale and design of the Avoiding Cardiovascular events through COMbination therapy in Patients LIving with Systolic Hypertension (ACCOMPLISH) trial. American Journal of Hypertension, Vol. 17, No.9, (September, 2004), pp. 793–801.

James, M.T.; Hemmelgarn, B.R.; Tonelli, M. (2010). Early recognition and prevention of chronic kidney disease. *Lancet,* Vol. 375. No. 9722, (April, 2010), pp. 1296-1309.

Johnson RJ, Segal MS, Srinivas T, Ejaz A, Mu W, Roncal C, Sanchez- Lozada LG, Gersch M, Rodriguez-Iturbe, B.; Kang, D.H.; Acosta, J.H. (2005). Essential hypertension, progressive renal disease, and uric acid: A pathogenetic link? *Journal of the American Society of Nephrology,* Vol. 16, (April, 2005), pp. 1909-1919.

Kamijo, A. et al. Urinary fatty acid-binding protein as a new clinical marker of the progression of chronic renal disease. *The Journal of the Laboratory and Clinical Medicine,* Vol. 143, No.1 (January, 2004), pp. 23-30 (2004).

Kamijo, A. et al. (2006). Urinary liver-type fatty acid binding protein as a useful biomarker in chronic kidney disease. *Molecular and Cellular Biochemistry,* Vol. 284, No.1-2, (March, 2006), pp. 175-182.

Kamijo-Ikemori A, Sugaya T, Yasuda T et al. (2011). Clinical significance of urinary liver-type fatty acid binding protein in diabetic nephroptahy of type 2 diabetic patients. *Diabetes Care,* Vol. 34, (July, 2011), pp. 691-696.

Kang DH, Nakagawa T, Feng L, Watanabe S, Han L, Mazzali M, et al. (2002). A role of uric acid in the progression of renal disease. *Journal of the American Society of Nephrology,* Vol. 13, (December, 2002), pp. 2888-2897.

Komlosi P, Fuson AL, Fintha A, Peti-Peterdi J, Rosivall L, Warnock DG, Bell PD. (2003) Angiotensin I conversion to angiotensin II stimulates cortical collecting duct sodium transport. *Hypertension,* Vol. 42, (August, 2003), pp.195-199.

Kobori H, Nangaku M, Navar LG, Nishiyama A. (2007), The intrarenal renin-angiotensin system: from physiology to the pathobiology of hypertension and kidney disease. *Pharmacological reviews,* Vol. 59, (September, 2007), pp. 251-287.

Kobori H, Urushihara M, Xu JH, Berenson GS, Navar LG. (2010). Urinary angiotensinogen is correlated with blood pressure in men (Bogalusa Heart Study). *Journal of Hypertension,* Vol. 28, (July, 2010), pp. 1422-1428.

Kronenberg, F. (2009). Emerging risk factors and markers of chronic kidney disease progression. *Nature Reviews Nephrology,* Vol. 5. (December, 2009) pp. 677-689.

Lee JE, Kim YG, Choi YH, Huh W, Kim DJ, Oh HY. (2006). Serum uric acid is associated with microalbuminuria in prehypertension. *Hypertension,* Vol. 47, (March, 2006), pp. 962-967.

Leemans JC, Butter LM, Pulskens WP, Teske GJ, Claessen N, et al. (2009). The role of Toll-like receptor 2 in inflammation and fibrosis during progressive renal injury. *Public Library of Science ONE,* Vol. 4. No.5, (May, 2009), pp. e5704.

Levey, A.S.; Coresh, J.; Greene, T.; Marsh, J.; Stevens, L.A.; Kusek, J.W.; Van Lente, F. (2007). Expressing the modification of diet in renal disease study equation for estimating glomerular filtration rate with standardized serum creatinine values. *Clinical Chemistry,* Vol. 53, (March, 2007), pp. 766-772.

Ljutic, D.; Kes, P. (2003). The role of arterial hypertension in the progression of non-diabetic glomerular diseases. *Nephrology Dialysis Transplantation,* Vol. 18. (July, 2003), Pp. v28-v30.

Locatelli, F.; Vecchio, L.D.; Pozzoni, P. (2002). The importance of early detection of chronic kidney disease, *Nephrology Dialysis Transplantation,* Vol. 17, Suppl. 11, pp. 2-7.

Lock, E.A. (2010). Sensitive and early markers of renal injury: where are we and what is the way forward? *Toxicology Sciences,* Vol. 116. No.1, (July, 2010), pp. 1-4.

Lockhart, C.J.; Hamilton, P.K.; Quinn, C.E.; McVeigh, G.E. (2009). End-organ dysfunction and cardiovascular outcomes: The role of the microcirculation. *Clinical Science,* Vol. 116, (February, 2009), pp. 175-190.

López-Novoa et al. (2011). Etiopathology of chronic tubular, glomerular and renovascular nephropathies: Clinical implications, *Journal of Translational Medicine,* Vol. 9, (January, 2011), pp. 13.

Ly NP, Komatsuzaki K, Fraser IP, Tseng AA, Prodhan P, et al. (2005) Netrin-1 inhibits leukocyte migration in vitro and in vivo. *Proceedings of the National Academy of Science of the United States of America,* Vol. 102, No.41, (October, 2005), pp. 14729- 14734.

Mai, M.; Geiger, H.; Hilgers, K.F. et al. (1993). Early interstitial changes in hypertension-induced renal injury. *Hypertension,* Vol. 22, (November, 1993), pp. 754-765.

Malyszko J, Koc-Zorawska E, Malyszko JS, Mysliwiec M. (2010). Kidney injury molecule-1 correlates with kidney function in renal allograft recipients. *Transplant Proceedings,* Vol. 42, No.10, (December, 2010), pp. 3957-3959.

Mancia G, De Backer G, Dominiczak A, Cifkova R, Fagard R, et al. (2007). The Task Force for the Management of Arterial Hypertension of the European Society of Hypertension (ESH) and of the European Society of Cardiology (ESC). European Heart Journal, vol. 28, No.12, (June, 2007), pp. 1462–1536.

Marangella, M. (2005). Uric acid elimination in the urine. Pathophysiological implications. *Contributions to Nephrology,* Vol. 147, pp. 132–148, DOI: 10.1159/000082551.

Marín R, Gorostidi M, Fernández-Vega F, Alvarez-Navascués R. (2005). Systemic and glomerular hypertension and progression of chronic renal disease: the dilemma of nephrosclerosis. *Kidney International,* vol.99, (December, 2005), pp. 52-56.

Marney, A.M.; Brown, N.J. (2007). Aldosterone and end-organ damage. *Clinical Sciences (Lond).* Vol. 113, (August, 2007), pp. 267-78.

Mattson Porth C. (2011). *Essentials of Pathophysiology,* 3rd Edition, Wolters Kluwer Health, Lippincott Williams & Wilkins, Philadelphia.

McMurray, M.D.; Trivax, J.E.; McCullough, P.A. (2009). Serum cystatin C, renal filtration function, and left ventricular remodeling, *Circulation. Heart failure,* vol. 2, no. 2, (March, 2009), pp. 86–89.

Mishra, J.; Dent, C.; Tarabishi, R.; et al. (2005). Neutrophil gelatinase-associated lipocalin (NGAL) as a biomarker for acute renal injury after cardiac surgery. *Lancet,* Vol. 365, pp. 1231–1238.

Mitchell KD, Braam B, Navar LG (1992). Hypertension mechanisms mediated by the renal actions of the renin-angiotensin system, *Hypertension,* Vol. 19, Suppl I, pp. I18-I27.

Montañés BR, Gràcia GS, Pérez SD, Martínez CA, Bover SJ. (2011). Consensus document. Recommendations on assessing proteinuria during the diagnosis and follow-up of chronic kidney disease, *Nefrologia,* (May, 2011), Vol. 31, No.3, pp. 331-45.

Nakamura T, Sugaya T, Kawagoe Y, Ueda Y, Osada S, Koide H. (2005). Effect of pitavastatin on urinary liver-type fatty acid-binding protein levels in patients with early diabetic nephropathy. *Diabetes Care,* Vol. 28, No.11, (November, 2005), pp. 2728- 2732.

National Kidney Foundation. (2002). K/DOQI clinical practice guidelines for chronic kidney disease: evaluation, classification, and stratification. *American Journal of Kidney Di*seases, Vol. 392, suppl 1, (February, 2002), pp. S1–266.

Navar LG and Hamm LL. (1999). The kidney in blood pressure regulation. In: Atlas of Diseases of the Kidney. Hypertension and the Kidney, edited by Wilcox CS. Philadelphia: Current Medicine, Inc., 1999, p. 1.1-1.22.

Navar LG, Harrison-Bernard LM, Nishiyama A, Kobori H. (2002). Regulation of intrarenal angiotensin II in hypertension. *Hypertension.* Vol. 39, pp. 316–*322.*

Nagakawa T, Kang DH, Feig D, Sanchez-Lozada LG, Srinivas TR, Sautin Y, Ejaz AA, Segal M, Johnson RJ. (2006). Unearthing uric acid: An ancient factor with recently found significance in renal and cardiovascular disease. *Kidney International,* Vol. 69, No.10. (May, 2006), pp. 1722–1725.

Noordzij, M.J.; Lefrandt, J.D.; Smit, A.J. (2008). Advanced glycation end products in renal failure: an overview, *Journal of Renal Care,* Vol. 34, No.4. (November, 2008), pp. 207- 212.

Plantinga, L.C.; Tuot, D.S.; Powe, N.R. (2010). Awareness of chronic kidney disease among patients and providers. *Advances in Chronic Kidney Disease,* Vol. 17. No.3, (May, 2010), pp. 225- 236.

Perticone, F., Maio, R., Perticone, M., Sciacqua, A., Shehaj, E., Naccarato, P. and Sesti, G. (2010). Endothelial dysfunction and subsequent decline in glomerular filtration rate in hypertensive patients. *Circulation,* Vol. 122, No.4, (July, 2010), pp. 379–384.

Pohl, M.A. (1999). Renovascular hypertension and ischemic nephropathy. *Atlas of Diseases of the Kidney,* 1st Ed., edited by Wilcox CS, Schrier RW, Philadelphia, Current Medicine, pp. 3.1–3.21.

Post TW, Rose BD. (2006). Urinalysis in the diagnosis of renal disease. *Up To Date,* Vol. 13, pp. 3.

Prunotto, M.; Gabbiani, G.; Pomposiello, S.; Ghiggeri, G., Moll, S. (2011). The kidney as a target organ in pharmaceutical research. *Drug Discovery Today,* Vol. 16. No. 5-6, (March 2011), pp. 244-259.

Ramesh G, Krawczeski CD, Woo JG, Wang Y, Devarajan P. (2010). Urinary netrin-1 is an early predictive biomarker of acute kidney injury after cardiac surgery. *Clinical Journal of American Society of Nephrology,* Vol. 5, No.3 (March, 2010), pp. 395–401.

Redon J, Rovira E, Miralles A, Julve R, Pascual JM. (2002). Factors related to the occurrence of microalbuminuria during antihypertensive treatment in essential hypertension. *Hypertension,* Vol. 39, No.3, (March, 2002), pp. 794–798.

Roldán, J.; Morillas, P.; Castillo, J; Andrade, H; Guillén S. (2010). Plasma aldosterone and glomerular filtration in hypertensive patients with preserved renal function, *Revista Española de Cardiología (English Edition),* Vol. 63. No.1, (January, 2010), pp. 103-106.

Romero JC and Reckelhoff JF. (1999). Role of angiotensin and oxidative stress in arterial hypertension. *Hypertension,* Vol. 34:, pp. 943-949.

Rosenberger P, Schwab JM, Mirakaj V, Masekowsky E, Mager A, et al. (2009) Hypoxia-inducible factor-dependent induction of netrin-1 dampens inflammation caused by hypoxia. *Nature Immunology,* Vol. 10, No.2, (February, 2009), pp. 195–202.

Ruilope, L.M. (2002). The kidney as a sensor of cardiovascular risk in essential hypertension. *Journal of the American Society of Nephrology,* Vol. 13, Suppl. 3, (November, 2002), pp. S165- S168.

Sacks FM, Svetkey LP, Vollmer WM, Appel LJ, Bray GA, Harsha D, et al. (2001). Effects on blood pressure of reduced dietary sodium and the Dietary Approaches to Stop Hypertension (DASH) diet. DASH-Sodium Collaborative Research Group. *New England Journal of Medicine,* (January, 2001), Vol. 344 , pp. 3–10.

Segura, J.; Christiansen, H.; Campo, C; Ruilope, L.M. (2003). How to titrate ACE inhibitors and angiotensin receptor blockers in renal patients: According to blood pressure or proteinuria? *Current Hypertension Reports,* Vol. 5, (October, 2003), pp. 426–429.

Singh, D.; Whooley, M.A.; Ix JH, Ali, S, Shlipak MG. (2007). Association of cystatin C and estimated GFR with inflammatory biomarkers: The Heart and Soul Study. *Nephrology Dialisis Transplant,* Vol. 22, (January, 2007), pp. 1087–1092.

Soni, S.S.; Ronco, C.; Katz, N.; Cruz, D.N. (2009). Early diagnosis of acute kidney injury: the promise of novel biomarkers. *Blood Purification,* Vol. 28, No.3., (July, 2009), pp. 165- 174.

Staples, A.; Wong, C.S.; (2010). Risk factors for progression of chronic kidney disease. *Current Opinion in Pediatrics,* Vol. 22, No. 2, (April, 2011), pp. 161–169.

Stuveling, E.M.; Hillege, H.L.; Bakker, S.J.; Gans, R.O.; De Jong, P.E.; De Zeeuw, D. (2003). C-reactive protein is associated with renal function abnormalities in a nondiabetic population. *Kidney International,* Vol. 63, (February, 2003), pp. 654–661.

Stuveling, E.M.; Bakker, S.J.; Hillege, H.L.; de Jong, P.E.; Gans, R.O.B., de Zeeuw, D. (2005) Biochemical risk markers: a novel area for better prediction of renal risk? *Nephrology Dialisis Transplantation,* Vol. 20, No.3. (Mars, 2005), pp. 497–508.

Taal, M.W.; Brenner, B.M. (2006). Predicting initiation and progression of chronic kidney disease: developing renal risk scores. *Kidney International,* Vol. 70, No. 10, (September, 2006), pp. 1694-1705.

Tesch, G.H., et al. (2010). Review: Serum and urine biomarkers of kidney disease: A pathophysiological perspective. *Nephrology,* Vol. 15, (August, 2010), pp. 609-616.

Tikellis C, Bernardi S, Burns WC (2011) Angiotensin-converting enzyme 2 is a key modulator of the renin-angiotensin system in cardiovascular and renal disease. *Current Opinion in Nephrology and Hypertension,* Vol. 20, No.1, (January, 2011), pp. 62–68.

Toto, R.D. (2005). Treatment of hypertension in chronic kidney disease. *Seminars in Nephrology*, Vol. 25, No. 6, (November 2005), pp. 435-439.

Ueda S, Yamagishi S, Kaida Y et al. (2007). Asymmetric dimethylarginine may be a missing link between cardiovascular disease and chronic kidney disease. *Nephrology* (Carlton), Vol. 12, No.6, (December, 2007), pp. 582–590.

Udani, S.; Lazich, I.; Bakris, G.L. (2011). Epidemiology of hypertensive kidney disease.*Nature Reviews Nephroogy.* Vol. 7, (January, 2011), pp. 11–21.

Vaidya VS, Ramirez V, Ichimura T, Bobadilla NA, Bonventre JV. (2006). Urinary kidney injury molecule-1: a sensitive quantitative biomarker for early detection of kidney tubular injury. *American Journal of Physiology Renal Physiology,* Vol. 290, (February, 2006), pp. F517–29.

van Guldener C. (2006). Why is homocysteine elevated in renal failure and what can be expected from homocysteine-lowering? *Nephrology Dialisis Transplant,* Vol. 21, No.5, (May, 2006), pp.1161–1166.

Vasan R, Evans JC, Larson MG, Wilson PWF, Meigs JB, Rifai N, Benjamin EJ, Ledy D. (2004). Serum aldosterone and the incidence of hypertension in nonhypertensive persons. *New England Journal of Med*icine, Vol. 351, (July, 2004), No.1, pp. 333–341.

Verma S, Li SH, Wang CH, Fedak PW, Li RK, Weisel RD, Mickle DA. (2003). Resistin promotes endothelial cell activation: further evidence of adipokine-endothelial interaction. *Circulation,* Vol. 108, No.6, (July, 2003). pp.736–740.

Wang W, Reeves WB, Ramesh G. Netrin-1 and kidney injury. I. (2008). Netrin-1 protected against ischemia-reperfusion injury of the kidney. *American Journal of Physiology Renal Physiology,* Vol. 294, No.4, (April, 2008), pp. F739-47.

Weiner, D.E.; Tighiouart, H.; Elsayed, E.F.; Griffith, J.L.; Salem, D.N.; Levey, A.S. (2008). Uric acid and incident kidney disease in the community. *Journal of American Society of Nephrology,* Vo. 19, (March, 2008), pp. 1204–1211.

Welch GN, Loscalzo J. (1998). Homocysteine and atherothrombosis. *New England Journal of Medicine,* Vol. 338, No.15, (Aprilie, 1998), pp. 1042–1050

8

Sickle Cell Disease and Renal Disease

Mathias Abiodun Emokpae and Patrick Ojiefo Uadia
University of Benin, Benin City
Nigeria

1. Introdution

The kidney of patients with sickle cell disease (SCD) is affected by both haemodynamic changes of chronic anaemia and by the consequences of vaso-occlusion which are especially marked within the renal medulla. There are many abnormalities in renal structure and function as a result of these changes. Functional changes occur with increasing age in subjects with sickle cell disease. Proteinuria, severe anaemia and haematuria are reliable markers and predictors of chronic renal disease in patients with sickle cell disease (Emokpae et al., 2010a). Sickle cell disease is characterized by chronic haemolytic anaemia due to adverse effects of oxygen transport by the red blood cells. This often leads to a decrease in oxygen supply to peripheral tissues.
The substitution of valine for glutamic acid at the sixth position of the β-globin polypeptide chain made haemoglobin S (HbS) different from normal adult haemoglobin A (HbA) (Reid *et al.*, 1984).The inheritance of HbS gene in the heterozygous state results in sickle cell trait while inheritance in the homozygous state results in sickle cell disease (SCD). The prevalence of Hb S gene in various parts of Africa varies between 20-40% (Arabs, 1970), while in Nigeria the prevalence is put at 20-25percent (Lindner *et al.*, 1974; Ukoli *et al.*, 1988). Sickling phenomenon occurs secondary to intra erythrocytic HbS polymerization because of low oxygen tension which becomes reversible with adequate re-oxygenation of the haemoglobin. But with repeated sickling and resultant deformation, the red cell membranes become fragile and haemolyse. Sickle cell disease often results in a severe disease, with profound anaemia and multiple organ involvement including cerebrovascular events, acute vaso-occlusive episodes, retinopathy, acute chest syndrome and renal damage (Guash *et al.*,2006).Haemoglobin S may coexist with other mutant beta globin chains (β^c or β^D) in a mixed heterozygous state leading to haemoglobin SC or SD disease. Haemoglobin SC disease is the most common mixed heterozygous form of sickle haemoglobinopathies occurring in one per 800 births in the African Americans (Guash *et al.*, 2006). Sickle cell anaemia (SCA) affects the kidney, causing defects in tubulomedullary function (Allon, 1990); and also causes proteinuria, progressive renal insufficiency and end stage renal disease (Pham *et al.*, 2000). The glomerulopathy is the cause of the proteinuria and progressive renal insufficiency (Guash *et al.*, 1996).

2. Origin of sickle cell disease

The origin of sickle cell disease is not known but a substantial evidence that the sickle cell mutation occurred as several independent events was reported (Serjeant, 1992).Two

theories of evolution were postulated, namely- single mutation theory and multiple mutation theory. A single mutation occurring in Neolithic times in the then fertile Arabian Peninsula was favoured by Lehmann (1954), who postulated that the changing climatic conditions and conversion of this area to a desert caused a migration of peoples that could have carried the gene to India, Eastern Saudi Arabia and to Africa. Lehmann and Hunstan (1974) supported this hypothesis by citing the distribution of certain agricultural practices and anthropological evidence as well as the geographical distribution of the gene within Africa which manifested a decline in gene frequency from East to West Africa together with higher levels on the north compared to the south bank of the Zambesi River. This is compatible with the fact that the river acted as a barrier to a southern migration (Serjeant, 1992). This theory was also supported by Gelpi (1973), who considered that the evidence from blood groups and other genetic markers was more compatible with an origin in Equatorial Africa and subsequent diffusion of the gene to India, Arabia and the Mediterranean by the East Africa slave trade (Kamel and Awny, 1965).
The multiple mutation theory recently received support from the studies of DNA polymorphism. The use of restriction endonucleases to recognize and cut DNA at specific sequence has identified variations in DNA structure (polymorphism) that are inherited and may be used as genetic markers (Serjeant, 1992). The first of such polymorphism to be reported was a variation in the recognition site of the restriction endonuclease HPa 1 to the 3′ side of the β-globin gene (Kan and Dozy, 1978). In most normal human DNA digested with HPa 1, the β-globin gene occurred on a DNA fragment 7.6 kd long. Polymorphism at this site in West African population resulted in β–gene occurring on the fragments 7.0 and 13.0 kd long. Subsequently the 13.0kd fragment was found to be relatively lightly linked to the β-gene, the frequency of the 13.0 kd fragment in the AS genotype being 0.31 and in the SS genotype 0.87(Kan and Dozy,1978). The immediate application of this observation was in antenatal diagnosis (Kan and Dozy, 1978), but it was also of potential value as a genetic marker in anthropological studies. The 13.0 kb fragment was found to be linked to the β^c gene (Feldenzer *et al.*, 1979).

3. Study of the kidney

The study of nephrology as a major discipline in medicine dates back to about five decades ago. The discipline has its origin in the writing of pioneers who used their observational skills to establish its basic framework. From their observations and analyses came the realization of the vital role of the kidney in the maintenance of health, particularly in relation to homeostasis of body fluids and electrolytes (Travis *et al.*, 1984). These pioneers recorded the profound changes in health that occurred with any of a variety of kidney disorders. While imaginative postulates about the physiology of the kidney in health and disease were beginning to evolve, detailed construct of the precise mechanisms by which various renal events took place were not easily obtainable. Opportunities to explore in detail the postulates were limited primarily by the primitive technology which was available then. Only recently when technological advances were made and applied that the theoretical bases and principles of renal physiology and molecular biology established and an understanding reached of the alterations that occurred in the disease state (Travis *et al.*, 1984). With technological advancement, there has been a deeper insight into the pathophysiologic mechanisms that interact to create renal disease.

The kidneys are essential for life. Normally more water and ions are ingested than the body requires. This excess intake is excreted in urine. The kidneys therefore regulate both the volume and the composition of the body fluids. As well as the surplus water and electrolytes, the urine contains metabolic waste products, foreign substances and their metabolic derivatives (Bray *et al.*, 1999).The kidneys also produce a variety of humoral agents, including erythropoietin, active metabolites of vitamin D, renin and prostaglandins. Each human kidney has about one million functional units- the nephrons; arranged in parellel (Risdon, 1985). The renal regulation of the volume and composition of the body fluids involves each of these nephrons in three processes: filtration at the glomerulus, tubular reabsorption and tubular secretion.

4. Renal manifestations in sickle cell disease

The kidney in SCD is affected by both the haemodynamic changes of a chronic anaemia and by the consequences of vaso-occlusion which are especially marked within the renal medulla. As a result, there are many abnormalities in renal structure and function (sergeant, 1992). Renal size in SCD varies with age of the patients and the method of examination. Renal weight at autopsy was normal in young children (Alleyne *et al.*, 1975), increased in older children and young adults and decreased in patients over 40years (Morgan *et al.*, 1987). In children, bilateral renal enlargement was common in intravenous urography (Minkin *et al.*, 1997; Odita *et al.*, 1983) and in adults; renal length exceeded 15cm in at least one kidney in about 10% Jamaicans (McCall *et al.*, 1987) and Nigerians (Odita *et al.*, 1983). In the Nigerian study, the mean kidney length in patients with SCD was significantly greater than in normal controls. Renal structure on imaging in SCD revealed that intravenous urography in 189 Jamaican adults showed mild cortical scarring, the frequency increasing from 8% in the 16-25years old, to 45% in those over 35years (McCall *et al.*,1987). Calyceal abnormalities included calyceal cysts, blunting and clubbing, which also increased with age. Radiological evidence of renal papillary necrosis occurred in 44 (26%) of adults patients in the Jamaican study. This high prevalence was also noted in Nigerians (Odita *et al.*, 1983). Functional changes occur with increasing age in patients with SCD. In children and young adults there are increases in effective renal blood flow (ERBF), effective renal plasma flow (ERPF) and glomerular filtration rate (GFR), although the filtration fraction is decreased (Hatch *et al.*, 1970). With age, there is a progressive decline in ERBF, ERPF and GFR and in patients over the age 40years; GFR and ERPF tend to decline (Morgan and sergeant, 1981). But normal or above normal values may persist in some patients (Alleyne *et al.*, 1975). Progressive renal failure at older ages is a major cause of illness and death (Morgan *et al.*, 1987). Glomerular disease is common (15 - 30 percent) in homozygotes for sickle cell disease. Glomerular hyperfiltration and hypertrophy occur within the first 5years of life. Approximately 15 - 30 % of patients develop proteinuria in the first three decades, and 5% develop ESRD. The glomerular pathology is usually focal segmental glomerulosclerosis, probably due to sustained glomerular capillary hypertension or membrane proliferative glomerulonephritis (MPGN). Predictors of chronic renal failure are worsening anaemia, proteinuria, nephrotic syndrome and hypertension (Powars *et al.*, 2005).

5. Sickle cell disease and glomerulopathy.

Patients with sickle cell anaemia (SCA) may develop glomerulopathy with proteinuria and progressive renal insufficiency leading to End Stage Renal Disease(ESRD) (Gausch *et al.*,

2006). These authors observed that the patients with sickle cell haemoglobin (Hb SS) have a more severe disease than individuals with other sickling haemoglobinopathies using clinical, haematologic and biochemical parameters in a group of patients with sickle cell haemoglobinopathies. It was reported that increased albumin excretion rate (AER) occurs in 68% of the patients; macroalbuminuria was present in 26% and microalbuminuria in 42% while only 32% of adults with 'SS' disease had normoalbuminuria. There was no gender differences reported in the prevalence of albuminuria. In a study of proteinuria among SCA patients in Nigeria, male predominance of sickle cell nephropathy was reported (Abdu et al., 2011). The concentration of 24hours urine protein in the SCA male subjects with proteinuria was significantly higher (0.25g/day;p<0.001) compared with the SCA female patients with proteinuria (0.09g/day)(Emokpae et al.,2010a). The sex differences in the mechanisms underlying renal injury suggest that androgens may permit or accelerate renal damage while estrogen may provide renoprotection (Ji et al., 2005; Standberg, 2008). The female sex hormone (estradiol) is thought to have antioxidant properties. Estradiol is capable of increasing superoxide dismutase and glutathione peroxidase expression as well as decreases NADPH oxidase enzyme activity and superoxide production (Lopez-Ruiz et al., 2008). The graded albuminuria according to age hence duration of disease showed that, in 'SS' disease the prevalence of abnormal AER increased from 61% in patients aged 18 to 30 years to as high as 79% in patients older than 40 years. Albumin excretion rate was reported to have increased as creatinine clearance decreased, but there was a large variability and a significant number of patients had increased AER despite a preserved creatinine clearance. In a four decade observational study of 1056 patients with sickle cell disease, Powars *et al.*,(2005) reported that 73% of the patients had one or more clinically recognized forms of irreversible organ damage. By the fifth decade, nearly one-half of the surviving patients (48%) had documented irreversible organ damage. ESRD (glomerulosclerosis), chronic pulmonary disease with pulmonary hypertension, retinopathy and cerebral micro infarctions were manifestations of arterial and capillary microcirculation obstructive vasculopathy. In an earlier report on chronic renal failure in sickle cell disease : risk factors, clinical course and mortality indicated that histologic studies showed characteristic lesion of glomerular "drop out" and glomerulosclerosis, in thirty six patients with sickle cell disease who developed sickle cell renal failure (Powards *et al.*, 1991; Powards *et al.*, 2002). Table 1 shows changes in biochemical parameters in sickle cell disease patients with or without proteinuria in northern Nigeria.

Renal insufficiency in SCA was defined as a creatinine clearance <90ml/min using Crockcroft- Gault, (1976) equation. It was reported that 21% of patients with SCA had renal insufficiency while 27% of patients with other sickling disorders also had renal insufficiency but the percentage of patients with renal insufficiency and advanced kidney failure (chronic kidney disease stage 3 or higher) was higher in SS disease than other sickling disorders (Guasch *et al.*, 2006). Guasch *et al.*(1997) previously showed renal insufficiency in SCA results from a glomerulopathy, which can be detected by the presence of albumin and other large molecular weight proteins in urine. Recently it was observed that glomerular involvement is extremely common in Nigerian sickle cell haemoglobinopathies (Abdu et al.2011). Increased AER occurs in approximately 70% of adults with haemoglobin SS disease and about 40% in adults with other sickling disorders. There was an indication of sickle cell glomerulopathy in a majority of older adults with SS disease and its prevalence was much higher than previously reported on the basis of a positive urinary dipstick for protein (Falk *et al.*, 1992).

	Males with no proteinuria	Males with proteinuria	p-value	Females with no proteinuria	Females with proteinuria	p-value
No of subjects	68	32		76	24	
Age (Years)	22.2 ± 3.8	26.4 ± 7.3	$P < 0.005$	21 ± 3.0	20.4 ± 7.6	NS
Weight (Kg)	45 ± 12.3	50 ± 7.2	$P < 0.001$	42 ± 7.6	47.4 ± 5.3	$P < 0.001$
Na+ mmol/l	134.7 ± 3.4	140 ± 3.8	$P < 0.001$	136 ± 5.4	141 ± 5.3	$P < 0.001$
K + mmol/l	4.2 ± 0.5	3.9 ± 0.5	$P < 0.05$	4.05 ± 0.35	3.9 ± 0.13	NS
Cl- mmo/l	97.4 ± 2.3	103 ± 4.1	$P < 0.001$	98.2 ± 5.3	101 ± 3.9	NS
Hco3- mmo/l	97.4 ± 2.3	103 ± 4.1	NS	22.3 ± 1.55	20.2 ± 3.0	$p < 0.05$
Urea mmol/l	2.46 ± 0.88	8.07 ± 2.2	$P < 0.001$	2.79 ± 1.77	2.46 ± 1.22	NS
CR µmol/l	59.2 ± 10.2	280 ± 22.3	$P < 0.001$	61.2 ± 12.4	67 ± 23.7	NS
eGFR ml/min	104 ± 22.8	70 ± 6.9	$P < 0.001$	97 ± 3.5	101 ± 2.5	NS

CR = creatinine, eGFR = estimated glomerular filtration rate, NS = not significant, Adapted from Abdu et al.,2011.

Table 1. Urea, electrolytes, creatinine and estimated glomerular filtration rates in sickle cell anaemia patients with proteinuria and those with no proteinuria.

The pathogenesis of glomerular damage in SCA is not well understood. Children with sickle cell anaemia have renal haemodynamic alterations characterized by renal hyperperfusion and glomerular hyperfiltration. These probably resulted from renal vaso-dilation associated with chronic anaemia. In some patients, these changes are followed by the development of glomerular proteinuria and progressive renal disease. Histologically, patients with SCA may develop glomerular hypertrophy and focal segmented glomerulosclerosis, features that are suggestive of haemodynamically mediated injury (Falk *et al.*, 1992). The causes of the haemodynamic injury to the glomerulus in SCA are unclear, but anaemia could cause glomerular damage by increasing blood flow. Other factors that are related to the rheology or stickness of sickle erythrocyte could cause glomerular damage independently or in conjunction with the haemodynamic changes that are associated with anaemia (Guasch *et al.*, 1999). In the analysis of significance of abnormal albuminuria in SCA, several authors demonstrated by physiologic and pathologic studies that macroalbuminuria is the clinical manifestation of an underlying glomerulopathy (Falk *et al.*, 1992; Guasch *et al.*, 1999; Emokpae et al., 2010a;Abdu et al.,2011). Twenty eight percent of patients with SCD patients were observed to have significant proteinuria in Nigerian SCD patients (Abdu et al.,2011), confirming the fact that proteinuria is a more sensitive marker than elevated serum creatinine values in detecting glomerular injury and early manifestation of sickle cell nephropathy. From that study, 50% of SCA male patients with proteinuria had CKD. However, it was observed that the high prevalence of CKD reported may be due to the fact that the study was conducted in a tertiary health care referral centre where there is likelihood of having patients population with more severe disease (Abdu et al., 2011). Table 2 shows haematological changes in SCD patients with or without proteinuria and those with chronic kidney disease in northern Nigeria.

	Control HbSS	Macroalbu minuria HbSS	*P*-value	CKD	*P*-value
No. of subjects	144	40	-	16	-
Age (years)	21.6±3.2	20.8±4.2	-	32.6	$P<0.001$
Haematocrit (%)	20.1±5.9	19.1±3.9	NS	18.7±1.19	NS
Haemoglobin (g/dl)	7.0±2.1	6.25±0.9	$P<0.001$	6.1±0.2	$P<0.001$
Total leukocyte Count ($x10^9/L$)	11.7±4.05	11.8±3.2	NS	11.9±1.04	NS
Red blood cells Count ($x10^{12}/L$)	2.43±0.6	2.19±1.0	NS	2.07±0.2	$P<0.001$
Platelet count ($x10^9/L$)	373±135	348±92	NS	428±221	$P<0.001$
Mean cell Hemoglobin (pg)	29.6±2.6	35.7±3.3	NS	36.6±1.5	NS
Mean cell volume(fl)	82.2±6.9	84.9±4.2	NS	87±0.9	$P<0.001$
Mean cell hemoglobin Conc. (g/dl)	36.4±2.1	35.7±3.3	NS	36.6±1.5	NS
Absolute lymphocyte Count ($x10^9/L$)	4.0±1.3	3.2±0.6	$P<0.001$	2.8±0.4	$P<0.001$
Absolute neutrophil Count ($x10^9/L$)	5.2±1.7	6.0±0.8	$P<0.001$	6.4±0.6	$P<0.001$
Absolute Monocyte Count ($x10^9/L$)	0.5±0.2	0.4±0.03	$P<0.001$	0.4±0.04	$P<0.001$
Absolute eosinophil Count ($x10^9/L$)	0.2±0.1	0.2±0.02	NS	0.2±0.1	NS

Adapted from Emokpae et al., 2010a

Table 2. Haematological indices in SCD patients with macroalbuminuria, CKD and controls

In patients with macroalbuminuria but preserved GFR, the glomerular ultrafiltration coefficient was reduced versus normalbuminuric sickle cell control subjects; indicating that macroalbuminuria irrespective of the level of GFR reflects an underlying glomerular pathology (Guasch *et al.*, 2006). It was reported that in children the development of microalbuminuria follows an age dependent manner. In a study by Dhranidharka *et al.*(1998) in a group of sicklers, It was observed that microalbuminuria was not present in children who were younger than 7years but reached 43 percent in the second decade of life. In another similar study, Wigfall *et al.*(2000) observed an age-dependent occurrence of dipstick proteinuria: proteinuria was not present in children who were less than 6years, but occurs in 7% of children aged 7-10years and 10% of children who were aged 13 to 17years. It was therefore speculated that sickle cell glomerulopathy could evolve in five clinical stages.

- A normoalbuminuric stage of variable duration followed by a stage of
- Microalbuminuria which could lead to
- Macroalbuminunnia but with preserved GFR and to
- Macroalbuminuna and progressive renal insufficiency and
- ESRD.

However, evidence of progression from micro to macroalbuminuria is lacking and such classification may remains a hypothesis (Guasch *et al* , 2006). It was concluded that the prevalence of glomerular damage in SCA is much higher than previously thought; a majority of patients with SS disease are at risk for the development of progressive renal insufficiency and late renal failure especially because the life expectancy in patients with SS disease has improved with better medical care. Secondly, in contrast to most glomerular disease, the glomerulopathy in SS disease is not accompanied by the development of significant systemic hypertension. Lastly, the haemodynamic changes that are associated with chronic anaemia per se are not solely responsible for the development of sickle cell glomerulopathy and indicate that other mechanisms are involved in the pathogenesis of the glomerular damage in this population.

There is a large variability in the severity of the clinical manifestation of sickle cell anaemia (SCA), including renal involvement. Some patients develop multiorgan failure while others have relatively few end-organ complications (Guasch *et al.*, 1999). Epigenetic and environmental factors have been implicated to explain these differences in clinical severity. In children, lower haemoglobin levels and a relatively high degree of haemolysis are associated with a poorer clinical outcome while the persistence of high levels of foetal haemoglobin (HbF) is associated with less aggressive clinical manifestation (Platt *et al.*, 1994). Epidemiologic studies in African and Asian countries have suggested that differences in the degree of clinical severity are related to the geographical origin of the sickle cell mutation (Adedeji, 1988). The β-globin gene cluster is located on chromosome 11 and consists of a long segment of DNA (approximately 60,000 bp) that contains the β-globin gene and other globin genes. Distinct polymorphism in this gene cluster can be identified by restriction endonucleases that cleave the DNA at specific sites. When the restriction sites patterns are arranged by alleles, they form a haplotype. In the African, specific haplotypes are associated with different groups from different geographic area and define an individual's origin from Benin, Central African Republic, Senegal, Saudi Arabia or Cameroun (Nagel *et al.*, 1985). Since substitution of valine for glutamic acid at position six arose on different haplotypes, it must have arisen in different ethnic groups (Guasch *et al.*, 1999). Some studies have suggested that the severity of SCA varied with haplotype, with the Central African Republic (CAR) haplotype associated with a higher incidence of stroke, leg ulcer, acute chest syndrome, bone infarcts and kidney failure compared with non-CAR haplotypes (Powars *et al.*, 1990; Powars *et al.*, 1991). Guasch *et al.*, (1996) have emphasized the development of proteinuria and progressive renal insufficiency, leading to end-stage renal disease in a subset of SCA patients. It was observed that glomerulopathy is the cause of the progressive renal insufficiency and can be detected as increased excretion of albumin in the urine.

The prevalence of renal insufficiency in patients with SCA has been reported to be low (<5%), based on the serum creatinine (Powars *et al.*, 1991). However, Guasch *et al* (1996) found that serum creatinine is a very insensitive marker of renal insufficiency in SCA, becoming abnormal only after GFR is reduced to <30 to 40mL/min per 1.73m^2

6. Renal matrix alterations in glomerulosclerosis

Progressive renal disease of many etiologies is characterized by increased accumulation of acellular material within the glomerular mesangium. Initially, this process is characterized by focal areas of glomerular hyalinosis, acellular material that stains with eosin but not with periodic acid Schiff, together with capillary collapse and adhesions of the glomerular tuft to Bowman's capsule. With time, the mesangial compartment is occupied by material that stains positively with both periodic acid Schiff and silver. Ultimately, the capillary tuft is replaced by this sclerotic material and ceases filtration (Rennke and Klein, 1989).Other features of progressive glomerulosclerosis are more variable. The mesangial compartment is in some cases occupied by an increased number of cells both mesangial cells and resident macrophages. In the case of diabetic nephropathy, there is an associated thickening and wrinkling of the glomerular basement membrane which contributes to compromised capillary lumens. In addition to an expanded mesangial compartment, some patients with diabetic nephropathy also exhibit a characteristic nodular glomerulosclerosis (Kimmelstiel-Wilson lesion)(Rennke and Klein, 1989).

The mesangial components that are expressed as a consequence of inflammation or the sclerotic process belong to two classes. First, normal mesangial matrix molecules accumulate in excess quantities. These include laminin, type IV collagen, heparin sulphate proteoglycan and fibronectin. Second, the sclerotic mesangium contains matrix molecules that are not usually present in this location. These include interstitial collagens, particularly type III collagen and the small proteoglycan decorion. These matrix consistuents are typical products of fibroblasts and related cell types. In a sense, the reappearance of these interstitial matrix products represents a return to biosynthethic activity of the embryonic renal interstitial mesenchyme (Yoshioka *et al.*, 1989).

Studies of matrix protein distribution in various primary renal diseases suggest that the proteins expressed and the regional pattern of expression differ considerably between different renal diseases (Oomura *et al.*, 1989; Yoshioka *et al.*, 1989). In all, with progressive glomerulosclerosis particularly with a mesangial proliferative component, the mesangial contains increased amounts of fibronectin, laminin, heparin sulphate proteoglycan and type III and IV collagen. Despite the widespread use in experimental animals of the nephron ablation model of progressive glomerulosclerosis, relatively little is known about the nature of or the mechanisms responsible for the accumulated glomerular matrix components.

Alterations in the renal expression of chondroitin sulphate proteoglycans are another component of the sclerosing process. The normal glomerulus expresses the small proteoglycan biglycan. In experimental glomerulonephritis induced by antibodies to the Thy-1-antigen, there is increased synthesis of biglycan as well as of another related proteoglycan, decorin by isolated glomeruli (Okuda *et al.*, 1990). Activated mesangial cells are a possible source for these proteoglycans.

Diabetes mellitus in humans and experimental animals is associated with evidence of deregulation of renal extracellular matrix proteins expression. More is known about the matrix alterations in this disorder than other forms of glomerulosclerosis, perhaps in part due to the availability of animal models. Biochemical investigation has shown increased accumulation of basement membrane components in diabetes glomeruli from experimental animals. Thus glomeruli from streptozotocin-diabetic rats contain more type IV collagen compared with glomeruli from normal rats (Hasslacher *et al.*, 1986). On the other hand, the data for glomerular content of heparin sulphate proteoglycan are conflicting, with an increase reported in streptozocin-diabetic rats and a decrease reported in diabetic human patients (Klein *et al.*, 1986; Shimonura and Spiro, 1987). The discrepancy underscores the need for caution in extrapolating from studies of diabetic rodents to mechanisms of human disease.

Immunohistochemical investigation of the sclerotic regions of human diabetic glomeruli show evidence of an increase in laminin, fibronectin and types IV and V collagen (Karttunen *et al.*, 1986).

While our understanding of the protein constituents of the sclerotic process has improved, the molecular mechanisms responsible for their accumulation are just being understood. It is likely that many factors including capillary physical forces, dietary constituents, metabolic injury and the effects of local growth factors and products of inflammation converge on a common pathway that generates matrix components within the glomerulus and mesangium. The process whereby matrix accumulates in response to injury, likely parallel the process of scarring and wound healing critical for the survival of other tissue types. In the kidney, however the generation of matrix may sufficiently disrupt the normal nephron architecture to render it useless. It may be possible in the future to modify the normal healing process in the glomerulus so that a loss of functioning nephrons does not hold the remaining glomeruli at increased risk for sclerosis.

7. Mechanisms whereby proteinuria cause progressive renal disease

The possibility that proteinuria may accelerate kidney disease progression to end stage renal failure has received support from the results of increasing numbers of experimental and clinical studies (Abbate *et al.*, 2006). Researches in nephrology in recent times have yielded substantial information on the mechanisms by which persisting dysfunction of an individual component cell in the glomerulus is generated and signaled to other glomerular cells and to the tubule. Spreading of disease is central to processes by which nephropathies of different types progress to end stage renal disease (ESRD). Independent of the underlying causes, chronic proteinuric glomerulopathies have in common a sustained or permanent loss of selectivity of the glomerular barrier to protein filtration. Glomerular sclerosis is the progressive lesion beginning at the glomerular capillary wall, the site of abnormal filtration of plasma proteins. Injury is transmitted to the intestitium favouring the self destruction of nephrons and eventually of the kidney (Abbate *et al.*, 2006). Baseline proteinuria was an independent predictor of renal outcome in patients with diabetes, non-diabetes as well as sickle cell nephropathies (Peterson *et al.*, 1995; Breyer *et al.*, 1996; Abdu et al.,2011). Clinical trials consistently showed renoprotective effects of proteinuric reduction and led to the recognition that, the antiproteinuric treatment is instrumental to maximize renoprotection (Peterson *et al.*, 1995; Wapstra *et al.*, 1996). Findings that the rate of GFR decline correlated negatively with proteinuria reduction and positively with residual proteinuria provided further evidence for a pathogenic role of proteinuria (Ruggenenti *et al.*, 2003). It was documented that whenever proteinuria is decreased by treatments, progression to ESRD is reduced (Brenner *et al.*, 2001).

7.1 Glomerular proteinuria as signal for interstitial inflammation

In vitro studies using proximal tubular cells as a model to assess effects of apical exposure to plasma proteins proved highly valuable to approaching direct casual relationships. In monolayers of proximal tubular cells, the load with plasma proteins (albumin, IgG and transferrin) induced the synthesis of the vasoconstrictor peptide endothelin-1 (ET-1), a mediator of progressive renal injury by virtue of ability to stimulate renal cell proliferation and extracellular matrix production and to attract monocytes (Zoja *et al.*, 1995). Other investigators confirmed and extended the stimulatory effects of a diversity of plasma proteins on the expression of proinflammatory and profibrotic mediators in renal tubular cells (Yard *et al.*, 2001; Tang *et al.*, 2003). Among molecules attracted are monocytes/macrophages and T-lymphocytes, monocyte chemoattractant protein-1 (MCP-1) and RANTES which were over-expressed in proximal tubular cells that were challenged with plasma proteins (Wang *et al.*, 1997; Zoja *et al.*, 1998). Albumin upregulated tubular gene expression and production of interleukin 8(IL-8), a potent chemotatic agent for lymphocytes and neutrophils (Tang *et al.*, 1999).The releases of ET-1 and chemokines in response to proteins was polarized mainly toward the basolateral compartment of the cell as to mirror a directional secretion that favoured the interstitial inflammatory reaction that was observed in-vivo. Protein overloading of human proximal tubular cells induced the synthesis of fractalkine, which in its membrane-anchored form promotes mononuclear cell adhesion via CX3CR1 receptor (Danadelli *et al.*, 2003). Fractalkine mRNA was overexpressed in kidneys of mice with protein overload proteinuria, and the gene product was detected in tubular epithelial cells mainly in the basal region. Treatment of mice with an antibody against CX3CR1 limited the interstitial accumulation of monocytes /macrophages (Danadelli *et al.*, 2003).

Investigation of the molecular mechanisms underlying chemokine upregulation in proximal tubular cells or protein challenge had initial focus on the activation of transcriptional NF-β (Zoja et al., 1998). Other studies confirmed the pathway and revealed reactive oxygen as a secondary messenger (Drumm *et al.*, 2003). Protein overload elicited rapid generation of hydrogen peroxide in human proximal tubular cells, an effect that together with NF-β activation was prevented by antioxidants (Morigi *et al.*, 2002). Specific inhibitors of proteins kinase C (PKC) prevented hydrogen peroxide generation, NF-β activation and MCP-1 and IL-8 genes up regulation that was induced by protein overload (Tang *et al.*, 2003), suggesting a cascade of signals from PKC- dependent oxygen radical generation to nuclear translocation of NF-β and consequent gene up regulation. A link also has been made between induction of NF-β activity by protein and mitogen-activated protein kinases, including p38 and extracellular signal-regulated kinase 1 and 2 (ERK1/ERK2) that are involved in chemokine synthesis (Dixon *et al.*, 2000; Danadelli *et al*, 2003). In support of the hypothesis of protein overload as a key activator of signaling in proximal tubule is the finding that albumin activated the signal transducer and activator of transcription (STAT) proteins in cultured proximal tubular cells. Because the STAT pathway is the principal mechanism that converts the signal from a wide array of cytokines and growth factors into gene expression programs that regulate cell proliferation, differentiation, survival and apoptosis, it was suggested that albumin may stimulate proximal tubular cells in the manner of a cytokine (Rawlings *et al.*, 2004; Brunskill *et al.*, 2004).

Despite evidence that albumin overload elicits several responses by tubular cells in-vitro, it has been argued that albumin per se may not be toxic to the proximal tubular epithelium. Compounds that are bound to albumin, such as free fatty acids (FFA), instead have been implicated to be causative in pro inflammatory activation or injury of cultured proximal tubular cells (Schreiner, 1995). It was also observed that among various fatty acids, oleic acid and linoleic acids exert the most toxic and profibrogenic effects in human proximal tubular cells in culture. These studies collectively indicate that the ability of albumin to act as a carrier enhances the pro inflammatory activation of proximal tubular cells. In addition, in-vivo gene expression profile analysis of proximal tubules from mice with protein overload proteinuria identified 2000 genes that were differentially regulated by excess proteins. More than half of them were upregulated (Nakajima *et al.*, 2002). They included thymic shared antigen -1, the fibroblast-associated gene GS188 and glia maturation factor-B, a protein that originally was purified as a neurotrophic factor (Kaimori *et al.*, 2003). The expression of glia maturation factor-β was induced in renal proximal tubular cells of mice with protein overload proteinuria (Kaimori et al., 2003). Proximal tubular cells that over expressed glia maturation factor-β acquired more susceptibility to death by sustained oxidative stress through p38 pathway activation.

There was a controversial issue relating to the concentration of albumin that was used in various in-vitro studies. Burton *et al.* (1999) discovered that the apical exposure of human proximal tubular cells to 1mg/ml albumin or transferrin did not increase MCP-1 or PDGF-AB release, an effect that was observed after exposure to a human serum fraction (40 to 100 KD) in the molecular weight range similar to albumin and transferrin. Studies that reported the effects of protein overload on NF-β activation showed responses from 0.5mg/mL in some experiments and usually >2.5 - >5mg/mL (Zoja *et al.*, 1995; Wang *et al.*, 1997). The latter concentration seems too far exceed the concentration reached in the proteinuric ultrafiltrate in-vivo (Gekle, 2005).

The proximal tubule bears other receptors for ultrafiltered proteins such as immunoglobulins and complement molecules (Braun *et al.*, 2004). The functional role of such receptors has not been established. It is likely that filtered proteins other than or in addition to albumin induces tubular dysfunction and injury in conditions of non selective proteinuria, in which large molecular weight proteins are a significant component. In contrast, relatively selective albuminuria induces delayed mononuclear cells infiltration and usually is associated with or mild chronic tubulo-interstitial injury. In this respect, the case of minimal-change disease has been considered sometimes an exception to the rule that interstitial infiltrates develop with time in proteinuric glomerulopathies. In addition, in minimal-change disease, a substantial percentage of patients respond to steroid and the regression of proteinuria prevents inflammation and renal function deterioration (Remuzzi and Giachelli, 1995).

7.2 Key role for the intra-renal activation of complement

Complement activation is a powerful mechanism underlying tubular and interstitial injury via cytotoxic, proinflammatory and fibrogenic effects. Abnormal complement, C_3 and C_5b-9 staining in proximal tubular cells and along the brush border is a long known feature both in human chronic proteinuric diseases and experimental models. Glomerular permeability dysfunction of proteinuric nephropathies allows complement factors to be ultrafiltered abnormally across the altered glomerular barrier into the Bowman's space and tubular lumen. Plasma- derived C_3 (molecular weight 180kd) is likely to reflect more loss of glomerular permselectivity and to enhance cell dysfunction in the presence of abnormally filtered plasma proteins. Renal tubular cells also synthesize C_3 and other complement factors in ways that may have critical importance in disease, as found in experimental renal transplant rejection and post ischemic acute renal failure (Pratt *et al.*,2002; Farrar *et al.*, 2006). Therefore both excess ultrafiltration and proximal tubular cell synthesis of complement could underlie complement - mediated injury in chronic proteinuric renal disease. Recent findings of C_3 mRNA upregulation and C_3 accumulation in proximal tubular cells in kidneys of mice with protein overload proteinuria are in support of a role for the local synthesis of complement (Abbate *et al.*, 2004). Complement is an important effector of interstitial mononuclear cell infiltration and fibrogenesis in this model as shown by significant attenuation of injury in C_3 deficient mice (Abbate *et al.*, 2004). A direct role for protein overload as a stimulus was indicated by findings that the exposure of cultured proximal tubular cells to total serum proteins at the apical surface upregulated C_3 mRNA expression and protein biosynthesis (Tang *et al.*, 1999).

7.3 Profibrogenic signal from proximal tubular cells in response to protein overload

Local recruitment of macrophages by tubular cells that are loaded with ultrafiltered plasma proteins may contribute to interstitial fibrosis by engaging matrix producing interstitial myofibroblasts. Macrophages also regulate matrix accumulation via release of growth factors such as TGF-β and PDGF, ET-1 and PAI-1, TGF-β stimulates the transformation of interstitial cells into myofibroblasts. In addition, proximal tubular epithelial cells communicate with interstitial fibroblasts to promote fibrogenesis via paracrine release of TGF-β. (Abbate *et al.*,2006).

8. Pathogenesis of lipoprotein abnormalities in chronic kidney disease

Regardless of the aetiology of renal disease, patients with CKD develop complex qualitative and quantitative abnormalities in lipid and lipoprotein metabolism. These damages and the underlying molecular mechanism has been the subject of some reviews (Vaziri, 2006; Chan *et al.*, 2006). Classical uraemic dyslipidaemia is characterized by raised triglyceride, low high density lipoprotein (HDL) and normal total cholesterol. These qualitative defects become more pronounced with advancing renal failure and modified by renal replacement therapy, renal transplantation, co-morbid conditions such as diabetes mellitus and concurrent medication (for example steroids, cyclosporine) (Vaziri,200) Lipoprotein metabolism is a dynamic system that can be disturbed owing to alterations in apolipoprotein receptors. When GFR falls below 60ml/min, there is a fall in the ratio of apolipoprotein AI (apo A) to apolipoprotein C - III (apo C - III) in spite of normal cholesterol and triglyceride concentrations (Batsta *et al.*, 2004). As renal function deteriorates in non- nephrotic patients with CKD, triglyceride concentrations increase while HDL concentrations decline (Farbekhsh and Kasiske, 2005) and there is accumulation of the more atherogenic small dense low-density lipoprotein (LDL) particles.

In advanced CKD, there is decreased concentration of apoA-containing lipoproteins, increased concentrations of triglyceride-rich apo B containing lipoproteins and serum lipoprotein(a). Reduced catabolism and clearance of triglyceride-rich apo B containing lipoproteins is a consequence of : (a) decreased activity of lipolytic enzymes, such as lipoprotein lipase (LPL)and hepatic lipase (HL), (b) reduced receptor- mediated uptake via hepatic LDL- receptor related protein(LRP) and VLDL receptors (c) accumulation of certain inhibitors of LPL such as pre - β HDL (Chan *et al.*, 2006). Impaired clearance of triglyceride-rich lipoproteins is further compounded by reductions in apolipoprotein C-11 (apo C- II) and apolipoprotein E (apo E). Impaired divalent ion metabolism arising from parathyroid gland hyperplasia in CKD (stage 3–4) may also adversely affect lipoprotein metabolism by suppressing LPL and hepatic lipase activities (Nishizawa *et al.*, 1997). Post prandial lipoprotein metabolism is also impaired in CKD, resulting in accumulation of chylomicron particles and their remnants. Reduction in the expression of HL and down regulation of LRP in uremia may also account for the accumulation of remnant lipoprotein (Kim and Vaziri, 2005). Maturation of HDL is impaired due to decreased plasma lecithin: cholesterol acyltransferase (LCAT) activity and gene expression. Plasma HDL concentration also falls in uremia due to decreased expression of both apo AI and AII. (Vaziri *et al.*, 2001). These abnormalities can lead to impaired HDL mediated cholesterol uptake from the vascular tissue and contribute to the cardiovascular disease. In addition, LCAT deficiency can in part, account for elevated serum free cholesterol, reduced HDL/total cholesterol and elevated pre - β HDL in CRF. The latter can in turn depress lipolytic activity and hinder triglyceride-rich lipoprotein clearance in CRF (Vaziri *et al.*, 2001; Emokpae et al.,2010a). Statistically significant decrease in LCAT and lipoprotein lipase (LPL) activities were observed in SCA subjects in steady state compared with HbAS and HbAA controls in both males and females. The activities of LCAT and LPL were lower in subjects with SCA than sickle cell trait and normal haemoglobin. It was concluded that this may contribute to the changes observed in lipid metabolism in SCA(Emokpae et al.,2010b) Although Dyslipidaemia is present in patients with SCD and patients with renal insufficiency irrespective of the haemoglobin genotype, it was reported that the lipoprotein levels observed in Nigerian adults with SCA patients were more lower compared with the lipid levels observed in both African Americans and Saudi Arabian patients with SCD. The potential effects of lipids on cardiovascular disease risk as measured by three predictor ratios were higher in SCA compared to HbAS and HbAA patients with kidney disease (Emokpae et al.,2010c).Plasma total cholesterol is frequently low to normal and only occasionally elevated in CRF patients. In addition 3-hydroxyl-3- methyl-glutaryl- coA (HMG COA) reductase, the rate-limiting step in cholesterol biosynthesis and cholesterol 7 α-hydrolase, the rate limiting step in cholesterol catabolism, are unaffected by CRF (Liang and Vaziri., 1997). Moreover, LDL receptor and scavenger receptor B1, the primary pathways of hepatic cholesterol uptake are normal in CRF (Vaziri *et al.*, 1999).

The dyslipidaemia of CKD has similar feature to the metabolic syndrome. The metabolic syndrome, including type 2 diabetes, is known to predispose to CKD (Kurella *et al.*, 2005), which in turn aggravates insulin resistance and promotes dyslipidaemia. Insulin resistance increases free fatty acid (FFA) supply from adipocytes to increase hepatic lipogenesis and this stimulates hepatic secretion of apo B-100 containing lipoprotein specifically large triglyceride rich VLDL particles (Prinsen *et al.*, 2004). Impaired insulin signaling in skeletal muscles and adipose tissue also slows the catabolism of all triglycerides-rich containing lipoproteins. Expansion in the VLDL particle pool size impacts on the remodeling of LDL and HDL in an atherogenic direction (Chang *et al.*, 2006). Table 3 indicates changes in lipoproteins, lecithin: cholesterol acyltransferase and lipoprotein lipase in subjects with sickle cell anaemia, sickle cell trait and normal haemoglobin in northern Nigeria.

	HbSS males	HbAS males	p-value	HbAA males	p-value
No of subjects	68	25	-	25	-
Age in years	22.2±3.8	28.7±7	-	28.8±7	-
Triglyceride (mmol/L)	1.10±0.4	1.19±0.18	NS	1.4±0.12	P<0.001
T. Cholesterol (mmol/L)	3.06±0.5	4.05±0.06	P<0.001	4.3±0.12	P<0.001
HDL Cholesterol (mmol/L)	0.72±0.17	1.18±0.03	P<0.001	1.2±0.06	P<0.001
LDL Cholesterol (mmol/L)	1.92±0.54	2.15±0.14	NS	2.52±0.16	P<0.001
VLDL Cholesterol (mmol/L)	0.48±0.06	0.42±0.07	NS	0.41±0.08	NS
LPL (umolglycerol liberated/hr/l Plasma)	4.12±1.2	5.12±0.4	P<0.001	5.56±0.23	P<0.001
LCAT (umolcholesterol liberated/hr/l Plasma)	66.8±2.8	69.2±3.0	P<0.001	70.2±2.96	P<0.001
Adapted from Emokpae et al.,2010b					

Table 3. Lipid, lipoproteins, LCAT and LPL in male sickle cell disease subjects compared with HbAS and HbAA controls.

9. Effect of oxidative stress

Reactive oxygen species or free radicals are highly reactive entity and very short-lived molecules which are constantly produced in a wide variety of normal physiological functions, they are however toxic when generated in excess (Parke and Sapota, 1996). The most important characteristic of toxic free radicals either in vivo or in vitro is peroxidation of lipid resulting in tissue damage and death of affected cells (Bandyopadhyay *et al.*, 1999). There are profound evidence implicating free radicals in induced lipid peroxidation in the pathogenesis of several pathological conditions including chronic inflammation (Vijayakumar *et al.*, 2006), renal disease (Dakshinamurty *et al.*, 2006; Suryawanshi *et al.*, 2006),sickle cell renal disease (Emokpae et al.,2010d) and cardiovascular disease (Kaysen *et al.*, 2004). Table 4 indicates changes in oxidative stress and lipid peroxide parameters in control SCD, proteinuria and chronic kidney disease while table 5 shows inflammatory markers in subjects with SCD in northern Nigeria.

The harmful effect of reactive oxygen species is neutralized by a broad species of protective agents termed antioxidants which prevent oxidative damage by reacting with free radicals before any other molecules can become a target. The non enzymatic antioxidants are vitamins E, C and reduced glutathione while the antioxidant enzymes include superoxide dismutase (SOD), catalase (CAT) and glutathione peroxidase (GPX). They all play important roles in the protection of cells and tissues against free radical mediated tissue damage (Yu *et al.*, 1994; Airede and Ibrahim, 1999; Ray and Hussain, 2002).There was a significant reduction in the activity levels of antioxidant enzymes in the serum of SCD patients compared with control sickle cell trait and normal haemoglobin (Emokpae et al.,2010d). This is an indication that SCA patients produce greater quantities of reactive oxygen species than controls. In SCD, the production of reactive oxygen species can be grossly amplified in response to variety of pathophysiological conditions such as inflammation immunologic disorders, hypoxia, metabolism of drugs or alcohol and deficiency in antioxidant enzymes. Sickle cell anaemia patients showed low activity levels of antioxidant enzymes which may be due to the consumption of these substances by pro-oxidants in SCA. This therefore place SCA patients at increased risk of oxidative stress and injury. The oxidative stress may contribute to sickling process with the formation of dense cells, the development of vaso-occlussive and shortened red blood cell survival. We also demonstrated increased serum levels of some acute phase proteins in SCA, which may be as a result of sub-clinical vaso-occlusion which in turn can lead to a hidden inflammatory response (Emokpae et al.,2010d). Based on the results of the study, increased level of malondialdehyde compared significantly with lower activities level of antioxidant enzymes and increased acute phase proteins. In SCD patients with CKD, it was observed that there were increases in stress and inflammatory markers. C-reactive protein and fibrinogen were increased in subjects with renal insufficiency and were associated with increased urea and creatinine levels. Proteinuria as observed in SCA patients with renal insufficiency may act in synergy with oxidative stress and inflammation to initiate and accelerate the progression of renal disease. Chronic exposure of renal tubular epithelium to high levels of filtered plasma proteins may cause tissue injury (Emokpae et al.,2010a).

In certain diseases such as renal disease and sickle cell disease, the toxic material produced by activated phagocytes during reaction can cause maximal damage to the membrane because they are active in the lipid phase. The damaging effects of elevated toxic radical are due to an increase in the formation of superoxide radicals within the cells which cause inactivation of superoxide dismutase enzyme (Suryawanshi *et al.*, 2006). Oxidative stress occurs when there is an imbalance between production and scavenging. Increase in lipid peroxidation in sickle renal disease is due to excess formation of free radicals. Glycosylated protein, auto-oxidation, reduced superoxide dismutase enzyme and ascorbic acid and lack of reduced glutathione are other causes for oxidative stress.

Oxidative stress Markers	Controls HbSS	Macroalbuminuria HbSS	*P*-value	CKD HbSS	*P*-value
No of subjects	144	40		16	
Age (years)	21.6±3.2	20.8±4.2	NS	32.6±3.0	*P*<0.001
Malondialdehyde (mmol/l)	2.5±0.4	3.82±1.0	*P*<0.01	5.8±0.4	*P*<0.001
Glutathione Peroxidase (mU/ml)	9.6±0.9	8.3±3.0	*P*<0.001	2.81±0.24	*P*<0.001
Superoxide Dismutase (ng/ml)	32.5±4.2	25.4±4.6	*P*<0.001	18.3±2.8	*P*<0.001
Catalase (µmol/min/ml)	156±5.9	152±1.9	*P*<0.001	148±1.06	*P*<0.001

Adapted from Emokpae et al., 2010a

Table 4. Oxidative stress markers in serum of SCD patients with macroalbuminuria, CKD and controls (mean ± SD)

Inflammatory Markers	Controls HbSS	Macroalbuminuria HbSS	*P*-value	CKD HbSS	*P*-value
No of subjects	144	40		16	
C-reactive protein (μg/ml)	1.120±0.02	1.23±0.1	*P*<0.001	1.81±0.05	*P*<0.001
Fibrinogen (mg/dl)	299±9.1	307±6.0	*P*<0.001	317±4.1	*P*<0.001
Urea (mmol/l)	2.6±0.25	3.4±0.2	NS	14.0±2.8	*P*<0.001
Creatinine (μmol/l)	59.2±10.2	63±27	NS	496±78	*P*<0.001
eGFR (ml/min)	103±22	101±2.5	NS	14.5±2.0	*P*<0.001

Adapted from Emokpae et al., 2010a

Table 5. Serum levels of inflammatory markers, urea, creatinine and eGFR in SCD patients with macroalbuminuria, CKD and controls (mean ± SD)

Oxidative stress Markers	Controls HbSS	Control Hb AA	CKD HbSS	CKD HbAA
No. of subjects	144	20	16	20
Age (years)	21.6±3.2	22.0±2.6	32.6±3.0*	48.6±15.2*
Malondialdehyde (mmol/l)	2.5±0.4	2.4±0.2	5.8±0.4*	5.03±0.8*
Glutathione Peroxidase (mU/ml)	9.6±0.9	10.3±2.7	2.81±0.24*	4.35±1.8*
Superoxide Dismutase (ng/ml)	32.5±4.2	34.5±1.6**	18.3±2.8*	17.2±12.0*
Catalase (μmol/min/ml)	156±5.9	163±5.8*	148±1.06*	153±3.0*
***P*<0.001**				

Adapted from Emokpae et al., 2010a

Table 6. Oxidative stress markers in controls HbSS, HbAA, CKD HbSS and CKD HbAA

Sickle cell anaemia patients in both steady state and renal impairments undergo constant inflammatory process which may in turn leads to inflammatory response (Bourantas et al.,1998; Emokpae et al., 2010d). Haemoglobin S containing red blood cells auto-oxidize faster thereby generating more superoxide, hydrogen peroxide, hydroxyl radicals and lipid peroxides than HbAA. Reactive oxygen species can cause damage to biological macromolecules and membrane lipids readily react and undergo peroxidation. Studies have shown that there were increases in stress and inflammatory markers in SCD patients with renal insufficiency.

The mechanisms by which inflammation may lead to decline in renal function is not clear but cytokine could act directly on the endothelium and mesangium of the glomerulus (Fried et al.,2004). Studies in animal model have shown that kidney in SCD is susceptible to hypoxia because of occlusion of blood flow in the vasa recta which may lead to medullary and papillary necrosis and fibrosis (Emokpae et al.,2010a). There are evidence to suggest that prolonged glomerular hyperfiltration due to any cause especially in SCD could lead to glomerular damage resulting to glomerular sclerosis, proteinuria and progressive renal disease. It was suggested that filtered plasma proteins taken up by tubular epithelium

stimulate inflammatory genes, release inflammatory and vaso-active substances into the renal interstitium that induce scarring and sclerosis (Remuzzi and Bertani,1998).We also showed a solid association of chronic inflammation with CKD in SCA and this observation supported the hypothesis that inflammatory and oxidative stress markers contribute to the pathophysiology of glomerulopathy in SCD. Other contributing factors to the pathophysiology of glomerulopathy in SCD are possible iatrogenic acceleration by analgesic medication. There are indication that morphine induces mesangial cell proliferation and glomerulopathy via kappa-opioid receptors as well as the effect of nonsteroidal anti-inflammatory drug-induced damage (Allon et al.,1998;Weber et al.,2005).
Lipid metabolism in SCA patients appears to be different from sickle cell trait and normal haemoglobin in both steady state and renal disease. Alterations in lipid metabolism are often observed in all three Hb genotypes with CKD but marked differences in pattern and severity of lipid disorder differ and thus appear to be more severe in SCD subjects with CKD. Since proteinuria is observed in the early stages of SCD nephropathy, it is the hallmark of future deterioration of renal failure. It is therefore important to detect this early so that intervention at this early stage may prevent or delay renal damage in SCD patients more so as this group of subjects do not do well with renal replacement therapies.

10. References

Abbate, M., Corna, D., Rottoli, D. *et al.* (2004) An intact complement pathway is not dispensable for glomerular and tubulointersititial injury induced by protein overload. J Am Soc Nephrol 15:479-484.

Abbate, M., Zoja, C and Remuzzi, G. (2006) How does proteinuria cause progressive Renal Damage? J Am Soc Nephrol 17:2974-2984.

Abdu A, Emokpae MA, Uadia PO, Kuliya-Gwarzo A (2011). Proteinuria among adult sickle cell anaemia patients in Nigeria. Annals Afri Med 10(1):34-37.

Adedeji, M.O. (1988) Complications of sickle cell disease in Benin City, Nigeria. East Afr Med J 65:3–7.

Airede, K.I and Ibrahim, M. (1999) Antioxidants in neonatal systemic disease. Sahel Med J 2:66-72.

Alleyne, G.A.O., Statius-Van EPs, L.W., Addae, S.K., Nicholson, G.D and Schouten, H.(1975). The kidney in sickle cell Anaemia. Kidney Int 7:371 - 379.

Allon, M. (1990). Renal abnormalities in Sickle cell disease. Arch Intern Med 150: 501-504.

Arab, A.B. (1979). A Survey of haematological variables in 600 healthy Nigerians. Nig Med J 6: 49-53.

Bandyopadhyay, U., Das, D. and Banerjee, R.K. (1999). Reactive oxygen species: oxidative damage and pathogenesis. Current sci 77:658-666.

Batista, M.C., Welty, F.K and Diffenderter, M.R. (2004). Apolipoprotein A-I, B-100 and B-48 metabolism in subjects with chronic kidney disease, obesity and metabolic syndrome. Metabolism 53:1255-1261.

Border, W.A., Okuda, S. and Nakamura, T. (1989). Extracellular matrix and glomerular disease. Semin Nephrol 9:307-311.

Boren, J., Rustaeus, S. and Olofsson, S.O. (1994). Studies on the assembly of apolipoprotein B-100-and B-48-containing very low density lipoproteins in McA-RH7777 cells. J Biol Chem 269:2587-2588.

Bourantas, K.L., Dalekos, G.N., Makis, A., Chaidos, A. Tsiara, S. and Mavridis, A.(1998). Acute phase proteins and interleukine in steady state sickle cell disease. Eur J haematol 61(1):49-54.

Brady, H.R., O'meara, Y.M. and Brenner, B.M. (1998). The major glomerulopathies In: Harrison's Principles of internal Medicine 14th ed Mcgraw-Hill companies p. 1536-1545

Brady, H.R and Brenner, B.M. (1998). Acute Renal Failure In: Harrison's Principles of internal Medicine 14th edition Mcgraw-Hill companies p.1504-1513

Braun, M.C., Reins, R.Y., Li, T.B. *et al.* (2004). Renal expression of the C3a receptor and function responses of primary human proximal tubular epithelial. J Immunol 173:4190-4196.

Bray, J.J., Cragg, P.A., Macknight, A.D.C. and Mills, G.G. (1999). Lecture notes on Human physiology, 4th edition Blackwell science p. 512- 540.

Brenner, B.M. (1985). Nephron adaptation to renal injury or ablation. Am J physiol 249:324 -329.

Brenner, B.M., Cooper, M.E., de Zeeuw, D. *et al.* (2001). Effects of losartan on renal and cardiovascular outcomes in patients with type 2 diabetes and nephropathy. N Engl Med 345:861-869.

Brenner, B.M. and Stein, J.H. (1984). Pediatric Nephrology, Chunchill Livingstone p. 1 – 19.

Breyer, J.A., Bain, R.P., Evans, J.K. *et al.*(1996). Predictors of the progression of renal insufficiency in patients with insulin-dependent diabetes and overt diabetic nephropathy. The Collaborative study Group. Kidney Int 50:1651-1658.

Dakshinamurty, K.V., Srinivasa Rao, P.V.L.N., Saibaba, K.S.S., *et al.* (2002). Antioxidant status in patients on maintenance haemodialysis. Ind J Nephrol 12:77-80.

Dharnidharka, V.R., Dabbagh, S., Afiyeh, B., Simpson, P. and Sarnaik, S. (1998). Prevalence of microalbuminuria in children with sickle cell disease. Paediatr Nephrol 12:475-478

Dixon, R. and Brunskill, N.J. (2000). Albumin stimulates p44/p42 extracellular-signal-regulated mitogen-activated protein kinase in opossum kidney proximal tubular cells. Clin Sci (Lond) 98:295-301.

Donadelli, R., Zanchi, C., Morigi, M., Buelli, S. *et al.* (2003).Protein overload induces fractlkine up-regulation in proximal tubular through nuclear factor kappaB- And p38 mitogen-activated protein kinase-dependent pathways. J Am Soc Nephrol 14:2436-2446.

Drumm, K., Lee, E., Stanners, S., Gassner, B. *et al.* (2003). Albumin and glucose effects on cell growth parameters, albumin uptake and Na^+/H^+ exchanger lsoform 3 in OK cells. Cell physiol Biochem 13:199-206.

Emokpae MA, Uadia PO, Gadzama AA (2010a). Correlation of oxidative stress and inflammatory markers with the severity of sickle cell nephropathy. Annals Afri Med 9(3):141-146.

Emokpae MA, Uadia PO, Osadolor HB (2010b). Lecithin:Cholesterol acyltransferase, lipoprotein lipase and lipoproteins in adult Nigerians with sickle cell disease. Afri J Biochem Res 4(2):17-20.

Emokpae MA, Abdu A, Uadia PO, Borodo MM (2010c). Lipid profile in sickle cell disease patients with chronic kidney disease. Sahel Med J 13(1):20-23.

Emokpae MA, Uadia PO, Kuliya-Gwarzo A (2010d). Antioxidant enzymes and acute phase proteins correlate with marker of lipid peroxide in adult Nigerian sickle cell disease patients. Iran J Basic Med Sci 13(4):177-182.

Falk, R.J., Scheinman, J., Phillips, G., Orringer, E., Johnson, A. and Jennette, R.J. (1992). Prevalence and pathologic features of sickle cell nephropathy and response to inhibition of angiotensin-converting enzyme. N Engl J Med 326:910-915

Farbakhsh, K. and Kasiske, B.L. (2005). Dyslipidaemia in patients who have chronic kidney disease. Med Clin North Am 89:689-699.

Farrar, C.A., Zhou, W., Lin, T.and Sacks, S.H. (2006). Local extravascular pool of C_3 is a determinant of post ischemic acute renal failure. FASEB J 20:217-226.

Feldenzer, J., Mears, J.G., Burns, A.L., Natta, C. and Bank, A. (1979).

Heterogeneity of DNA fragments associated with the sickle - globin gene. J Clin Invest 64:751 - 755.

Gekle, M. (2005). Renal tubule albumin transport. Annu Rev Physiol 67:573-594.

Gelpi, A.P. (1973). Migrant Populations and the diffusion of the sickle cell gene. Ann intern Med 79: 258 - 264.

Guasch, A., Cua, M. and Mitch, W.E. (1996). Extent and the course of glomerular injury in patients with sickle cell anaemia. Kidney Int 49:826-833

Guasch, A., Cua, M., You, W. and Mitch, W.E. (1997). Sickle cell anaemia causes a distinct pattern of glomerular dysfunction. Kidney Int 51:826-833

Guasch, A., Zayas, C.F., Eckman, J.R., Muralidharan, K., Zhang, W. and Elsas, L.J.(1999). Evidence that microdeletions in the alpha globulin gene protect against the development of sickle cell glomerulopathy in humans. J Am Soc Nephrol 10:1014-1019

Guasch, A., Navarrete, J., Nass, K. and Zayas, C. (2006). Glomerular involvement in Adults with Sickle cell hemoglobinopathies: Prevalence and Clinical correlates of progressive renal failure. J Am Soc Nephrol 17:2228-2235.

Hasslacher, C., Reichenbacher, R., Gechter, F. and Timpl, R. (1986). Glomerular basement membrane synthesis and serum concentration of hype IV collagen in stretozotocin - diabetic rats. Diabetologia 26:150-155.

Hatch, F.E., Azar, S.H., Ainsworth, T.E., Nardo, J.M. and Culbertson, J.W. (1970). Renal circulatory studies in young adults with sickle cell anaemia J Lab Clin Med 76:632- 640.

Ji H, Pesce C, Zheng W et al.(2005) Sex differences in renal injury andnitric oxide production in renal wrap hypertension. Am J Physiol Heart Circ Physiol 288(1):43-47.

Kaimori, J.Y., Takenaka, M., Nakajima, H. *et al.* (2003). Induction of gla maturation factor-beta in proximal tubular leads to vulnerability to oxidative injury through the p38 pathway and changes in antioxidant enzyme activities. J Biol Chem 278:33519-33527.

Kamel ,K. and Arony, A.Y. (1965). Origin of the sickling gene. Nature 205:919

Kan, Y.W. and Dozy, A.M. (1978). Polymorphisms of DNA sequence adjacent to human β globin structural gene: relationship to sickle mutuation. Proc Natl Acad Sci, USA 75:5631:5635.

Karttunen, T., Risteli, J., Autio-Harmainen, H. and Risteli, L. (1986). Effect of age and diabetes on type IV collagen and laminin in human kidney cortex. Kidney Int 30:586-589.

Kaysen, G.A. and Eiserich, J.P. (2004). The Role of oxidative stress- Altered lipoprotein structure and function and micro inflammation on cardiovascular risk in patients with minor Renal dysfunction. J Am Soc Nephrol 15:538-548.

Kelley, D.E., Mokan, M., Simoneau, J.A. and Mandarino, L.J. (1993). Interaction between glucose and free fatty acid metabolism in human skeletal muscle. J Clin Invest 92:91-98.

Kim, C. and Vaziri, N.D. (2005). Down regulation of hepatic LDL receptor related protein (LRP) in chronic renal failure. Kidney Int 67:1028-1032.

Klein, D.J., Brown, D.M. and Oegema, T.R. (1986). Glomerular proteoglycan in diabetes. Diabetes 35:1130-1135.

Kurella, M., LO, J.C., Chertow, G.M. *et al.* (2005). Metabolic syndrome and the risk for chronic Kidney disease among non diabetes adults. J Am Soc Nephrol 16:2134-2140.

Lechleitner, M. (2000). Dyslipidaemia and renal disease - pathophysiology, lipid lowering therapy in patients with impaired renal function. J Clin Basic Cardiol 3 (1): 3 -6.

Lehmann, H. (1954). Distribution of the sickle cell gene. A new light on the origin of the East Africans. Eugenics Review 46:101 - 121.

Lehmann, H. and Huntsman, R.G. (1974). Man's Haemoglobins 2nd edition, North Holland Publishing Company, Amsterdam Holland p. 5 - 20.

Liang, K. and Vaziri, N.D. (1997). Gene expression of LDL receptor, HMG-coA reductase and cholesterol -7 alpha- hydrolase in chronic renal failure. Nephrol Dial Transplant 12:1381-1386.

Llach, F. (1993). Pappers Clinical Nephrology 3rd ed. little, Brown and Company p. 25-28

Lopez-Ruiz A, Sartori-Valinotti J, Yanes LL, Iliescu R, Reckelhoff JF (2008). Sex differences in control of blood pressure: role of oxidative stress in hypertension in females. Am J Physiol Heart Circ Physiol 295(2):H466-474

Manfredini, V., Lazzaretti, L.L., Griebeler, I.H.*et al.* (2008). Blood Antioxidants parameters in sickle cell Anaemia Patients in steady state.J National Med Ass 100(8):897-902.

McCall, I.W., Moule, N., Desai, P. and Sergeant, G.R.(1978). Urographic findings in homozygous sickle cell disease. Radiology 126: 99 - 104.

Minkin, S.D., Oh, K.S., Sanders, R.C. and Siegeman, S.S.(1979). Urologic manifestations of sickle haemoglobinopathies. Southern Med 72: 23 - 28.

Morgan, A.G. and Sergeant, G.R. (1981). Renal function in patients over 40 with homozygous sickle cell disease. Br med J 282:1181 - 1183.

Morgan, A.G., Shah, D.J. and Williams, W.(1987). Renal Pathology in Adults over 40 with sickle cell disease. West Ind Med J 36:241 - 250.

Morigi, M., Macconi, D., Zoja, C. *et al.* (2002). Protein overload-induced NF-KappaB activation in proximal tubular requires H_20_2 through a PKC-dependent pathway. J Am Soc Nephrol 13:1179-1189.

Nagel, R.L., Fabry, M.E., Pagnier, J. *et al.* (1985). Haematologically and genetically distinct forms of sickle cell anaemia in Africa: The Senegal type and the Benin type. N Engl J Med 312: 880 - 884.

Nakajima, H., Takenaka, M., Kaimori, J.Y. *et al.* (2003). Gene expression profile of renal proximal tubules regulated by proteinuria. Kidney Int 61:1577-1587.

Nishizawa, Y., Shoji, T., Kawagishi, T. and Moril, H. (1997). Atherosclerosis in uremia possible roles of hyperparathyroidism and intermediate density lipoprotein accumulation. Kidney Int Suppl 62: 590-592.

Odita, J.C., Ugbodaga, C.I., Okafor, L.A., Ojugwu, L.I. and Ogisi, A.O. (1983). Urographic changes in homozygous sickle cell disease. Diag Imaging 52:259 - 263.

Okuda, S., Languino, L.R., Ruoslahti, E. and Border, W.A. (1990). Elevated expression of transforming growth factor b and proteoglycan production in experimental glomerulonephritis. J Clin Invest 86:453-456.

Oomura, A.,Nakamura, T., Arakawa, M. *et al.* (1989). Alteractions in the extracellular matrix components in human glomerular disease. Virchows Arch 415:151-154.

Parke, D.V. and Sopota, A. (1996). Chemical toxicity and reactive oxygen species. Int J Occup Med Environ Health. 9:331-340.

Peterson, J.C., Adler, S., Burkart, J.M. *et al.* (1995). Blood pressure control, proteinuria, and the progression of renal disease. The Modification of Diet in Renal Disease study. Ann Intern Med 123;754-762.

Pham, P.T., Pham, P.T., Wilkinson, A.H. and Lew, S.Q. (2000). Renal abnormalities in sickle cell disease. Kidney Int 57:1-8

Platt, O.S., Brambilla, D.J., Rosse, W.F. *et al.* (1994). Mortality in sickle cell disease: Life expectantly and risk factors for early death. N Engl J Med 330:1639 - 1644.

Powars, D., Chan, L.S. and Schroeder, W.A. (1990). The variable expression of sickle cell disease is genetically determined. Semin Hematol 27: 360 - 376.

Powars, D.R., Elliott-Mills, D.D., Chan, L. *et al.* (1991). Chronic renal failure in sickle cell disease:risk factors,clinical course and mortality. Ann Intern Med 115 (8):614-620

Powars, D.R., Hiti, A., Ramicone, E., Johnson, C. and Chan, L. (2002). Outcome in haemoglobin SC disease: a four decade observational study of clinical, haematologic and genetic factors. Am J Haematol 70(3):206-215

Powars, D.R., Chan, L.S., Hiti, A., Ramicone, E. and Johnson, C. (2005). Outcome of Sickle cell anaemia: a four decade observational study of 1056 patients. Medicine (Baltimore) 84 (6): 363-376

Pratt, J.R., Basheer, S.A. and Sacks, S.H. (2002). Local synthesis of complement component C_3 regulates acute renal transplant rejection. Nat Med 8:582-587.

Rawlings, J.S. and Harrison, D.A. (2004). The JAK/STAT signaling pathways. J Soc 117:1281-1283.

Ray, G. and Husain, S.H. (2002). Oxidants, antioxidants and carcinogenesis Ind J Exp Biol 40:1213-1232.

Reid, H.J., Photiades, D.P., Ukponmwan, V.O. and Osamo, O. (1984). Concurrent diabetes mellitus and the haemoglobinopathies: A Nigerian Study, IRCS Med. Sci. 12:853

Remuzzi, G. and Bertaini, T. (1998). Pathophysiology of progressive nephropathies. N Engl J Med 339:1448-1456.

Rennke, H.A. and Klein, P.S. (1989). Pathogenesis and significance of non primary focal and segmental glomerlosclerosis. Am J Kidney Dis 6:443-447.

Risdon, A. (1985). The anatomy of Nephrology ed. F.P Marsh, William Heinemann Medical books Ltd, London p.1-20

Ruggenenti, P., Perna, A. and Remuzzi, G. (2003). Retarding progression of chronic renal disease; the neglected issue of residual proteinuria. Kidney Int 63:2254-2261.

Saborio, P. and Scheinman, J.I. (1999). Sickle Cell Nephropathy. J Am Soc Nephrol 10:187-192

Schreiner, G.F. (1995). Renal toxicity of albumin and other lipoproteins. Curr Opin Nephrol Hypertens 4:369-373.

Serjeant, G. R. (1992). Renal Manifestation in Sickle cell Disease 2nd edition (oxford university press) p. 261 - 281

Shimonura, H. and Spiro, R.G. (1987). Studies on the macromolecular components of human glomerular basement membrane and alterations in diabetes. Diabetes 36:374-378.

Shlipak, M.G., Heidenreich, P.A., Noguchi, H. *et al.* (2002). Association of renal insufficiency with treatment and outcomes after myocardial infarction in elderly patients. Ann Int Med. 137:555-562.

Suryawanshi, N.P., Bhutey, A.K., Nagdeote, A.N., Jadhav, A.A. and Manoorkar, G.S. (2006). Study of lipid peroxide and lipid profile in Diabetes mellitus. Ind J Clin Biochem 21:126-130.

Tang, S., Sheerin, N.S., Zhou, W., Brown, Z. and Sacks, S.H. (1999). Apical proteins stimulate complement synthesis by cultured human proximal tubular epithelial. J Am Soc Nephrol 10:69-76.

Tang, S., Leung, J.C.K., Abe, K., Wah-Chan, K., Chan, T. and Neng, L. K.(2003). Albumin stimulates interleukin-8 expression in proximal tubular epithelia in vitro and in vivo. J Clin Invest 111:515-527.

Travis, L.B., Brouhard, B.H. and Kalia, A. (1984). Overview with special emphasis on epidemiologic considerations in: Pediatric Nephrology eds. S.A Mendoza and B.M Tune. Churchill Livingstone p. 1-19

Ukoli, F.A.M., Adedeji, M.O. and Reid, H.J. (1988). The prevalence of anaemia among school children in Benin City, South western Nigeria. Health and Hygiene 9:103-106

Vassalli, P., Simon, G. and Rouiller, C. (1963). Electron microscopic study of glomerular lesions resulting from intravascular fibrin formation. Am J Pathol 43:579-616

Vaziri, N.D., Deng, G. and Liang, K. (1999). Hepatic HDL receptor, SR- B1 and APO A-1 expression in chronic renal failure. Nephrol Dial Transplant 14: 1462-1466.

Vaziri, N.D. and Parks, J.S. (2001). Down-regulation of hepatic lecithin: cholesterol acyltransferase gene expression in chronic renal failure. kidney Int 59:2192-2196.

Vaziri, N.D. (2006). Dyslipidaemia of chronic renal failure: the nature, mechanism and potential consequences. Am J Physiol Renal physiol 290:F262-F272.

Vaziri, N.D. (2008). Managing lipid disorders in chronic kidney disease: An expert commentary. Medscape Nephrology, Cleveland clinic workshop on Innovation in uremia therapy p. 1-4

Wang, Y., Chen, J., Chen, L., Tay, Y.C., Rangan, G.K. and Harris, D.C. (1997). Induction of monocyte chemoattractant protein- in proximal tubule by urinary protein. J Am Soc Nehrol 8:1537-1545.

Wapstra, F.H., Navis, G., de Jong, P.E. and de Zeeuw, D. (1996). Prognostic value of the short-term antiproteinuric response to ACE inhibition for prediction of GFR decline in patients with non diabetic renal disease. Nephrol 4(suppl 1) :47-52.

Wigfall, D.R., Ware, R.E., Burchinal, M.R., Kinney, T.R. and Foreman, J.W. (2000). Prevalence and clinical correlates of glomerulopathy in children with sickle cell disease. J Paediatr 136:749-753

Yard, B.A., Chorianopoulos, E., Herr, D. and Van der woude, F.J. (2001). Regulation of endothelin-1 and transforming growth factor-beta 1 production in cultured proximal tubular by albumin and heparin sulphate glycosaminoglcans. Nephrol Dial Transplant 16:1769-1775.

Yu, B.P. (1994). Cellular defences against damage from reactive oxygen species. Biol Rev 74:139-163.

Zoja, C., Donadelli, R., Colleoni, S., Figlizzi, M. *et al.* (1998).Protein overload stimulates RANTES production by proximal tubular depending on NF- KappaB Activation. Kidney Int 53:1608-1615.

Zoja, C., Morigi, M., Figliuzzi, M. *et al.* (1995). Proximal tubular synthesis and secretion of endothelin-1 on challenge with albumin and other proteins. Am J Kidney Dis 26:934-941.

9

Renal Cortical Neoplasms and Associated Renal Functional Outcomes

Gina M. Badalato, Max Kates, Neda Sadeghi and James M. McKiernan
Department of Urology, Columbia University Medical Center
USA

1. Introduction

In 2010 alone there were an estimated 54,000 new diagnoses and 12,000 deaths attributable to renal cell carcinoma (RCC), with the vast majority of these tumors consituting small renal masses incidentially detected on cross-sectional imaging.(2010; Chow, Dong, and Devesa, 2010) Renal cortical tumors include a complex family of neoplasms with unique histology, cytogenetic effects, and metastatic potential; the differential presentation of symptomatic, locally advanced disease as opposed to small renal tumors (median tumor size <4cm, T1a) evokes different management paradigms.(Lee et al., 2010; McKiernan et al., 2002b; Mitchell et al., 2006; Russo et al., 2002) This large subcategory of patients with localized RCC have historically been treated with radical nephrectomy, and this management has continued in many regions of the United Stes and the world.(Hollenbeck et al., 2006) Nevertheless, a paradigm shift has occured in the surgical management of renal cortical tumors over the last 10 years, favoring nephron-sparing surgery or partial nephrecotmy whenever this approach is feasible from a technical and oncologic standpoint. The rationale underpinning this shift has involved the observed *non-inferiority* in terms of cancer control and operative morbidity as well as the *superior* renal functional outcomes. Within the neprhology and urology communities, the last decade has also witnessed a increased understanding of how renal volume effects renal function, and how this in turn affects cardiovascular competence. It now is evident that having less renal parenchyma does not only worsen renal function, but it also is a poor prognosticator of cardiac function and overall survival. It is within this context that a review of renal functional outcomes following surgery for renal coritcal tumors can be undertaken.

2. Renal cancer: Changing epidemiology

Approximately 75-80% of patients in the United States with renal cancer are now diagnosed incidentally and with organ-confined disease. This shift is largely attributable to the increasing use of cross-sectional imaging with the utilization of CT and MRI increasing by 73% during 1986-1994 among the Medicare population. Furthermore, depending on the histologic sub-type, the prognosis ranges from 75-100% of patients achieving long-term survival, and an estimated 30% of patients over 70 years of age dying of unrelated causes within 5 years of surgery for a renal cortical neoplasm.(Jewett and Zuniga, 2008) The increased incidence and detection of these cancers is largely due to the diagnosis of small localized renal lesions, many of which have low metastatic potential. This finding is reflected in the fact that mortality as a result of renal cancer has not changed over time despite the increased incidence. (Figure 1)

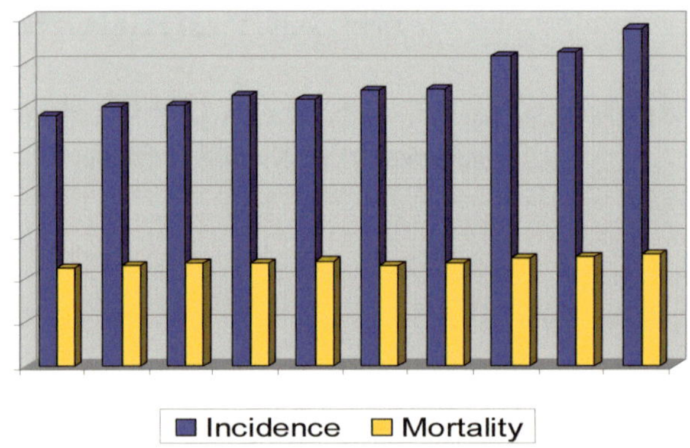

Fig. 1. Trends in Renal Cancer Over Time, American Cancer Society, Facts & Figures, 1997-2006

In parallel with the impetus underlying the increased detection of renal neoplasms, the detection of benign renal lesions, defined chiefly as oncocytoma, angiomyolipoma, and simple renal cysts, has also increased. In fact, a contemporary review of the Columbia University experience identified 775 patients with a tumor diameter of less than or equal to 7.0 cm. Of these patients the proportion of patients undergoing renal surgery for benign tumors increased annually: 5% before 1998, 15.2% from 1998-2003, and 21.2% from 2004 to 2007. The mean tumor diameter was found to decrease significantly during the study period ($p=0.006$) and year of surgery and tumor diameter were found to be independent predictors of benign histologic features ($p<0.05$).(Murphy et al., 2009)
This combination of observations thus underscores the changing phenomenology of renal cortical lesions, as an increase in the use of cross-sectional imaging has resulted in a higher proportion of patients with incidentally detected small renal masses and in turn the clinical recognition of benign renal pathology.

2.1 Renal cortical tumors: Heterogeneous presentations and oncologic implications

Renal cortical tumors are members of a complex category of histologic entities which includes the benign oncocytoma, the indolent papillary and chromophobe carcinomas, and also the potentially aggressive clear cell carcinoma. While published urological series consist predominantly of small, localized renal masses, approximately 90% of the medical oncology series reporting metastatic renal cancers consist of tumors of conventional clear cell histology. In fact, a retrospective review by McKiernan et al featured 246 consecutive partial nephrectomy specimens, and characterized the relative distribution of histologic subtypes in small renal masses.(McKiernan et al., 2002b) Within this series from Memorial Sloan Kettering Cancer Center, the most frequent finding was conventional clear cell carcinoma in 148 cases (51%), followed by papillary carcinoma in 54 (18%), oncocytoma in 32 (11%), and chromophobe in 21 (7%).

The World Health Organization (WHO)/ Heidelberg classification subdivides renal cell tumors into benign and malignant neoplasms based on documented genetic abnormalities.(Kovacs et al., 1997) In fact, studies focusing on sporadic and hereditary forms of renal cancer have suggested that abnormalities in the von Hippel-Lindau (chromosome 3p) and *met* genes are among the earliest alterations in conventional clear cell and papillary renal cancers, respectively. Table 1 highlights the major chromosomal alterations that have been implicated in different renal cortical neoplasms.

Histological Subtype	Early Genetic/ Molecular Defects	Late Genetic/ Molecular Defects	Associated Syndromes
Conventional	LOH 3p Mutation of 3p25 (VHL)	+5p -8p, -9p, -14q P53 mutationC-erB-1 Oncogene	Von Hippel-Lindau Sporadic RCC Hereditary RCC
Papillary	+7, +17 -Y Met gene mutation	+12, +16, +20 -9p, -11q, -14q, -17p, -21q PRCC-TFE3 gene fusion	Hereditary Papillary (HPRC) Sporadic Papillary
Chromophobe	-1	-1p, -2p, -6p, -13q, -21q, -Y p53 Mutation	
Collecting Duct	-18, -Y	-1q, -6p, -8p, -11, -13q, -21q C-erB-1	Renal Medullary Carcinoma
Oncocytoma	-1, -Y, 11q rearrangement		Familial Oncocytoma

Table. 1. Genetic Findings in Renal Carcinoma Subtypes. Zambrano et al. *J Urol* 1999; 163 (4): 1246-58 adapted by P. Russo, MD.

Later work demonstrated that pathologic tumor diameter may be useful in the prediction of conventional subtype in small renal cortical lesions. One retrospective review involved 393 patients who underwent radical or partial nephrectomy at one institution; logistic regression analysis demonstrated that for every 1cm increase in tumor diameter up to 4cm, the renal cortical lesion was 1.27 times more likely to be conventional clear cell (p=0.020).(Laudano et al., 2008) These findings were extrapolated to show that a 4cm renal cortical tumor was approximately 2 times more likely to be conventional clear cell than tumors 0.6-1.5cm in size. (Figure 2)

3. Partial nephrectomy is the standard of care for small renal masses (T1a)

Radical nephrectomy became the standard of care for renal cortical neoplasms approximately 40 years ago. In the 1980s this approach was challenged by reports demonstrating favourable results of partial nephrectomy in imperative cases (i.e. cases in which nephron-sparing surgery was mandatory to conserve adequate renal function such as in patients with a solitary kidney).(Novick et al., 1989; Zincke et al., 1985) During the last 10 years partial nephrectomy

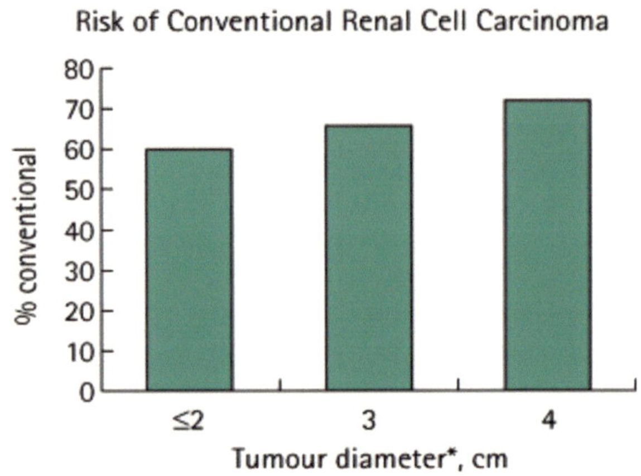

Fig. 2. The percentage of conventional clear cell renal carcinomas based on largest tumor diameter (*rounded to the nearest cm). Laudano et al. *BJU Int.* 2008; 102 (10): 1385-8.

has become the standard of care for the management of most small renal masses even in the presence of a normal contralateral kidney.(Becker et al., 2006b; Huang et al., 2006; Patard et al., 2004; Thompson et al., 2005) In addition to the benefits of preserving renal function and preventing cardiovascular complications, topics discussed in detail in the ensuing sections, evidence strongly supports the notion that cancer control and risk of cancer-related death are not compromised when a partial nephrectomy is performed instead of a radical procedure.(Dash et al., 2006; Leibovich et al., 2004)

Although data from the National Cancer Institute SEER program demonstrated that partial nephrectomy was underutilized at the beginning of this century (2000-2002), with only 20% of patients with tumors 2-4cm in size receiving this procedure, these rates are changing in favour of a nephron-sparing approach.(Hollenbeck et al., 2006; Miller et al., 2006) In fact, a retrospective review of 1,533 patients treated with partial or radical nephrectomy between 2000-2007 at Memorial Sloan Kettering Cancer Center reported that nephron-sparing surgery was performed in approximately 90% of patients with T1a tumors.(Thompson et al., 2009) A similar analysis at the national level is documented in Figure 3, demonstrating that the use of partial nephrectomy is increasing, albeit at a relatively modest rate, with 66% of patients presenting with a renal cortical tumor ≤2cm in size receiving a partial nephrectomy in 2007.

3.1 Partial nephrectomy is increasingly being utilized in medium-sized tumors (T1b)

The current size determination for renal tumors that forms the basis for the 2010 TNM staging classification was founded on the basis of several studies demonstrating improved survival in patients undergoing surgery for tumors less than 4cm as opposed to those that exceeded this dimension.(Gofrit et al., 2001; Hafez, Fergany, and Novick, 1999) More contemporary analyses have shown that regardless of the form of surgical intervention, namely partial or radical nephrectomy, patients with tumors larger than 4cm have a higher risk of relapse.(Lau et al., 2000; Lesage et al., 2007; Margulis et al., 2007; Mitchell et al., 2006; Zini et al., 2009) On the basis of these precedents, there has been a clear impetus to determine whether elective nephron-sparing surgery may be an option for patient with localized T1b (4-7cm) tumors.

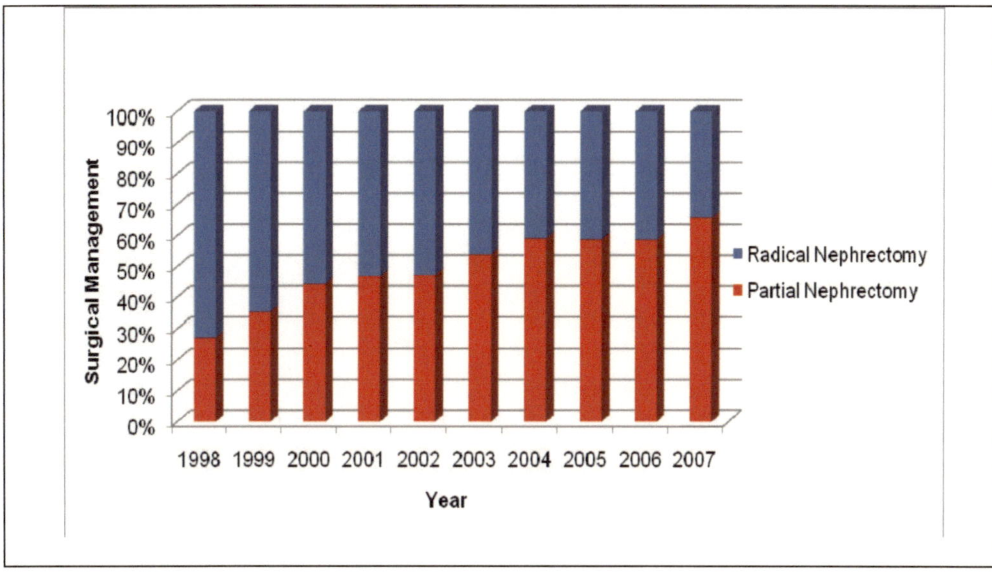

Fig. 3. The Current Standard of Care for the Treatment of Tumors ≤2cm based on Surveillance, Epidemiology, and End Results (SEER) estimates. The use of PN steadily increased over the study period, from 27% of all cases in 1998 to 66% in 2007. Kates et al. *J Uro* 2011 *IN PRESS.*

In fact, several antecedent investigations have indicated partial nephrectomy can safely be expanded to include patients with T1bN0M0 tumors.(Becker et al., 2006a; Kim et al., 2010; Mitchell et al., 2006; Patard et al., 2004) Leibovich and colleagues reported cancer-specific survival rates at 5 years of 98% for those receiving nephron-sparing surgery and 86% for patients treated with radical nehrectomy; and, after adjusting for several covariates including tumor grade and histologic subtype, this difference was found to no longer be statistically significant (risk ratio 1.60, 95% CI 0.50-5.12, p=0.430).(Leibovich et al., 2004) In a similar vein, Patard et al noted that 3 year disease-specific survival rates were comparable at 98% and 97% (p=0.8) when partial nephrectomy patients were stratified by tumor size less than and greater than 4cm, respectively.(Patard et al., 2007) Last, recent work has expounded upon these findings as it pertains to the laparoscopic management of T1bN0M0 tumors, documenting comparable cancer-specific mortality (3% vs 3%) and recurrence rates RN 3% vs PN 6%, p-0.40) for both procedures over a median follow-up of 57 months.(Simmons, Weight, and Gill, 2009) These studies thus set the precedent that nephron-sparing surgery is a viable option form an oncologic standpoint in an appropriately selected subset of patients with a medium-sized tumors when treated at centers experienced with these techniques.

Last, a subsequent investigation by Badalato et al. extended these findings regarding nephron-sparing surgery for T1b patients to the population level, utilizing data from the Surveillance, Epidemiology, and End Results (SEER) registry.(Badalato et al., 2011) Using propensity scoring, a statistical test that controls for measured variables between partial and radical nephrectomy cohorts, this study determined that no overall survival difference was noted within a matched cohort of pT1bN0M0 patients treated with either surgical alternative. (Figure 4) These findings thus lend support to the aforementioned growing body of evidence that partial neprhectomy may become the preferred management alternative for T1b renal tumors.

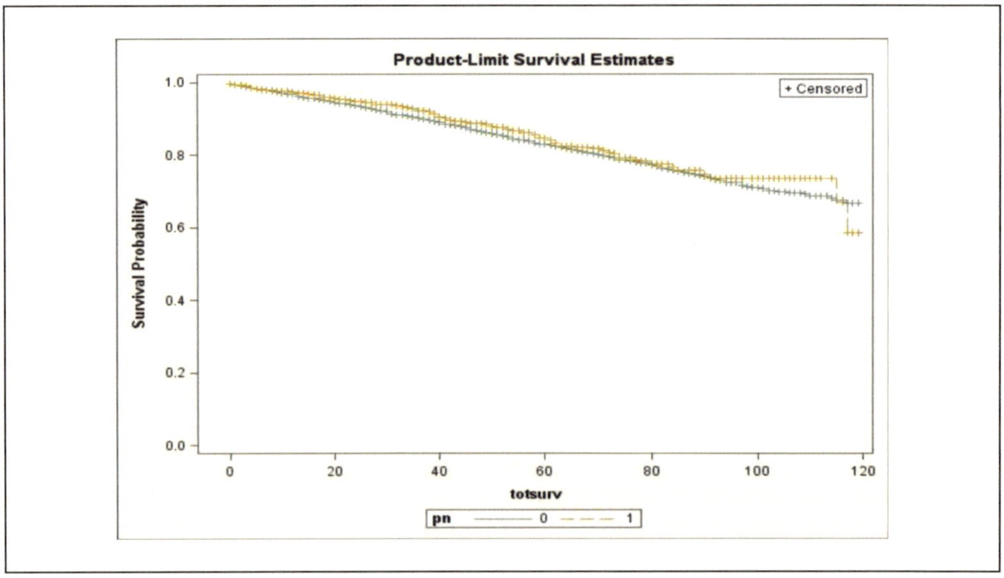

Fig. 4. Overall survival in a propensity-matched cohort of SEER patients receiving partial versus radical nephrectomy. For the entire cohort, there was no difference in survival when groups were divided based on surgical treatment. Badalato et al. *BJU Int.* 2011 *IN PRESS*

4. Renal tumor patients may have unrecognized medical renal disease before intervention

Patients with renal tumors are not a screened population and tend to be older (mean age 61 years) with cardiovascular comorbidities. Accordingly, clinical and pathological evidence has shown that this population of patients has a greater degree of underlying renal disease than previously appreciated.(Bijol et al., 2006; Kaplan et al., 1975) In fact, a retrospective cohort study of patients with small renal tumors by Huang et al. showed that 26% of their patients with T1a RCC and normally functioning kidneys had pre-existing chronic kidney disease (CKD), defined as GFR <60 mL/min per 1·73 m^2. (Huang et al., 2006)

The most common renal diseases found in patients with renal tumors are due to hypertension and diabetes. Bijol and colleagues reported that up to 60% of nephrectomy specimens show features of renal disease, most of which are due to changes from hypertension or diabetes. (Bijol et al., 2006) Other causes of renal disease include smoking, glomerulonephritis, cystic kidney diseases, congenital malformations, immune diseases, obstruction, and infection.

Moreover, many of the risk factors that are implicated in the pathogenesis of renal disease overlap with the risk factors that contribute to renal cell carcinoma. For example, although the pathophysiologic mechanism for this relationship is still unclear, there is a progressive increase in the risk of renal cell carcinoma in correlation with worsening hypertension. (Chow, Dong, and Devesa, 2010; Schlehofer et al., 1996; Setiawan et al., 2007) With regard to diabetes, the pre-surgical incidence of this disease ranges from 6.8% to 23%. (Hepps and

Chernoff, 2006; Lindblad et al., 1999; Schlehofer et al., 1996) Since diabetic nephropathy affects approximately one-third of patients with this condition, it is reasonable to extrapolate that a significant proportion of patients diagnosed with a renal cortical tumor will have pre-existing diabetic nephropathy. Last, smoking is another well-known risk factor prevalent within the population that contributes to an increased risk for the development of both renal disease and renal cell carcinoma. (Ejerblad et al., 2004; Hunt et al., 2005)

Recent evidence by Donin et al. also demonstrated renal tumor diameter independently predicted decreased preoperative estimated GFR when controlling for hypertension and race on multivariable analysis. (Donin et al., 2011) This study thus suggests that the growth of a renal neoplasm and perhaps the replacement of healthy renal parenchyma independently modulates renal functional deterioration to some degree.

Cumulatively, the presence of underlying renal disease in patients diagnosed with a renal cortical neoplasm is significant because renal function plays an important role in the surgical management and overall survival associated with management. Therefore, it remains prudent to be aware of the risk of underlying renal disease in patients with RCC.

4.1 Chronic kidney disease poses and independent risk factor for cardiovascular-related death

Approximately 26 million adults in the United States have CKD. CKD is most commonly seen among African-Americans, Hispanics, Pacific Islanders, Native Americans, and the elderly. The National Kidney Foundation, American Heart Association, and the Seventh Joint National Committee on prevention, Detection, Evaluation, and Treatment of High Blood Pressure deemed CKD as an independent risk factor for cardiovascular disease.(2002; Chobanian et al., 2003; Sarnak et al., 2003) Similarly, cardiovascular disease is the leading cause of morbidity and mortality among patients with CKD.

The criteria for CKD is defined by The National Kidney Foundation - Kidney Disease Outcomes Quality Initiative (NKF-K/DOQI) workgroup (See Table 2).

Criteria
1. Kidney damage for ≥3 months, as defined by structural or functional abnormalities of the kidney, with or without decreased GFR, manifest by *either*: • Pathological abnormalities; or • Markers of kidney damage, including abnormalities in the composition of the blood or urine, or abnormalities in imaging tests
2. GFR <60 mL/min/1.73 m^2 for ≥3 months, with or without kidney damage

Table 2. Criteria for Definition of Chronic Kidney Disease. *Am J Kidney Dis 2002* 39 (2 Suppl 1), S1-266.

Many studies have provided evidence that renal damage, assessed by markers of renal function such as serum creatinine, GFR, and albuminuria, is an independent risk factor for cardiovascular disease and cardiovascular mortality.

In a study of 1,120,295 patients in the San Francisco Bay Area, Go and colleagues demonstrated a progressively increased risk of death and/or a cardiovascular event as renal function declined. They reported that the adjusted risk of a cardiovascular event increased by 43% with an estimated GFR of 45 to 59 ml/minute/1.73 m^2 (HR 1.4; CI 1.4-1.5) and by 343% with an estimated GFR of less than 15 ml/minute/1.73 m^2 (HR 3.43; CI 3.1-3.8). The presence of proteinuria was also an independent factor that predicted the risk of a cardiovascular event (HR1.3; CI 1.2-1.3). (Go et al., 2004)

Level I evidence from the Heart Outcomes Prevention Evaluation (HOPE) trial demonstrated that the presence of kidney disease, defined as an increased serum creatinine >1.4 mg/dL and/or microalbuminuria, independently increased the risk of cardiovascular death, myocardial infarction, or stroke (HR, 1.40; CI, 1.16-1.69 for serum creatinine) (HR 1.59; CI 1.37- 1.84 for microalbuminuria). Moreover, compared to patients with neither risk factor, patients with both increased serum creatinine and microalbuminuria were at increased risk of having a cardiovascular death or cardiovascular event (28.6% vs 13.6%); this suggests the additive nature of these risk factors. (Mann et al., 2001)

Cumulatively, the findings from these and similar studies qualify CKD alone as a risk factor for cardiovascular disease.

5. Partial nephrectomy preserves renal function

Emerging evidence strongly favors partial nephrectomy (PN), as opposed to radical nephrectomy (RN), for tumors that are 7cm or smaller as the best approach to preserve postoperative renal functional outcomes. The data in support of this position stemmed from early work examining the prevalence and onset of CKD among postoperative renal cancer patients. Then, as now, there is not standardized metric of renal function, although some precise mechanisms of assaying such function have gradually permeated the urologic literature. McKiernan et al published one of the early papers on this subject, selecting a cohort of 290 patients with T1a (<4cm) renal cell carcinoma and a pre-operative serum creatinine of less than 1.5mg/dl and then longitudinally tracking the onset of chronic renal insufficiency (defined in the study as creatinine >2mg/dl) following surgical intervention.(McKiernan et al., 2002a) In fact, at 5 years of follow-up the rate of freedom from CRI was 100% in the partial nephrectomy grouping and 84.8% in the radical nephrectomy cohort. Huang et al. Later validated these findings in a level 2 prospective study using eGFR of less than 60mL/min per 1.73m^2 as the index defining CKD Stage III or greater.(Lane et al., 2010b) In a total of 662 patients with a normal serum creatinine prior to surgery for RCC, freedom from new onset CKD was determined to be 80% after partial nephrectomy as opposed to just 35% following radical nephrectomy.(Huang et al., 2006) (Figure 5) Moreover, after controlling for relevant clinical and pathological differences between surgical groups, patients receiving a radical nephrectomy were found to be a t a four-fold higher risk of having CKD post-operatively as compared to their counterparts undergoing nephron-sparing surgery. These findings were substantiated in similar work using creatinine clearance as an alternative measure of renal function.(Clark et al., 2008)

Despite controversy related to the best metric for renal functional outcomes in the perioperative setting, the fact that partial nephrectomy results in improved long-term renal function compared to radical nephrectomy has continued to be validated in the literature.(Jeon et al., 2009; Lane et al., 2010c; Malcolm et al., 2009; Miller et al., 2008) In fact, although there was initially concern that vascular clamping at the renal hilum during partial nephrectomy might increase the rate of renal insufficiency due to the prolonged cold ischemia time, clamp time was shown not to be associated with long-term renal functional measures in patients who had a normal renal function at baseline. Yossepowitch et al. went on to demonstrate that in healthy patients with two renal units, renal insufficiency is primarily a transient, postoperative entity.(Yossepowitch et al., 2006) While non-modifiable factors such as preoperative eGFR as well as the amount and quality of the renal parenchyma left in situ may be prognostic of postoperative renal function, there is no level 1 evidence to further inform these notions.(Lane et al., 2011; Thompson and Blute, 2007)

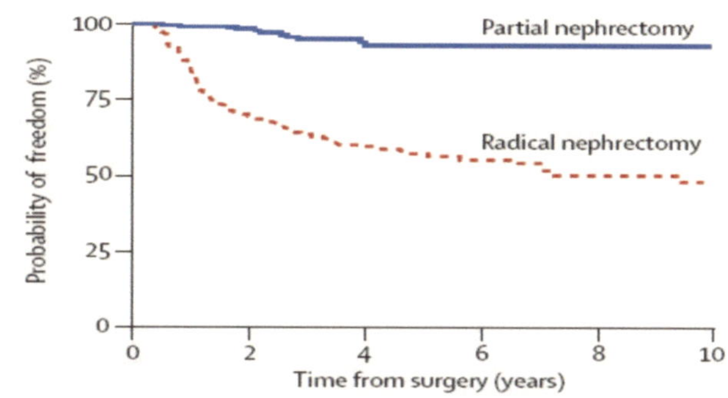

Number at risk						
Partial nephrectomy	385	187	84	33	13	6
Radical nephrectomy	262	130	86	56	33	21

Fig. 5. Probability of freedom from new onset of GFR lower than 45 mL/min per 1.72m^2 by operation type. Huang et al. *Lancet Oncol* 2006; 7: 735-40.

5.1 Poor renal functional outcomes following nephrectomy increases the risk of cardiovascular sequelae and death

Several prior studies have demonstrated the increase in non-cancer related deaths among patients undergoing radical as opposed to partial nephrectomy.(Thompson et al., 2008; Weight et al., 2010b) Although it has been postulated that this increase in mortality was attributable to an increased rate of CKD and by extension cardiovascular disease, this theory had not been proven prior to the publication of recent work. In fact, Weight, Novick, and colleagues examined the overall and disease-specific survival outcomes in 1,004 patients with T1b RCC (4-7cm) who underwent either partial or radical nephrectomy. Over a median follow-up period of 4 years, a significantly decreased level of real function was observed in the radical nephrectomy cohort.(Weight et al., 2010a) Furthermore, this difference in renal function correlated with a 25% increase in the risk of cardiovascular death and a 17% risk of death from any cause. In subsequent work, Huang et al corroborated the results of this single-institution study with a population-level investigation involving Medicare beneficiaries; they found that radical nephrectomy was associated with an increased risk of cardiovascular events and non-cancer mortality within this grouping.(Huang et al., 2009) Table 1 summarizes data that continues to emerge in contemporary work, substantiating the worsened overall and cardiovascular survival associated with radical as compared to nephron-sparing surgery. (Table 2)

Study	Year	Age	Tumor Size	Patients (*n*) RN	PN	Overall Death HR	CV Events/Death HR
Thompson [22]	2008	<65	≤4cm	140	187	2.16	–
Huang [25]	2009	>65	≤4cm	2547	556	1.38	1.4
Weight [24]	2010	–	4-7cm	480	525	1.17	1.25
Weight [23]	2010	–	≤7cm	111	388	2.5	–

Table 2. Open series outcomes: Overall and Cardiovascular Mortality. Kates et al. *Curr Opin Urol 2011 IN PRESS*

5.1.1 Partial nephrectomy is underutilized, within certain populations: case in point – the elderly

In the seminal articles on post-nephrectomy renal function published by McKiernan et al. and Huang et al., most of the with decompensating function were diagnosed less than 3 years following their initial surgery.(Huang et al., 2006; McKiernan et al., 2002a) Thus the concept of "long-term" benefit from a nephron-sparing approach is a fallacy, as this advantage is noted within a few years following surgical intervention. An older patient, albeit with a shorter life expectancy may thus benefit from a partial nephrectomy. This finding is especially pertinent since it has already been demonstrated that the risk of complication from a partial nephrectomy is no greater for patients over 75 years of age as compared to younger counterparts.(Lowrance et al., 2010) This understanding is especially important due to urologists' hesitation to perform a nephron-sparing procedure in the elderly - cumulatively a historic disparity which is not substantiated by an evidence-based approach and has persisted to this decade.(Hollenbeck et al., 2006; Kates et al., 2011) (Figure 6) Recently, Lane and colleagues demonstrated that a decline in renal function associated with a radical procedure in patients 75 years of age and older resulted in a corresponding increase in the risk of cardiovascular death.(Lane et al., 2010a) In a cohort of elderly patients with local renal cell cancer 7cm or less, there was no statistically significant difference in survival for those receiving surgery, namely radical or partial nephrectomy, as opposed to those on active surveillance. This finding suggests that no surgery or the proverbial "maximal nephron-sparing procedure" may be indicated for a carefully selected subset of the elderly patient population.

6. Preoperative risk stratification schemata

Comprehensive pre-operative risk stratification is important for patients undergoing kidney surgery in order to help approximate the best renal functional outcomes. Remarkably, recent estimates have reported that up to one-third of patients with pre-existing Stage I or II CKD will progress to Stage II (GFR<60).(Clark et al., 2011) Accordingly, several risk factors for the post-operative development of stage III CKD have been well described; chief among them involves having a prior diagnosis of diabetes.(Lane et al., 2011) Composite risk profiles have been well-elucidated to predict a patients' risk of CKD based on preoperative clinical parameters. One such method is the Screening for Occult Renal Disease (SCORED) tool, a modified example of which is demonstrated in figure 7. This prediction tool utilizes factors such as patient age, gender, and clinical characteristics (such as anemia, proteinuria, and cardiovascular comorbidities) to stratify patient into risk

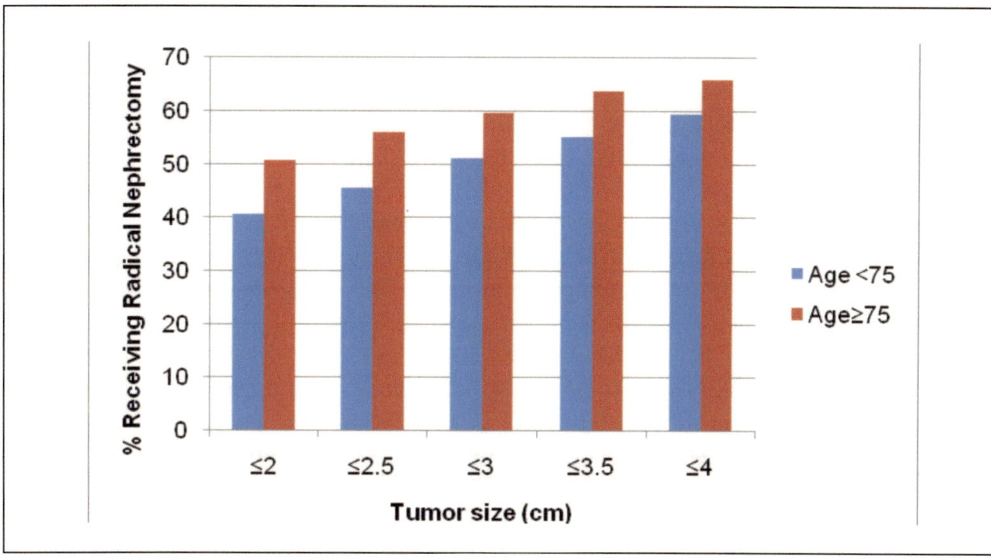

Fig. 6. Percentage of patients receiving radical nephrectomy for T1a RCC between 1998-2007 according to tumor size. A higher percentage of elderly patients consistently receive a radical nephrectomy for a given tumor size. Kates et al. *Urology 2011 IN PRESS.*

Do You Have Kidney Disease? Take This Test and Know Your Score.

Find out if you might have silent chronic kidney disease now. Check each statem that is true for you. **If a statement is not true or you are not sure, put a zero.** Tl add up all the points for a total.

- Age:
  1. I am between 50 and 59 years of age....................Yes 2 ______
  2. I am between 60 and 69 years of age....................Yes 3 ______
  3. I am 70 years old or older....................Yes 4 ______
- I am a woman....................Yes 1 ______
- I had/have anemia....................Yes 1 ______
- I have high blood pressure....................Yes 1 ______
- I am diabetic....................Yes 1 ______
- I have a history of heart attack or stroke....................Yes 1 ______
- I have a history of congestive heart failure or heart failure.......Yes 1 ______
- I have circulation disease in my legs....................Yes 1 ______
- I have protein in my urine....................Yes 1 ______

Total ______

If You Scored 4 or More Points

You have a 1 in 5 chance of having chronic kidney disease. At your next office vi a simple blood test should be checked. Only a professional health care provider determine for sure if you have kidney disease.

If You Scored 0-3 Points

You probably do not have kidney disease now, but at least once a year, you shou take this survey.

Your total score from SCORED	Probability of having chronic kidney disease no	
	In general healthy individuals	In cardiovascul patients
≤1	<2 %	<6 %
2	<2 %	~10 %
3	2-3 %	10-15 %
4	5-6 %	10-15 %
5	10-15 %	20-25 %
6	15-25 %	~30 %
7	25-35 %	40-45 %
8	35-45 %	45-65 %
≥9	>40 %	>60 %

Fig. 7. Risk assessment chart for CKD using the SCORED model from Bang et al. *Arch Intern Med* 167(4), 374-81.

groupings for the development of CKD. During the course of validating this instrument in the setting of patients with small renal masses undergoing surgery, Lucas et al determined that patients in high risk categories (SCORED$\geq$4) were 3 times more likely to develop Stage III CKD.(Bang et al., 2007; Lucas et al., 2008) Other groups have followed suit with the proposal of alternative nomograms. For example, Sorbellini et al have described a mechanism to predict renal insufficiency, which was defined as 2 or more values of a creatinine of 2.0mf/dl at least one month following surgery.(Sorbellini et al., 2006) Nevertheless, while this nomogram accounts for the change in renal volume, it relies on creatinine and does not include known predictors of CKD such as preoperative comorbidity information.

Other systems of risk stratification have looked at the renal parenchyma in and of itself as a tool for predicting postoperative outcomes. Notably, the presence and extent of glomerolosclerosis in normal parenchyma has been shown to be commensurate with deterioration in postoperative renal function, although this trend was not noted for features such as arteriosclerosis or interstitial fibrosis/ tubular atrophy.(Gautam et al., 2010; McCann et al., 2009)

7. Conclusion

Among patients diagnosed with a renal cortical neoplasm, those having a radical nephrectomy are at an increased risk for the development of CKD compared to those receiving nephron-sparing surgery or no surgery. In parallel with these findings, the implications of radical nephrectomy and CKD also translate into adverse cardiovascular events and eventual end stage renal disease. Accordingly, in patients presenting with a renal cortical mass, a comprehensive assessment of current and projected renal function is paramount in determining preferred management options.

8. References

(2002). K/DOQI clinical practice guidelines for chronic kidney disease: evaluation, classification, and stratification. *Am J Kidney Dis* 39(2 Suppl 1), S1-266.

(2010). Cancer Facts and Figures 2010.

Badalato, G., Kates, M., Wisnivesky, J., RoyChoudhury, A., and McKiernan, J. (2011). Survival Following Partial and Radical Nephrectomy for the Treatment of Stage T1bN0M0 Renal Cell Carcinoma in the United States: A Propensity Scoring Approach. *BJU Int* In Press.

Bang, H., Vupputuri, S., Shoham, D. A., Klemmer, P. J., Falk, R. J., Mazumdar, M., Gipson, D., Colindres, R. E., and Kshirsagar, A. V. (2007). SCreening for Occult REnal Disease (SCORED): a simple prediction model for chronic kidney disease. *Arch Intern Med* 167(4), 374-81.

Becker, F., Siemer, S., Hack, M., Humke, U., Ziegler, M., and Stockle, M. (2006a). Excellent long-term cancer control with elective nephron-sparing surgery for selected renal cell carcinomas measuring more than 4 cm. *Eur Urol* 49(6), 1058-63; discussion 1063-4.

Becker, F., Siemer, S., Humke, U., Hack, M., Ziegler, M., and Stockle, M. (2006b). Elective nephron sparing surgery should become standard treatment for small unilateral renal cell carcinoma: Long-term survival data of 216 patients. *Eur Urol* 49(2), 308-13.

Bijol, V., Mendez, G. P., Hurwitz, S., Rennke, H. G., and Nose, V. (2006). Evaluation of the nonneoplastic pathology in tumor nephrectomy specimens: predicting the risk of progressive renal failure. *Am J Surg Pathol* 30(5), 575-84.

Chobanian, A. V., Bakris, G. L., Black, H. R., Cushman, W. C., Green, L. A., Izzo, J. L., Jr., Jones, D. W., Materson, B. J., Oparil, S., Wright, J. T., Jr., and Roccella, E. J. (2003). Seventh report of the Joint National Committee on Prevention, Detection, Evaluation, and Treatment of High Blood Pressure. *Hypertension* 42(6), 1206-52.

Chow, W. H., Dong, L. M., and Devesa, S. S. (2010). Epidemiology and risk factors for kidney cancer. *Nat Rev Urol* 7(5), 245-57.

Clark, A. T., Breau, R. H., Morash, C., Fergusson, D., Doucette, S., and Cagiannos, I. (2008). Preservation of renal function following partial or radical nephrectomy using 24-hour creatinine clearance. *Eur Urol* 54(1), 143-49.

Clark, M. A., Shikanov, S., Raman, J. D., Smith, B., Kaag, M., Russo, P., Wheat, J. C., Wolf, J. S., Jr., Matin, S. F., Huang, W. C., Shalhav, A. L., and Eggener, S. E. (2011). Chronic kidney disease before and after partial nephrectomy. *J Urol* 185(1), 43-8.

Dash, A., Vickers, A. J., Schachter, L. R., Bach, A. M., Snyder, M. E., and Russo, P. (2006). Comparison of outcomes in elective partial vs radical nephrectomy for clear cell renal cell carcinoma of 4-7 cm. *BJU Int* 97(5), 939-45.

Donin, N. M., Suh, L. K., Barlow, L. J., Hruby, G., Newhouse, J., and McKiernan, J. (2011). Tumour diameter and decreased preoperative estimated glomerular filtration rate are independently correlated in patietns with renal cell carcinoma. *BJU Int* In Press.

Ejerblad, E., Fored, C. M., Lindblad, P., Fryzek, J., Dickman, P. W., Elinder, C. G., McLaughlin, J. K., and Nyren, O. (2004). Association between smoking and chronic renal failure in a nationwide population-based case-control study. *J Am Soc Nephrol* 15(8), 2178-85.

Gautam, G., Lifshitz, D., Shikanov, S., Moore, J. M., Eggener, S. E., Shalhav, A. L., and Chang, A. (2010). Histopathological predictors of renal function decrease after laparoscopic radical nephrectomy. *J Urol* 184(5), 1872-6.

Go, A. S., Chertow, G. M., Fan, D., McCulloch, C. E., and Hsu, C. Y. (2004). Chronic kidney disease and the risks of death, cardiovascular events, and hospitalization. *N Engl J Med* 351(13), 1296-305.

Gofrit, O. N., Shapiro, A., Kovalski, N., Landau, E. H., Shenfeld, O. Z., and Pode, D. (2001). Renal cell carcinoma: evaluation of the 1997 TNM system and recommendations for follow-up after surgery. *Eur Urol* 39(6), 669-74; discussion 675.

Hafez, K. S., Fergany, A. F., and Novick, A. C. (1999). Nephron sparing surgery for localized renal cell carcinoma: impact of tumor size on patient survival, tumor recurrence and TNM staging. *J Urol* 162(6), 1930-3.

Hepps, D., and Chernoff, A. (2006). Risk of renal insufficiency in African-Americans after radical nephrectomy for kidney cancer. *Urol Oncol* 24(5), 391-5.

Hollenbeck, B. K., Taub, D. A., Miller, D. C., Dunn, R. L., and Wei, J. T. (2006). National utilization trends of partial nephrectomy for renal cell carcinoma: a case of underutilization? *Urology* 67(2), 254-9.

Huang, W. C., Elkin, E. B., Levey, A. S., Jang, T. L., and Russo, P. (2009). Partial nephrectomy versus radical nephrectomy in patients with small renal tumors--is there a difference in mortality and cardiovascular outcomes? *J Urol* 181(1), 55-61; discussion 61-2.

Huang, W. C., Levey, A. S., Serio, A. M., Snyder, M., Vickers, A. J., Raj, G. V., Scardino, P. T., and Russo, P. (2006). Chronic kidney disease after nephrectomy in patients with renal cortical tumours: a retrospective cohort study. *Lancet Oncol* 7(9), 735-40.

Hunt, J. D., van der Hel, O. L., McMillan, G. P., Boffetta, P., and Brennan, P. (2005). Renal cell carcinoma in relation to cigarette smoking: meta-analysis of 24 studies. *Int J Cancer* 114(1), 101-8.

Jeon, H. G., Jeong, I. G., Lee, J. W., Lee, S. E., and Lee, E. (2009). Prognostic factors for chronic kidney disease after curative surgery in patients with small renal tumors. *Urology* 74(5), 1064-8.

Jewett, M. A., and Zuniga, A. (2008). Renal tumor natural history: the rationale and role for active surveillance. *Urol Clin North Am* 35(4), 627-34; vii.

Kaplan, C., Pasternack, B., Shah, H., and Gallo, G. (1975). Age-related incidence of sclerotic glomeruli in human kidneys. *Am J Pathol* 80(2), 227-34.

Kates, M., Badalato, G., Pitman, M., and McKiernan, J. (2011). The Persistent Overuse of Radical Nephrectomy in the Elderly. *Urology* In Press.

Kim, J. M., Song, P. H., Kim, H. T., and Park, T. C. (2010). Comparison of Partial and Radical Nephrectomy for pT1b Renal Cell Carcinoma. *Korean J Urol* 51(9), 596-600.

Kovacs, G., Akhtar, M., Beckwith, B. J., Bugert, P., Cooper, C. S., Delahunt, B., Eble, J. N., Fleming, S., Ljungberg, B., Medeiros, L. J., Moch, H., Reuter, V. E., Ritz, E., Roos, G., Schmidt, D., Srigley, J. R., Storkel, S., van den Berg, E., and Zbar, B. (1997). The Heidelberg classification of renal cell tumours. *J Pathol* 183(2), 131-3.

Lane, B. R., Abouassaly, R., Gao, T., Weight, C. J., Hernandez, A. V., Larson, B. T., Kaouk, J. H., Gill, I. S., and Campbell, S. C. (2010a). Active treatment of localized renal tumors may not impact overall survival in patients aged 75 years or older. *Cancer* 116(13), 3119-26.

Lane, B. R., Demirjian, S., Weight, C. J., Larson, B. T., Poggio, E. D., and Campbell, S. C. (2010b). Performance of the chronic kidney disease-epidemiology study equations for estimating glomerular filtration rate before and after nephrectomy. *J Urol* 183(3), 896-901.

Lane, B. R., Fergany, A. F., Weight, C. J., and Campbell, S. C. (2010c). Renal functional outcomes after partial nephrectomy with extended ischemic intervals are better than after radical nephrectomy. *J Urol* 184(4), 1286-90.

Lane, B. R., Russo, P., Uzzo, R. G., Hernandez, A. V., Boorjian, S. A., Thompson, R. H., Fergany, A. F., Love, T. E., and Campbell, S. C. (2011). Comparison of cold and warm ischemia during partial nephrectomy in 660 solitary kidneys reveals predominant role of nonmodifiable factors in determining ultimate renal function. *J Urol* 185(2), 421-7.

Lau, W. K., Blute, M. L., Weaver, A. L., Torres, V. E., and Zincke, H. (2000). Matched comparison of radical nephrectomy vs nephron-sparing surgery in patients with unilateral renal cell carcinoma and a normal contralateral kidney. *Mayo Clin Proc* 75(12), 1236-42.

Laudano, M. A., Klafter, F. E., Katz, M., McCann, T. R., Desai, M., Benson, M. C., and McKiernan, J. M. (2008). Pathological tumour diameter predicts risk of conventional subtype in small renal cortical tumours. *BJU Int* 102(10), 1385-8.

Lee, D. J., Hruby, G., Benson, M. C., and McKiernan, J. M. (2010). Renal function and oncologic outcomes in nephron sparing surgery for renal masses in solitary kidneys. *World J Urol.*

Leibovich, B. C., Blute, M. L., Cheville, J. C., Lohse, C. M., Weaver, A. L., and Zincke, H. (2004). Nephron sparing surgery for appropriately selected renal cell carcinoma between 4 and 7 cm results in outcome similar to radical nephrectomy. *J Urol* 171(3), 1066-70.

Lesage, K., Joniau, S., Fransis, K., and Van Poppel, H. (2007). Comparison between open partial and radical nephrectomy for renal tumours: perioperative outcome and health-related quality of life. *Eur Urol* 51(3), 614-20.

Lindblad, P., Chow, W. H., Chan, J., Bergstrom, A., Wolk, A., Gridley, G., McLaughlin, J. K., Nyren, O., and Adami, H. O. (1999). The role of diabetes mellitus in the aetiology of renal cell cancer. *Diabetologia* 42(1), 107-12.

Lowrance, W. T., Yee, D. S., Savage, C., Cronin, A. M., O'Brien, M. F., Donat, S. M., Vickers, A., and Russo, P. (2010). Complications after radical and partial nephrectomy as a function of age. *J Urol* 183(5), 1725-30.

Lucas, S. M., Nuss, G., Stern, J., Lotan, Y., Sagalowsky, A. I., Cadeddu, J. A., and Raj, G. V. (2008). The screening for Occult Renal Disease (SCORED) value is associated with a higher risk for having or developing chronic kidney disease in patients treated for small, unilateral renal masses. *Cancer* 113(10), 2681-6.

Malcolm, J. B., Bagrodia, A., Derweesh, I. H., Mehrazin, R., Diblasio, C. J., Wake, R. W., Wan, J. Y., and Patterson, A. L. (2009). Comparison of rates and risk factors for developing chronic renal insufficiency, proteinuria and metabolic acidosis after radical or partial nephrectomy. *BJU Int* 104(4), 476-81.

Mann, J. F., Gerstein, H. C., Pogue, J., Bosch, J., and Yusuf, S. (2001). Renal insufficiency as a predictor of cardiovascular outcomes and the impact of ramipril: the HOPE randomized trial. *Ann Intern Med* 134(8), 629-36.

Margulis, V., Sanchez-Ortiz, R. F., Tamboli, P., Cohen, D. D., Swanson, D. A., and Wood, C. G. (2007). Renal cell carcinoma clinically involving adjacent organs: experience with aggressive surgical management. *Cancer* 109(10), 2025-30.

McCann, T., Barlow, L., Knight, M., Benson, M., and McKiernan, J. (2009). Evidence of Medical Renal Disease in Surrounding Renal Parenchyma and Its Effect on Onset of Chronic Renal Insufficiency after Renal Surgery. *In* "Presented data, American Urologic Association".

McKiernan, J., Simmons, R., Katz, J., and Russo, P. (2002a). Natural history of chronic renal insufficiency after partial and radical nephrectomy. *Urology* 59(6), 816-20.

McKiernan, J., Yossepowitch, O., Kattan, M. W., Simmons, R., Motzer, R. J., Reuter, V. E., and Russo, P. (2002b). Partial nephrectomy for renal cortical tumors: pathologic findings and impact on outcome. *Urology* 60(6), 1003-9.

Miller, D. C., Hollingsworth, J. M., Hafez, K. S., Daignault, S., and Hollenbeck, B. K. (2006). Partial nephrectomy for small renal masses: an emerging quality of care concern? *J Urol* 175(3 Pt 1), 853-7; discussion 858.

Miller, D. C., Schonlau, M., Litwin, M. S., Lai, J., and Saigal, C. S. (2008). Renal and cardiovascular morbidity after partial or radical nephrectomy. *Cancer* 112(3), 511-20.

Mitchell, R. E., Gilbert, S. M., Murphy, A. M., Olsson, C. A., Benson, M. C., and McKiernan, J. M. (2006). Partial nephrectomy and radical nephrectomy offer similar cancer outcomes in renal cortical tumors 4 cm or larger. *Urology* 67(2), 260-4.

Murphy, A. M., Buck, A. M., Benson, M. C., and McKiernan, J. M. (2009). Increasing detection rate of benign renal tumors: evaluation of factors predicting for benign tumor histologic features during past two decades. *Urology* 73(6), 1293-7.

Novick, A. C., Streem, S., Montie, J. E., Pontes, J. E., Siegel, S., Montague, D. K., and Goormastic, M. (1989). Conservative surgery for renal cell carcinoma: a single-center experience with 100 patients. *J Urol* 141(4), 835-9.

Patard, J. J., Pantuck, A. J., Crepel, M., Lam, J. S., Bellec, L., Albouy, B., Lopes, D., Bernhard, J. C., Guille, F., Lacroix, B., De La Taille, A., Salomon, L., Pfister, C., Soulie, M., Tostain, J., Ferriere, J. M., Abbou, C. C., Colombel, M., and Belldegrun, A. S. (2007). Morbidity and clinical outcome of nephron-sparing surgery in relation to tumour size and indication. *Eur Urol* 52(1), 148-54.

Patard, J. J., Shvarts, O., Lam, J. S., Pantuck, A. J., Kim, H. L., Ficarra, V., Cindolo, L., Han, K. R., De La Taille, A., Tostain, J., Artibani, W., Abbou, C. C., Lobel, B., Chopin, D. K., Figlin, R. A., Mulders, P. F., and Belldegrun, A. S. (2004). Safety and efficacy of partial nephrectomy for all T1 tumors based on an international multicenter experience. *J Urol* 171(6 Pt 1), 2181-5, quiz 2435.

Russo, P., Goetzl, M., Simmons, R., Katz, J., Motzer, R., and Reuter, V. (2002). Partial nephrectomy: the rationale for expanding the indications. *Ann Surg Oncol* 9(7), 680-7.

Sarnak, M. J., Levey, A. S., Schoolwerth, A. C., Coresh, J., Culleton, B., Hamm, L. L., McCullough, P. A., Kasiske, B. L., Kelepouris, E., Klag, M. J., Parfrey, P., Pfeffer, M., Raij, L., Spinosa, D. J., and Wilson, P. W. (2003). Kidney disease as a risk factor for development of cardiovascular disease: a statement from the American Heart Association Councils on Kidney in Cardiovascular Disease, High Blood Pressure Research, Clinical Cardiology, and Epidemiology and Prevention. *Circulation* 108(17), 2154-69.

Schlehofer, B., Pommer, W., Mellemgaard, A., Stewart, J. H., McCredie, M., Niwa, S., Lindblad, P., Mandel, J. S., McLaughlin, J. K., and Wahrendorf, J. (1996). International renal-cell-cancer study. VI. the role of medical and family history. *Int J Cancer* 66(6), 723-6.

Setiawan, V. W., Stram, D. O., Nomura, A. M., Kolonel, L. N., and Henderson, B. E. (2007). Risk factors for renal cell cancer: the multiethnic cohort. *Am J Epidemiol* 166(8), 932-40.

Simmons, M. N., Weight, C. J., and Gill, I. S. (2009). Laparoscopic radical versus partial nephrectomy for tumors >4 cm: intermediate-term oncologic and functional outcomes. *Urology* 73(5), 1077-82.

Sorbellini, M., Kattan, M. W., Snyder, M. E., Hakimi, A. A., Sarasohn, D. M., and Russo, P. (2006). Prognostic nomogram for renal insufficiency after radical or partial nephrectomy. *J Urol* 176(2), 472-6; discussion 476.

Thompson, R. H., and Blute, M. L. (2007). At what point does warm ischemia cause permanent renal damage during partial nephrectomy? *Eur Urol* 52(4), 961-3.

Thompson, R. H., Boorjian, S. A., Lohse, C. M., Leibovich, B. C., Kwon, E. D., Cheville, J. C., and Blute, M. L. (2008). Radical nephrectomy for pT1a renal masses may be associated with decreased overall survival compared with partial nephrectomy. *J Urol* 179(2), 468-71; discussion 472-3.

Thompson, R. H., Kaag, M., Vickers, A., Kundu, S., Bernstein, M., Lowrance, W., Galvin, D., Dalbagni, G., Touijer, K., and Russo, P. (2009). Contemporary use of partial nephrectomy at a tertiary care center in the United States. *J Urol* 181(3), 993-7.

Thompson, R. H., Leibovich, B. C., Lohse, C. M., Zincke, H., and Blute, M. L. (2005). Complications of contemporary open nephron sparing surgery: a single institution experience. *J Urol* 174(3), 855-8.

Weight, C. J., Larson, B. T., Fergany, A. F., Gao, T., Lane, B. R., Campbell, S. C., Kaouk, J. H., Klein, E. A., and Novick, A. C. (2010a). Nephrectomy induced chronic renal insufficiency is associated with increased risk of cardiovascular death and death from any cause in patients with localized cT1b renal masses. *J Urol* 183(4), 1317-23.

Weight, C. J., Lieser, G., Larson, B. T., Gao, T., Lane, B. R., Campbell, S. C., Gill, I. S., Novick, A. C., and Fergany, A. F. (2010b). Partial nephrectomy is associated with improved overall survival compared to radical nephrectomy in patients with unanticipated benign renal tumours. *Eur Urol* 58(2), 293-8.

Yossepowitch, O., Eggener, S. E., Serio, A., Huang, W. C., Snyder, M. E., Vickers, A. J., and Russo, P. (2006). Temporary renal ischemia during nephron sparing surgery is associated with short-term but not long-term impairment in renal function. *J Urol* 176(4 Pt 1), 1339-43; discussion 1343.

Zincke, H., Engen, D. E., Henning, K. M., and McDonald, M. W. (1985). Treatment of renal cell carcinoma by in situ partial nephrectomy and extracorporeal operation with autotransplantation. *Mayo Clin Proc* 60(10), 651-62.

Zini, L., Perrotte, P., Capitanio, U., Jeldres, C., Shariat, S. F., Antebi, E., Saad, F., Patard, J. J., Montorsi, F., and Karakiewicz, P. I. (2009). Radical versus partial nephrectomy: effect on overall and noncancer mortality. *Cancer* 115(7), 1465-71.

10

The Role of B-Cells and B-Cell Targeted Therapies in Lupus Nephritis

Irene Blanco, Saakshi Khattri and Chaim Putterman
Albert Einstein College of Medicine
Division of Rheumatology
Bronx, NY
USA

1. Introduction

Systemic Lupus Erythematosus (SLE) is a multi-systemic autoimmune disorder that can have severe and potentially life-threatening manifestations. One such manifestation is lupus nephritis. While survival rates have improved significantly, SLE, and in particular lupus nephritis, continues to be associated with significant morbidity and mortality.

The incidence of SLE varies greatly among different populations. As a whole, rates are highest in non-Caucasians. Estimated incidence rates of SLE are similar in the US and in Europe where Caucasians have rates of 3.5-4 per 100,000 and those of African descent have significantly higher rates of 9.2-11.4 per 100,000.[1,2] While the disease is present to a certain degree in all populations, SLE affects primarily women in their child-bearing years with a ratio of 9:1 compared to men.[3,4] When men do present with SLE there is evidence that they have worse disease outcomes including increased mortality.[5,6] Regardless of race or gender, mortality in SLE has improved significantly since the 1950's, where the 5-year survival rate was approximately 50%.[7]

Currently, 10-year survival rates range between 85% and 95%.[7] Despite improved overall survival, lupus nephritis (seen in upwards of 60% of all SLE patients) continues to significantly affect morbidity and mortality.[8] While 5-year survival for those without nephritis is approximately 92%, those with this complication have a much lower rate of 82%.[8] Both in the US and in Europe, non-Caucasians have increased rates of nephritis, where not only is the condition more prevalent in these groups, it also tends to be more severe.[5,9] In the US, risk factors for progression to end-stage renal disease include: being African American, Hispanic, male, less than 24 years old and having high activity and chronicity on renal biopsy.[10] Risk factors notwithstanding, it has been shown that patients that receive early treatment have better outcomes.[11,12]

However, even with early and aggressive treatment, one study has found no change in the incidence of end-stage renal disease from lupus nephritis.[13] Therefore, it appears that while medications are usually effective in controlling renal inflammation, a substantial amount of patients fail treatment. In addition, conventional therapies are not target-specific and can lead to significant toxicity. Therefore, given that B cells play such an integral role in the pathogenesis of SLE and lupus nephritis, these cells are potential targets for more specific therapies.

2. Pathogenesis of lupus

The etiology of SLE and specifically lupus nephritis is multi-factorial involving environmental, genetic and hormonal factors to name a few. Loss of tolerance and interactions between the innate and adaptive immune system, as well as T cells and B cells, all play a role in the development of SLE and lupus nephritis.

2.1 Genetics

SLE is a genetically complex disease that generally does not exhibit straightforward mendelian modes of inheritance. In several cases, SLE is associated with rare but highly penetrant mutations: homozygous deficiencies of the complement components C1q, C2 or C4, complete FcγRIIIb deficiency, and mutations in the DNA exonuclease *TREX1*.[14-17] Genes in the human leukocyte antigen (HLA) region of the short arm of chromosome 6 exhibit the strongest association with the risk of developing SLE. Graham et al. identified HLA class II haplotypes containing DRB1 and DQB1 alleles as strong risk factors for human disease.[18]

In a majority of cases, however, SLE genetic susceptibility is probably determined by relatively common variants that are found throughout the population. Each only contributes modestly to the risk of disease; hence the finding of 34% concordance rate in monozygotic twins and 3% in dizygotic twins.[19,20] Genome-wide association studies have found hundreds of single nucleotide polymorphisms associated with SLE. A recent meta-analysis shows a total of 17 well-validated common SLE risk variants including: HLA-DR3, DR2, PTPN22 and STAT4. These variants account for a fraction of the total genetic contribution to SLE. Initial pathway analyses of these risk alleles indicate an important role for B cell development and signalling, signaling through toll-like receptors 7 and 9, and neutrophil function.[21]

2.2 Role of B-cells in SLE

B cells play a major role in the development of SLE, where loss of B cell tolerance is presumed to be the basis of disease. The most common alteration seen is B cell hyperactivity and subsequent autoantibody production. The presence of autoantibodies, particularly anti-nuclear antibodies, anti-Smith and anti-double stranded DNA (anti-DNA) antibodies, form part of the diagnostic criteria for SLE.

Immunoglobulin genes undergo rearrangement during B cell development in the bone marrow, where many autoreactive B cell receptors (BCR) are generated. In lupus patients, many, if not all of the checkpoints that eliminate autoreactive B cells are breached.[22] SLE patients also exhibit high levels of B cell activating factor (BAFF), a survival factor that contributes to the survival of these autoreactive cells. There is also overexpression of CD40L on B cells which results in excessive T cell co-stimulation, another mechanism for the survival of autoreactive B cells.[23,24] However, they not only generate autoantibodies; B cells also act as antigen presenting cells (APC's) providing costimulatory signals necessary for T cell activation, differentiation and expansion. In addition, B cells also produce cytokines like IL-10, IL-16, TNF-α and INF-γ that influence other cells in the immune system.[25] (Figure 1.)

2.3 Toll like receptors in SLE

Toll-like receptors (TLRs) play a key role in innate responses to infections. When bound by endogenous or exogenous ligands, they are involved in acute and chronic inflammatory

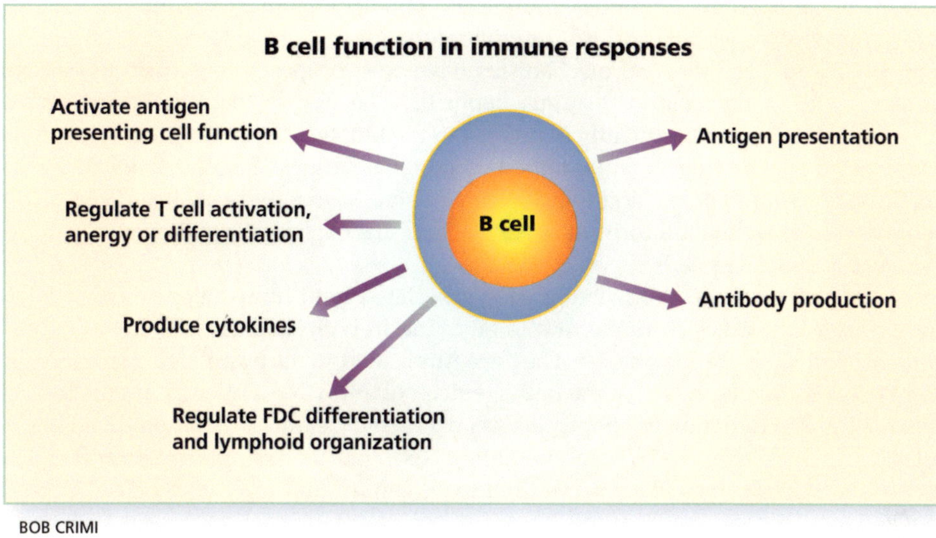

Fig. 1. B cell Function in Immune Responses.
Figure reproduced with permission from *Nature Immunology* and Bob Crimi, 2001;2:764-6

processes. Numerous *in vitro* studies have established that TLR-7 and TLR-9 are involved in immune complex recognition. It is hypothesized that nucleic acid-containing immune complexes are engaged simultaneously by both the BCR and TLR.[27] This engagement of TLR-7 or TLR-9 by an immune complex induces a MYD88-dependent pathway that activates inflammatory transcription factors, including IRF-7, NF-κB and AP-1. This leads to B cell and plasmacytoid dendritic cell (PDC) activation. The activation of PDC's stimulates the inappropriate production of many cytokines, particularly type I IFN which is intimately involved in the pathogenesis of SLE.[26]

How TLRs gain access to nuclear antigens in SLE can be explained by two mechanisms. The first suggests that pre-existing anti-Smith and anti-DNA antibodies form immune complexes with endogenous RNA and DNA, that are then taken up by APCs via Fc receptors. In endosomes, these complexes are degraded into nucleic acid components. These exposed nucleic acids then interact with TLR-7 or TLR-9 resulting in type I IFN production from PDC's and B cell activation. Another model hypothesizes that type I IFN production is induced by TLR recognition of nucleic acids from aberrant degradation of apoptotic cells.[29] Regardless of the mechanism of upregulation of type I IFN, once increased it induces upregulation of TLRs in B cells and subsequent maturation into IgG-secreting plasma cells.[30,31]

3. Pathogenesis of lupus nephrtitis

The serologic hallmark of SLE is the presence of autoantibodies against nuclear antigens.[3] Several antibodies, such as anti-DNA and anti-nucleosome antibodies, are highly specific for the disease.[3,32] There is evidence to suggest that they play a significant role in the pathogenesis of lupus nephritis.

While there are several different classes of lupus nephritis, what all have in common is renal deposition of antibodies, immune complexes and complement.[10] Immunofloresence typically shows staining for various immunoglobulins, where IgG is predominant, in addition to C3 and C1q.[33] Several mechanisms have been proposed to explain the presence of immune complex disposition in lupus nephritis. The first is that extra-renal immune complexes form and are subsequently deposited in the kidney. The second theory postulates that there is direct binding of autoantibodies to renal targets. Finally, there is also the possibility that autoantibodies bind to autoantigens that have previously been bound to the glomerulus. It is likely that all three of these mechanisms explain the pathogenesis of lupus renal disease to some degree.[34]

The antibody that has most consistently been associated with lupus nephritis is anti-DNA antibody. These antibodies were the first to be found in both humans with lupus nephritis and animal models of the disease.[35,36] They are implicated in all postulated mechanisms of disease; however the true extent of the pathogenicity of anti-DNA antibodies is unclear. SLE patients have a dysregulation in apoptosis with decreased clearance of apoptotic bodies that are released in the serum.[37,38] These circulating apoptotic bodies, double-stranded DNA fragments and nucleosomes likely serve as autoantigen for autoreactive B cells.[39] Exposure to these antigens, subsequently causes the generation of anti-nuclear antibodies such as anti-DNA.[40] It is possible that anti-DNA antibodies and the above antigens form complexes in the serum that then deposit in the kidney.

While interesting, several researchers have not been able to confirm the presence of substantial amounts of DNA-anti-DNA complexes in the serum or that these complexes are formed extra-renally and are then significantly deposited in the kidneys.[41,42] Immune complexes injected into normal mice can cause transient depositions in the glomeruli resulting in the activation of mesangial cells, but this is unlikely to cause disease.[43] If extra-renal immune complexes are involved in lupus nephritis, they likely amplify inflammation as opposed to initiating it.

What may in fact happen is that DNA fragments and nucleosomes bind to proteins in the glomerular basement membrane. They then act as "planted antigens" to which previously formed anti-nuclear antibodies can bind.[43,44] Collagen, fibronectin and laminin all have binding sites for DNA. In addition, DNA may bind to previously captured immune complexes and nucleosomes in the basement membrane. Anti-DNA antibodies can then bind, leading to *in situ* immune complex formation.[33,39]

Finally, there is significant evidence to show that anti-DNA antibodies bind directly to glomerular basement membrane proteins. Alpha-actinin, laminin, collagen and heparan sulfate can all directly bind anti-DNA antibodies.[45] The pathogenicity of these antibodies that bind to planted antigens on the basement membrane and/or directly to glomerular antigens is likely the same. Both can cause direct renal toxicity via complement fixation and via FcR expression on infiltrating leukocytes.[43] Neutrophils, macrophages and renal parenchymal cells are subsequently activated releasing inflammatory mediators and upregulating adhesion molecules, subsequently recruiting more leukocytes into the kidney.[46]

Despite the role that B cells play in lupus nephritis through the generation of auto-antibodies, they also exert their influence through immunoglobulin independent mechanisms. Several experiments using MRL-*lpr/lpr* (MRL-*lpr*) mice show that in the setting of B cell deficiency, mice do not develop nephritis while those with altered antibody production continue on to develop disease. Also B cell deficient lupus mice fail to activate CD4 T cells.[47] Therefore, B cells can participate in the pathogenesis of nephritis by acting as highly-efficient APC's thereby activating T cells.[48] CD4 T cells are activated through the MHC II molecule/T cell receptor interaction as well as through CD40/CD40 ligand co-stimulation. When these interactions are blocked, significant improvement in SLE disease activity is observed.[49] B/T cell interactions lead to an amplification of the immune response where activated CD4 T cells activate macrophages and drive autoreactive B cells to undergo somatic hypermutation and affinity maturation.[50]

With the increased understanding of the role of B cells in SLE, new therapies have been developed to specifically target this cell type. Over the course of the next few sections we will discuss the current, less selective, standard of care for the treatment of lupus nephritis and move on to novel, more specific B cell targeted therapies.

4. Current immunosuppressive therapy in lupus nephritis

Treating lupus nephritis involves an induction period of intensive immunosuppressive therapy aimed at halting disease progression. This is followed by a period of maintenance therapy to maintain the response. The treatment of lupus nephritis has undergone a dramatic change from steroids as initial therapy to immunosuppressive therapy like cyclophosphamide.

Steroids were the mainstay of treatment of lupus and lupus nephritis in the early 1960's but such an approach was often unable to control the progression to renal failure and was associated with significant morbidity and mortality.[51] Felson et al. conducted a pooled analysis of all published clinical trials where prednisone alone, or prednisone plus cyclophosphamide or azathioprine was used. They showed that patients receiving immunosuppressive therapy had less renal deterioration, were less likely to have end-stage renal disease, and had better survival rates compared to patients receiving steroids alone. When cyclophosphamide and azathioprine were considered separately, both were associated with a 40% reduction in the rates of adverse renal outcomes.[52]

4.1 Cyclophosphamide

Cyclophosphamide (CYP), an alkylating and cytotoxic agent, depletes both T and B cells reducing the production of pathogenic autoantibodies. Since the publication of studies by Austin et al. and Boumpas et al., CYP has become a mainstay for the treatment of lupus nephritis.

Patients with lupus nephritis enrolled in trials at the NIH between 1969 and 1981 were randomized into one of five treatment protocols: (1) high-dose prednisone; (2) azathioprine + low-dose prednisone; (3) oral CYP + low-dose prednisone; (4) combined oral azathioprine and oral CYP; and (5) intravenous CYP + low-dose oral prednisone. This study showed that renal function was better preserved in patients receiving immunosuppressive therapy, but the difference was statistically significant only for the intravenous CYP plus low-dose prednisone group as compared to the high-dose prednisone group.[53] Boumpas et al. later showed that an extended course of pulse CYP is more effective than 6 months of pulse methylprednisolone in preserving renal function in patients with severe nephritis. The addition of a quarterly intravenous CYP maintenance regimen to monthly pulses also reduced exacerbation rates.[54] These and several other studies established the NIH protocol for the treatment of lupus nephritis. However, this protocol can lead to significant morbidity with complications such infertility, and an increased risk of severe infections.

In response to increased morbidity rates attributable to CYP, the Euro-Lupus Nephritis Trial was developed to test lower doses of intravenous CYP (500 mg every 2 weeks for a total of 6 doses) against the typical NIH protocol for induction. Houssiau et al. found that there was no significant difference between the high dose and low dose patients in renal remission rates, or in developing recurrent renal flares or renal failure. Severe infection was more than twice as frequent in the high-dose group, though the difference was not statistically significant.[55] Ten year follow up data shows that death, sustained doubling of serum creatinine and end-stage renal disease rates did not differ between the low-dose and high-dose group nor did mean serum creatinine, 24 h proteinuria and damage score at last follow-up.[56]

4.2 Mycophenolate mofetil

Mycophenolate mofetil (MMF), the prodrug of mycophenolic acid, inhibits inosine monophosphate dehydrogenase which then suppresses DNA synthesis and the proliferation of T and B cells. Inspired by MMF's efficacy in preventing renal transplant rejection, investigators began to evaluate the drug's use in lupus nephritis. Several small trials showed that MMF was comparable to CYP in the treatment of proliferative LN.[57,58] Ginzler et al. conducted a 24-week randomized, open-label, non-inferiority trial comparing oral MMF with monthly intravenous CYP as induction therapy. They showed that MMF was more effective in inducing remission of lupus nephritis and had a better safety profile.[59]

A study by Chan et al. showed that for the treatment of diffuse proliferative lupus nephritis, one year of MMF therapy was as effective as a six months of CYP followed by six months of azathioprine. The MMF regimen was also found to be less toxic.[60] In the long-term extension trial, serum creatinine in both groups remained stable and comparable. Creatinine clearance increased in the MMF group, but the difference was not statistically significant. MMF treatment was also associated with fewer severe infections. This study showed that MMF constitutes an effective continuous induction and maintenance therapy for lupus nephritis.[61]

Given the reassuring data for the use of MMF, the Aspreva Lupus Management Study (ALMS), a large multicenter, randomized clinical trial, was developed to determine if MMF was in fact better than CYP therapy. They found no difference in response rates when comparing MMF to CYP pulse + azathioprine for maintenance. However, MMF was noted to be better in Hispanic and African American patients. Over the course of the maintenance phase, there was a higher failure rate in the azathioprine group versus in the MMF group (32% v 16%) at 3 years.[62]

Induction therapy with MMF is associated with fewer side effects than with CYP. MMF may be particularly suitable as induction therapy in women of child bearing age where there are less concerns for infertility as compared to CYP treatment. It also may work particularly well in African American and Hispanic patients, two groups with a large burden of disease. Nevertheless, while often better tolerated than CYP, MMF can cause significant morbidity. Many patients experience gastro-intestinal side effects such as diarrhea, nausea and vomiting. Patients treated with MMF are at risk for severe and possibly lethal infections, and are at a higher risk for the development of lymphoma and skin malignancies.Also, while MMF may not affect fertility, the drug had been associated with an increased risk of birth defects.

4.3 Azathioprine

Azathioprine (AZA) is used as a steroid sparing agent in patients with active SLE and as an alternative to CYP for maintenance therapy in lupus nephritis. It is a purine analog and inhibits nucleic acid synthesis thereby affecting both cellular and humoral immune function.

In 1975, Hahn et al. found that there was no significant effect of the addition of AZA to steroids for the early treatment of lupus nephritis.[63] In 2006, Grootscholten et al. showed that CYP pulse therapy was superior to AZA plus methylprednisolone with regards to relapses and short-term infections but renal function at the last visit did not differ between the 2 groups.[64] Although the MAINTAIN nephritis trial showed that MMF was not inferior to AZA in maintaining remission, there were fewer renal flares in patients on MMF.[65] Therefore AZA remains an option for therapy, particularly during pregnancy when other medications are contraindicated. Nevertheless, CYP and MMF continue to be the preferred treatment modalities for lupus nephritis.

5. B-cell targeted therapies

5.1 Rituximab

Rituximab (RTX) is a chimeric antibody directed against CD20, a cell surface protein expressed on certain B cell subsets but not plasma cells. The mechanisms by which it induces B cell depletion is likely through the induction of apoptosis as well as through cell mediated toxicity.[66] Initially used in non-Hodgkin's lymphoma, off-label use in lupus has shown potential efficacy in SLE and lupus nephritis.[67, 68]

Looney et al. conducted one of the first trials investigating the role of RTX in SLE. Eighteen SLE patients were recruited into a phase I/II dose escalation trial, where 7 of 18 patients had nephritis. Although those on CYP at baseline were excluded, the cohort overall had moderately active disease at baseline. Of the 10 patients that successfully depleted their B cells, all experienced some disease improvement. The SLE manifestations that experienced the most improvement were: rashes, mucositis, arthritis and alopecia. The authors do not comment on the overall efficacy in the nephritis patients but do mention one patient with class IV nephritis that entered remission, with remission, with resolution of proliferative changes on repeat biopsy.[69]

An open label trial was then conducted looking at the combination of CYP and RTX in the treatment of refractory SLE. Although 21 of 32 patients had lupus nephritis, the authors do not comment on these patients specifically. Overall, 12 remained disease free after one cycle of RTX. Global British Isles Lupus Assessment Group (BILAG) scores significantly improved at 6 months. Therefore we assume that the nephritis patients did well after RTX, given the entire group did well post treatment. However we do not know if they responded to the same magnitude as the non-nephritis patients.[70]

Jonsdottir et al. showed decreased disease activity scores at 6 months in 16 patients treated with RTX combined with CYP and steroids for refractory SLE. Of these 16 patients, 9 had nephritis, where 8 of 9 had failed treatment with CYP prior to starting RTX. All of the nephritis patients had BILAG scores of A before being given RTX. Response in these 16 patients was good. Five of 9 nephritis patients had BILAG renal scores of C or D at 6 months.[71] Other small trials showed similar efficacy in both treating lupus as well as lupus nephritis.[72-74]

Nevertheless, the results from recent randomized control trials were not as promising. The 52-week Exploratory Phase II/III SLE Evaluation of Rituximab trial, (EXPLORER), tested the efficacy and safety of RTX plus immunosuppressive therapy versus placebo plus immunosuppressive therapy in patients with moderate to severe extra-renal SLE.[75] This study showed that overall, there was no difference between the two groups in terms of both the primary or secondary efficacy endpoints. In subgroup analyses, Africans

Americans and Hispanics (approximately one-third of the study population), who received RTX had significantly better rates of both major and partial responses compared to placebo.

A second large trial, the LUpus Nephritis Assessment with Rituximab trial (LUNAR) was conducted to specifically look at the role RTX therapy in the treatment of class III/IV lupus nephritis. In this trial 144 patients on MMF and corticosteroids were randomized to either the addition of RTX or placebo. Although there were more renal responders in the RTX group (57% v 45.9%), the difference was not statistically significant. Again, though under-powered to detect a difference, the African American group had a higher proportion of patients that responded to RTX versus placebo (70% v 45%).[76] While there may be some benefit to the addition of RTX in African Americans, the medication overall does not seem to grant any additional benefit to current regimens.

Despite the failure of RTX for SLE as well as lupus nephritis in randomized clinical trials, data from the French Autoimmunity and Rituximab registry shows that overall 80 of 113 patients in the cohort responded to RTX therapy. Of those patients with renal disease, 74% showed at least a partial, if not complete response.[67] At the Hôpital Necker in Paris, good results were reported at 22 months of follow-up in the treatment of nephritis patients with concomitant RTX where 60% had a renal response.[77] Recently, Roccatello et al. found that a regimen of 4 doses of RTX with 2 intravenous pulses of CYP in eight patients with severe multi-organ SLE involvement, including nephritis, led to significant improvements in proteinuria at 3,6, and 12 months of follow-up.[78] While the use of RTX as first-line treatment or in patients with a mild form of the disease is not recommended, its off-label use in severe, refractory SLE appears to be sufficiently positive to warrant its use.

5.2 Epratuzumab

Another potential B cell depleting agent is epratuzumab (EPR), a humanized recombinant monoclonal antibody that targets CD22. CD22 is a co-receptor of the BCR and is present throughout B cell maturation, disappearing from the cell surface once it develops into a plasma cell.[79] CD22 has two functions on B cells: it is a negative regulator of BCR signaling and it also acts as an adhesion molecule for the homing of IgD B cells to the bone marrow.[80, 81] Although EPR appears to be cytotoxic to B cells, particularly CD27 negative cells, the depletion is not as pronounced as with RTX.[82,83] Therefore, the mechanism of action may be through the modification of action of CD22.[83,84]

Fourteen moderately active SLE patients were included in the initial clinical trial of EPR. It was infused intravenously every other week for 4 doses, while the patients continued on their baseline immunosuppression. Patients did well; where most decreased their BILAG score ≥50% at 6 weeks, and 38% had a sustained decrease at 18 weeks.[82] Although only four nephritis patients were included in this initial study, 3 of the 4 did show some improvement in BILAG scores.

Data from the phase IIb, EMBLEM trial, shows that EPR continues to be a promising regimen for moderate to severe SLE. A group of 227 patients were randomized to either placebo or one of several doses of EPR where the primary endpoint was the reduction of baseline BILAG scores. A cumulative dose of 2400 mg, either given as 600 mg weekly or 1200 mg every other week, was associated with significant improvements in general BILAG scores over placebo.[85] It remains to be seen what effect the drug will have on lupus nephritis given that the phase III, EMBODY trial excludes patients with active renal disease.[86]

5.3 Belimumab

B cell activating factor (BAFF), also known as B-lymphocyte stimulator (BLyS), and its homologue APRIL (a proliferation-inducing ligand), are members of the TNF-superfamily critical in the development of B cells. They are both widely expressed by neutrophils, macrophages, monocytes and dendritic cells as well as B and T cells.[87] BAFF binds to three receptors: BAFF-R, transmembrane activator and calcium modulator ligand interactor (TACI), and B cell maturation antigen (BCMA). Where BAFF-R only binds BAFF, APRIL can bind to both TACI and BCMA.[87] These receptors are expressed at different times of B cell development. BAFF-R is expressed by all B cells with the exception of plasma cells in the bone marrow. TACI is expressed by naïve and activated B cells, as well as CD27-positive memory B cells, and plasma cells. BCMA is found on tonsillar memory cells, germinal center B cells and plasma cells.[87] Binding of BAFF to its receptor promotes B cell survival and development, allowing for progression past the T1 stage into follicular and marginal zone cells.[88,89] Binding of BAFF and APRIL to TACI and BCMA allows for further survival and progression to class switching and somatic hypermutation, although BAFF is not necessary for this to occur.[90] For further details regarding the effects of BAFF on B cell biology, please refer to a recent review by Liu and Davidson.[88]

BAFF as well as BAFF-R and TACI have been implicated in murine models of SLE and nephritis. NZB/NZW mice have increased levels of circulating BAFF with increased B and T cell activation as well as short and long lived plasma cells.[91] Early inhibition of BAFF-R and TACI in these mice leads to improved mortality, decreased renal inflammation and decreased glomerular immune complex deposition.[92] Young MRL-*lpr* mice treated early with anti-TACI-Ig did not develop anti-DNA antibodies while older mice treated after the onset of disease had improved anti-DNA antibody levels.[93]

BAFF levels have been found to be elevated in patients with SLE compared to normal controls.[94] Whereas serum protein levels may be variable in patients, serum BAFF mRNA levels are less so and correlate better with disease activity.[95] Nevertheless, in a group of 245 patients followed over the course of 2 years, serum BAFF levels were significantly correlated with both disease activity scores and anti-DNA antibodies. In multivariate analyses, changes in disease activity were associated with changes in BAFF levels.[96]

There is data indicating that targeting B cell survival factors may be a potential treatment in lupus nephritis. Neusser et al. recently found on microdissected renal biopsies of lupus nephritis patients that BAFF and APRIL mRNA levels were significantly increased in the glomeruli of patients with class III and IV nephritis when compared to pre-transplant living donor kidneys. There was also increased tubulointerstitial expression of BAFF, APRIL, BCMA and TACI.[97]

Since BAFF levels correlate with disease activity, belimumab was designed as a recombinant fully human antibody, with a high affinity to soluble BAFF. In a phase II, 52 week placebo-controlled trial, 449 SLE patients were randomized to several doses of belimumab versus placebo. Although patients had moderate disease activity at entry, active nephritis patients were excluded from this trial. The medication was well tolerated; however, this study failed to meet its primary end points of reduction of disease activity scores and decreased time to flare at 24 weeks.

However a significant amount of these patients (38.5%) were ANA negative at enrollment. In subgroups analyses, seropositive patients performed significantly better on belimumab than on placebo with regards to disease activity, physician's global assessment (PGA), and

Short Form-36 (SF-36) physical component score.[98] There were also decreases in IgM levels as well as anti-DNA antibody titers, in addition to increased C4 levels in those on belimumab.[92]

Two multi-national phase III trials were conducted in ANA positive, SLE patients with a similar study design to the phase II study. One trial followed patients for 52 weeks (BLISS-52) while the other for 76 weeks (BLISS-76). In both studies, all patients were seropositive for anti-nuclear antibodies and had moderate to severe disease activity. Patients were randomized to either standard of care + placebo, standard of care + belimumab 1 mg/kg, or standard of care + belimumab 10 mg/kg. Again, patients with active nephritis were excluded, and less than 15% of the patients randomized had a history of nephritis. The primary end point was the response rate at 52 weeks, as measured by the SLE Responder Index (SRI).[89,99]

In both studies a total of 1684 patients were randomized to the 3 groups. In the combined results for both BLISS-52 and BLISS-76, SRI was significantly improved by week 52; however, the difference when compared to placebo was modest: belimumab 1 mg/kg v placebo: 46.2% v 38.8%, belimumab 10 mg/kg v placebo: 50.6% v 38.8%. In both belimumab groups, there was significant improvement in the PGA compared to placebo, and time to flare was prolonged in both treatment groups. Moreover, belimumab-treated patients were able to modestly reduce their prednisone dose as compared to placebo. Further details are given in Table 1.

Although there was significant improvement in the SRI in both treatment groups at 52 weeks, the effect appeared to wane. In BLISS-76, the SRI at 76 weeks was no longer significantly different in the treatment groups compared to placebo.[89,99,100] In subgroup analyses by organ system, there was improvement and/or less worsening in several systems; however, renal parameters did not show any significant changes. This was likely due to the fact that lupus nephritis patients were under-represented in these studies.[101]

Despite the modest improvement in disease activity, belimumab is the first medication for SLE approved by the Food and Drug Administration in 50 years. It remains to be seen though what role this drug will play in the treatment of lupus nephritis given that active nephritis patients were excluded from these studies. There is also a possibility that patients of African descent do not respond as well to belimumab. These patients, in both BLISS 52 and 76, had less efficacy as measured by SRI compared to placebo. It is possible though that these are spurious results given the small amount of patients of African descent that were recruited into the BLISS trials. Yet, these results are worrisome given that this population tends to have a worse prognosis with regards to SLE and lupus nephritis.

5.4 Atacicept

As noted, both BAFF and APRIL bind to the TACI receptor. To inhibit the action of both, a fully human fusion protein of the extracellular domain of TACI and the Fc portion of IgG was created as a potential therapy for SLE.[102] Binding of BAFF and APRIL to TACI contributes to short-lived plasma cell survival, resulting in decreased IgM and IgA levels.[103,104] In a phase I trial of atacicept in SLE patients, subcutaneous administration of the medication was well tolerated. As expected, IgM and IgA levels were reduced by approximately 50% and 33% respectively. Both mature and total B cells counts were also reduced.[105] Pena-Rossi et al. found similar findings in their phase I trial investigating the safety of intravenous and subcutaneous preparations of atacicept versus placebo.[106] In these phase I trials, atacicept was well tolerated and appeared to be effective in suppressing B cell function. Two trials are

Endpoints	SOC+ Placebo (N=562)	SOC+ Belimumab 1mg/kg (N=559)	p-value	SOC+ Belimumab 10mg/kg (N=563)	p-value
SRI at Week 52, n(%)	218 (38.8)	258 (46.2)	<0.01	285 (50.6)	<0.0001
• SS≥4-point reduction (%)	230 (40.9)	269 (48.1)	<0.01	297 (52.8)	<0.05
• ≤0.3-point PGA worsening (%)	372 (66.2)	424 (75.8)	<0.001	420 (74.6)	<0.01
• No new 1A/2B BILAG (%)	389 (69.2)	429 (76.7)	<0.01	425 (75.5)	<0.05
Mean % PGA improvement at week 24	24.3	28.8	ns	32.3	<0.01
Mean % PGA improvement at week 52	27.1	36.7	<0.01	37.8	<0.001
SFI flare %(HR)/median time to first flare, days	81.5/84	74.6 (0.82)/110	<0.01	74.6 (0.84)/110	<0.05
Severe SFI flare, %(HR)	23.7	17.0 (0.71)	<0.05	15.6 (0.64)	<0.01
New 1A/2B BILAG, % (HR)	32.0	27.2 (0.83)	ns	24.9 (0.75)	<0.05
New 1A BILAG, % (HR)	23.1	19.0 (0.81)	ns	16.2 (0.67)	<0.01
Prednisone dose reduction from >7.5mg/day baseline by 25% or to ≤7.5mg/day, during weeks 40-52, n (%)	39 (12.3)	67 (20.1)	<0.01	58 (17.9)	<0.05
Prednisone dose increase from ≤7.5 to >7.5mg/day at week 52, n (%)	82 (33.6)	58 (25.8)	ns	62 (25.9)	ns
SF-36 PCS change from baseline at week 52, mean (SD)	+2.9 (0.3)	+4.3 (0.4)	<0.01	+3.8 (0.3)	<0.05
FACIT-fatigue score change from baseline at week 52, mean (SD)	+2.5 (0.4)	+4.8 (0.4)	<0.001	+4.7 (0.4)	<0.001

Table 1. Combined Efficacy Results Of Bliss-52 And Bliss-76**
Abbreviations: BLISS: Belimumab International SLE Study: SRI: Systemic Response Index: SS: SELENA-SLEDAI; PGA, Physician's Global Assessment; HR, Hazard Ratio; SD: Standard Deviation; SFI: SS Flare Index; SF-36, Short Form-36; PCS, Physical Component Score; SOC: Standard of Care.
**Table reprinted from Biologics: Target and Therapy, Volume 5, Thanou-Stavraki, Sawalha AH, "An Update on Belimumab for the Treatment of Lupus", 2011 with permission from Dove Medical Press Ltd, and with additional permission from John Wiley and Sons.

currently underway to study the potential efficacy in the treatment of SLE. The first is a phase II/III trial in SLE patients with moderate disease activity; active nephritis patients are excluded from this study. However, a phase Ib trial in active lupus nephritis patients failing MMF treatment is currently recruiting patients.[86]

6. Possible future therapies

6.1 Abatacept

Binding of CD28 on T cells to its ligand CD80/86 on APCs and activated B cells provides the major costimulatory activation signal to T cells. Endogenous CTLA-4 is an inhibitory molecule on previously activated T cells that binds CD80/86 with higher affinity than CD28. Abatacept, a fusion protein of the extracellular portion of CTLA-4 with the Fc portion of IgG, takes advantage of this and blocks the interaction of CD28 with CD80/86, blocking T cell activation.[107]

Abatacept has been studied extensively in mouse models of lupus. Administration of CTLA-4 Ig to female NZB/NZW lupus-prone mice prevented the development of autoantibody production and kidney disease resulting in prolonged survival.[108] Administration of CTLA-4 Ig also prevented the onset of disease in SLE-prone NZB/NZW F1 mice.[109] Schiffer et al. showed that short-term administration of CTLA-4 Ig and CYP induced remission of nephritis in NZW/W mice with the resolution of proteinuria.[110] Treatment with abatacept increased lifespan of mice treated with CTLA-4 Ig plus CYP compared with those treated with CYP alone.

A phase IIb, multicenter, randomized, placebo controlled trial was conducted to evaluate the efficacy and safety of abatacept versus placebo for the treatment of SLE. This study included only patients with non-life threatening manifestations where the primary endpoint was a new BILAG flare A or B over 12 months. 118 patients were randomized to receive abatacept and 57 to receive placebo. The percentage of new BILAG A/B flares over 12 months did not different significantly between the groups (79.7% in the abatacept group and 82.5% in the placebo group). Consequently, this study failed to meet its primary endpoints. However, improvements in certain measures were noted in the study. At each visit throughout the trial, investigators were asked to state if the patient was experiencing a disease flare. By this measure, a difference in flare rates between the abatacept group (63.6%) and placebo group (82.5%) was noted.[111] Adverse events were comparable in the abatacept and placebo groups but serious adverse events were higher in the abatacept group.

Abatacept potentially has some efficacy in SLE and is being studied in two ongoing trials for the treatment of lupus nephritis, one in conjunction with MMF and the other in conjunction with CYP.[86]

6.2 TLR inhibitors

As previously mentioned, there are several studies that point to Toll-like receptors as possible contributors to the pathogenesis of SLE. While there are multiple TLRs, there are two that are of particular interest: TLR-7 that recognizes single stranded viral RNA and TLR-9 that recognizes bacterial hypomethylated DNA.[112] These two TLRs are implicated in both the activation of B cells in murine models and SLE patients, as well as in the generation of type I IFN, which can in turn also upregulate B cells.[112]

TLR-9 recognizes hypomethylated CpG-oligodeoxynucleotides (CpG-ODN), a motif present in bacterial DNA which has been found to induce T cell independent activation of B cells as well as the activation of other APCs such as dendritic cells.[113] Humans recognize foreign DNA as foreign because it is not methylated as is human DNA. SLE patients though have abnormalities in DNA methylation leading to segments of hypomethylated DNA.[112] Theoretically, when SLE patients release apoptotic bodies and create immune complexes with chromatin, they are exposing this hypomethylated DNA to TLR-9.[112] This has been shown *in vitro* where immune complexes containing DNA and IgG were bound to autoreactive B cells and induced the activation of the cell through TLR-9.[114]

Administration of CpG-ODN in several murine models of SLE is associated with worse disease activity. In MRL-*lpr* mice, CpG-ODN precipitated the progression to cresenteric nephritis and an increase in anti-DNA antibodies where TLR-9 localized to glomerular, tubulointerstitial and perivascular infiltrates.[115,116] TLR-9 localizes to the proximal tubules in NZB x NZW mice and is associated with increased proteinuria and tubular fibrosis when stimulated with CpG DNA and serum from lupus patients.[117]

In mononuclear cells of SLE patients with moderate disease activity, TLR-9 expression is higher than in those with inactive disease or healthy controls. The percentage of memory B cells and plasma cells expressing TLR-9 is higher in those with active disease and correlates with anti-DNA antibody titers.[118, 119] When B cells from active SLE patients were cultured with CpG-ODN, not only was there increased expression of TLR-9 but there was also increased anti-DNA antibody production.

In patients with lupus nephritis, TLR-9 and the other TLRs that bind nucleic acids (TLR-3, -7, and -8) are expressed throughout the kidney: in the glomeruli, proximal and distal tubules as well as in the capillaries.[120] In proliferative disease, TLR-9 expression co-localizes to areas with immune complex deposition, and is increased in those with higher disease activity on pathology and with increased serum anti-DNA antibodies.[26]

Autoimmunity via TLR-7 seems to function in a manner analogous to that of TLR-9. The RNA associated Smith and RNP proteins are common targets for auto-antibodies in SLE patients. RNA bound to these proteins are bound to immune complexes by anti-RNP antibodies causing activation of B cells through BCR as well as TLR signaling.[121] Activation by late apoptotic thymocytes generates anti-DNA antibodies via TLR-7 in B6 mice. In the Yaa murine lupus model, where autoimmunity is caused by a duplication of TLR-7 gene, when the receptor is deleted there is an improvement in auto-antibody levels and glomerulonephritis.[122] Although TLR-7 has not been as extensively studied in human disease, there is increased TLR-7 mRNA expression relative to healthy controls and it is correlated with type I IFN levels.[119] In patients with lupus nephritis there is moderate TLR-7 expression in the distal tubules and in Bowman's capsule.[120]

Given the apparent role that TLRs play in SLE and the likely role they play in nephritis, TLR inhibitors are now being investigated as possible treatments for SLE. This is especially important in light of recent findings that glucocorticoids in murine lupus models fail to inhibit TLR signaling in plasmacytoid dendritic cells.[123] This may partially explain why certain patients do not respond sufficiently to steroid therapy.

Several synthetic inhibitory oligonucleotides (INH-ODN) have been generated with the goal of blocking the activation of TLR-9 and TLR-7.[124,125] These INH-ODNs have proven to be effective in various mouse models. In NZB/NZW mice, treatment with an INH-ODN expressing either a TTAGGG motif or GpG not only delays the signs of nephritis but leads to increased survival.[126,127] Treatment of MRL-*lpr* mice with INH-ODNs that are specific for TLR-7 (IRS 661) and TLR-7 and -9 (IRS 954) leads to improvement of nephritis and in the case of IRS 661, reduced levels of anti-dsDNA antibodies, and anti-Smith antibodies.[116,128] NZBxNZW mice injected twice weekly with IRS 954 from age 4-9 months showed lower levels of autoantibodies as compared to controls as well reduced proteinuria and nephritis on pathology.[129]

Lenert et al. recently developed restricted activity-INH-ODNs (R-INH-ODN). They modified several INH-ODN constructs so that they no longer formed configurations, such as the G4 stack, that may have non-specific immune properties. *In vitro,* R-INH-ODNs were found to be 10 to 30 fold less potent in murine and human B cells. However, when encountering autoreactive B cells in vivo, R-INH-ODN were more potent than broad acting-INH-ODN. MRL-*lpr* mice treated with R-INH-ODN showed less proteinuria, improved renal score, and decreased renal IgG deposits as well as decreased anti-DNA and anti-Smith antibodies. Therefore R-INH-ODN are potentially more effective than other INH-ODNs when the BCR is activated in conjunction with either TLR-7 or TLR-9.[130]

Although promising, there are currently no clinical trials looking at the safety and efficacy of INH-ODNs in the treatment of SLE. It is unknown what role these potential medications will play with regards to current regimens, given that blocking TLRs may cause a significantly increased risk of infection. Only time will tell if these molecules will be developed further for potential use in humans.

7. Conclusion

Lupus nephritis causes significant morbidity and mortality. While current regimens have reduced the burden of disease, many patients continue on to end-stage renal disease despite treatment with aggressive immunosuppression. Given that B cells play such an integral role in nephritis through the generation of pathogenic autoantibodies and by acting as APCs, they are a natural target for therapy. Despite the fact that rituximab causes profound B cell depletion, two phase III clinical trials have failed to show increased efficacy in SLE. Epratuzumab, on the other hand, also causes some level of B cell depletion and may possibly modify the actions of CD22 on B cells. So far early trials are positive for this medication, however lacking nephritis specific data, it is difficult to say if epratuzumab will add significantly to current nephritis regimens.

Belimumab, while showing modest efficacy for the treatment of SLE, has also not been tested in patients with active lupus nephritis. Now that it has been approved by the FDA, it will be important to follow reports of its use in active nephritis patients, and to conduct nephritis specific trials to evaluate its use in this population. Nevertheless, belimumab is an exciting addition to our anti-B cell armamentarium.

Abatacept failed to meet primary endpoints in a phase IIb clinical trial. Despite this there is sufficient positive data that clinical trials in lupus nephritis are currently being conducted. Hopefully this medication proves to have significant efficacy in the nephritis population. Lastly, TLR inhibitors such as INH-ODNs, may eventually become an option for the treatment of lupus nephritis. Currently data is limited to mouse lupus models; however, studies are showing promise in that they limit the progression of renal disease in these animals.

Figure 2 summarizes some of the possible B cell directed therapies that can be used in lupus nephritis. All in all, while B cells seem to be a logical target for the treatment of lupus nephritis, the best way to target them remains elusive. Further studies and medication development will hopefully lead to an optimal treatment regimen where end-stage renal disease will become a rarely seen complication of nephritis.

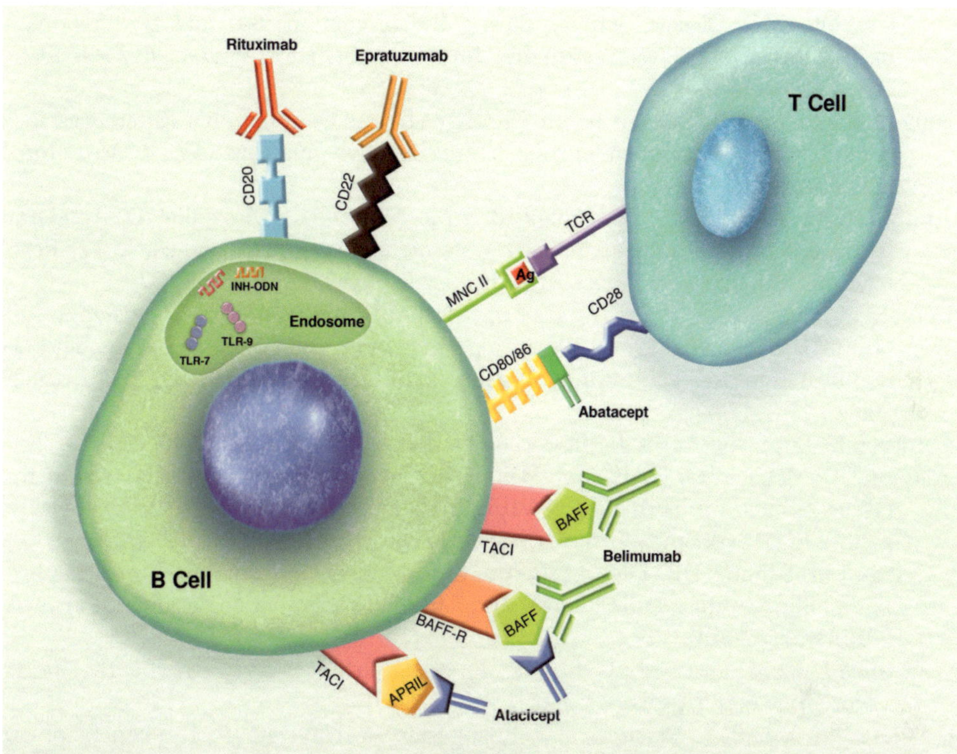

Fig. 2. Potential B cell Targeted Therapies for SLE and Lupus Nephritis.*
Rituximab: Chimeric, anti-CD20 monoclonal antibody; **Epratuzumab**: Humanized anti-CD 22 monoclonal antibody; **Belimumab**: Humanized monoclonal antibody targeting soluble BAFF; **Atacicept**: Recombinant fusion protein of the extracellular portion of the TACI receptor to the Fc portion of IgG targeting both soluble BAFF and soluble APRIL; **Abatacept**: Recombinant fusion protein of the extracellular portion of the CTLA-4 inhibitory molecule to the Fc portion of IgG targeting interaction of CD80/86 with CD28, inhibiting T cell co-stimulation; **INH-ODN**: Synthetic oligonucleotides that inhibit Toll-like Receptors, particularly TLR-7 and TLR-9.
*For the sake of simplicity BCMA, a receptor that also binds to both BAFF and APRIL, has been left off of the schematic.

8. References

[1] Hopkinson ND, Doherty M, Powell RJ. Clinical features and race-specific incidence/prevalence rates of systemic lupus erythematosus in a geographically complete cohort of patients. *Ann. Rheum. Dis.* Oct 1994;53(10):675-680.

[2] McCarty DJ, Manzi S, Medsger TA, Jr., Ramsey-Goldman R, LaPorte RE, Kwoh CK. Incidence of systemic lupus erythematosus. Race and gender differences. *Arthritis Rheum.* Sep 1995;38(9):1260-1270.
[3] Rahman A, Isenberg DA. Systemic lupus erythematosus. *N. Engl. J. Med.* Feb 28 2008;358(9):929-939.
[4] Sanchez-Guerrero J, Villegas A, Mendoza-Fuentes A, Romero-Diaz J, Moreno-Coutino G, Cravioto MC. Disease activity during the premenopausal and postmenopausal periods in women with systemic lupus erythematosus. *Am. J. Med.* Oct 15 2001;111(6):464-468.
[5] Seligman VA, Lum RF, Olson JL, Li H, Criswell LA. Demographic differences in the development of lupus nephritis: a retrospective analysis. *Am. J. Med.* Jun 15 2002;112(9):726-729.
[6] Andrade RM, Alarcon GS, Fernandez M, Apte M, Vila LM, Reveille JD. Accelerated damage accrual among men with systemic lupus erythematosus: XLIV. Results from a multiethnic US cohort. *Arthritis Rheum.* Feb 2007;56(2):622-630.
[7] Cervera R, Khamashta MA, Font J, et al. Morbidity and mortality in systemic lupus erythematosus during a 10-year period: a comparison of early and late manifestations in a cohort of 1,000 patients. *Medicine (Baltimore).* Sep 2003;82(5):299-308.
[8] Cameron JS. Lupus nephritis. *J. Am. Soc. Nephrol.* Feb 1999;10(2):413-424.
[9] Alarcon GS, McGwin G, Jr., Bastian HM, et al. Systemic lupus erythematosus in three ethnic groups. VII [correction of VIII]. Predictors of early mortality in the LUMINA cohort. LUMINA Study Group. *Arthritis Rheum.* Apr 2001;45(2):191-202.
[10] Ortega LM, Schultz DR, Lenz O, Pardo V, Contreras GN. Review: Lupus nephritis: pathologic features, epidemiology and a guide to therapeutic decisions. *Lupus.* Apr 2010;19(5):557-574.
[11] Zabaleta-Lanz ME, Munoz LE, Tapanes FJ, et al. Further description of early clinically silent lupus nephritis. *Lupus.* 2006;15(12):845-851.
[12] Esdaile JM, Joseph L, MacKenzie T, Kashgarian M, Hayslett JP. The benefit of early treatment with immunosuppressive agents in lupus nephritis. *J. Rheumatol.* Nov 1994;21(11):2046-2051.
[13] Ward MM. Changes in the incidence of endstage renal disease due to lupus nephritis in the United States, 1996-2004. *J. Rheumatol.* Jan 2009;36(1):63-67.
[14] Pickering MC, Walport MJ. Links between complement abnormalities and systemic lupus erythematosus. *Rheumatology (Oxford).* Feb 2000;39(2):133-141.
[15] Lee-Kirsch MA, Gong M, Chowdhury D, et al. Mutations in the gene encoding the 3'-5' DNA exonuclease TREX1 are associated with systemic lupus erythematosus. *Nat Genet.* Sep 2007;39(9):1065-1067.
[16] Walport MJ, Davies KA, Botto M. C1q and systemic lupus erythematosus. *Immunobiology.* Aug 1998;199(2):265-285.
[17] Fanciulli M, Norsworthy PJ, Petretto E, et al. FCGR3B copy number variation is associated with susceptibility to systemic, but not organ-specific, autoimmunity. *Nat Genet.* Jun 2007;39(6):721-723.
[18] Graham RR, Ortmann WA, Langefeld CD, et al. Visualizing human leukocyte antigen class II risk haplotypes in human systemic lupus erythematosus. *Am J Hum Genet.* Sep 2002;71(3):543-553.

[19] Block SR, Winfield JB, Lockshin MD, D'Angelo WA, Christian CL. Studies of twins with systemic lupus erythematosus. A review of the literature and presentation of 12 additional sets. *Am J Med.* Oct 1975;59(4):533-552.

[20] Deapen D, Escalante A, Weinrib L, et al. A revised estimate of twin concordance in systemic lupus erythematosus. *Arthritis Rheum.* Mar 1992;35(3):311-318.

[21] Graham RR, Hom G, Ortmann W, Behrens TW. Review of recent genome-wide association scans in lupus. *J Intern Med.* Jun 2009;265(6):680-688.

[22] Yurasov S, Wardemann H, Hammersen J, et al. Defective B cell tolerance checkpoints in systemic lupus erythematosus. *J Exp Med.* Mar 7 2005;201(5):703-711.

[23] Liu K, Mohan C. Altered B-cell signaling in lupus. *Autoimmun Rev.* Jan 2009;8(3):214-218.

[24] Hostmann A, Jacobi AM, Mei H, Hiepe F, Dorner T. Peripheral B cell abnormalities and disease activity in systemic lupus erythematosus. *Lupus.* Dec 2008;17(12):1064-1069.

[25] Moura R, Agua-Doce A, Weinmann P, Graca L, Fonseca JE. B cells from the bench to the clinical practice. *Acta Reumatol Port.* Apr-Jun 2008;33(2):137-154.

[26] Papadimitraki ED, Tzardi M, Bertsias G, Sotsiou E, Boumpas DT. Glomerular expression of toll-like receptor-9 in lupus nephritis but not in normal kidneys: implications for the amplification of the inflammatory response. *Lupus.* Aug 2009;18(9):831-835.

[27] Kim WU, Sreih A, Bucala R. Toll-like receptors in systemic lupus erythematosus; prospects for therapeutic intervention. *Autoimmun Rev.* Jan 2009;8(3):204-208.

[28] Marshak-Rothstein A. Toll-like receptors in systemic autoimmune disease. *Nat Rev Immunol.* Nov 2006;6(11):823-835.

[29] Barton GM, Kagan JC, Medzhitov R. Intracellular localization of Toll-like receptor 9 prevents recognition of self DNA but facilitates access to viral DNA. *Nat Immunol.* Jan 2006;7(1):49-56.

[30] Lovgren T, Eloranta ML, Kastner B, Wahren-Herlenius M, Alm GV, Ronnblom L. Induction of interferon-alpha by immune complexes or liposomes containing systemic lupus erythematosus autoantigen- and Sjogren's syndrome autoantigen-associated RNA. *Arthritis Rheum.* Jun 2006;54(6):1917-1927.

[31] Eloranta ML, Lovgren T, Finke D, et al. Regulation of the interferon-alpha production induced by RNA-containing immune complexes in plasmacytoid dendritic cells. *Arthritis Rheum.* Aug 2009;60(8):2418-2427.

[32] Muller S, Dieker J, Tincani A, Meroni PL. Pathogenic anti-nucleosome antibodies. *Lupus.* May 2008;17(5):431-436.

[33] Foster MH. T cells and B cells in lupus nephritis. *Semin. Nephrol.* Jan 2007;27(1):47-58.

[34] Su W, Madaio MP. Recent advances in the pathogenesis of lupus nephritis: autoantibodies and B cells. *Semin. Nephrol.* Nov 2003;23(6):564-568.

[35] Ceppellini R, Polli E, Celada F. A DNA-reacting factor in serum of a patient with lupus erythematosus diffusus. *Proc. Soc. Exp. Biol. Med.* Dec 1957;96(3):572-574.

[36] Krishnan C, Kaplan MH. Immunopathologic studies of systemic lupus erythematosus. II. Antinuclear reaction of gamma-globulin eluted from homogenates and isolated glomeruli of kidneys from patients with lupus nephritis. *J. Clin. Invest.* Apr 1967;46(4):569-579.

[37] Courtney PA, Crockard AD, Williamson K, Irvine AE, Kennedy RJ, Bell AL. Increased apoptotic peripheral blood neutrophils in systemic lupus erythematosus: relations with disease activity, antibodies to double stranded DNA, and neutropenia. *Ann. Rheum. Dis.* May 1999;58(5):309-314.

[38] Williams RC, Jr., Malone CC, Meyers C, Decker P, Muller S. Detection of nucleosome particles in serum and plasma from patients with systemic lupus erythematosus using monoclonal antibody 4H7. *J. Rheumatol.* Jan 2001;28(1):81-94.

[39] Clatworthy MR, Smith KG. B cells in glomerulonephritis: focus on lupus nephritis. *Semin Immunopathol.* Nov 2007;29(4):337-353.

[40] Mevorach D, Zhou JL, Song X, Elkon KB. Systemic exposure to irradiated apoptotic cells induces autoantibody production. *J. Exp. Med.* Jul 20 1998;188(2):387-392.

[41] Izui S, Lambert PH, Miescher PA. Failure to detect circulating DNA--anti-DNA complexes by four radioimmunological methods in patients with systemic lupus erythematosus. *Clin. Exp. Immunol.* Dec 1977;30(3):384-392.

[42] Hahn BH. Antibodies to DNA. *N. Engl. J. Med.* May 7 1998;338(19):1359-1368.

[43] Shlomchik MJ, Madaio MP. The role of antibodies and B cells in the pathogenesis of lupus nephritis. *Springer Semin. Immunopathol.* May 2003;24(4):363-375.

[44] Berden JH, Licht R, van Bruggen MC, Tax WJ. Role of nucleosomes for induction and glomerular binding of autoantibodies in lupus nephritis. *Curr. Opin. Nephrol. Hypertens.* May 1999;8(3):299-306.

[45] Yung S, Chan TM. Anti-DNA antibodies in the pathogenesis of lupus nephritis--the emerging mechanisms. *Autoimmun Rev.* Feb 2008;7(4):317-321.

[46] Nimmerjahn F, Ravetch JV. Fcgamma receptors: old friends and new family members. *Immunity.* Jan 2006;24(1):19-28.

[47] Chan OT, Madaio MP, Shlomchik MJ. The central and multiple roles of B cells in lupus pathogenesis. *Immunol. Rev.* Jun 1999;169:107-121.

[48] Pierce SK, Morris JF, Grusby MJ, et al. Antigen-presenting function of B lymphocytes. *Immunol. Rev.* Dec 1988;106:149-180.

[49] Kalled SL, Cutler AH, Datta SK, Thomas DW. Anti-CD40 ligand antibody treatment of SNF1 mice with established nephritis: preservation of kidney function. *J. Immunol.* Mar 1 1998;160(5):2158-2165.

[50] Shlomchik MJ, Craft JE, Mamula MJ. From T to B and back again: positive feedback in systemic autoimmune disease. *Nat Rev Immunol.* Nov 2001;1(2):147-153.

[51] Pollak VE. Treatment of the Nephritis of Systemic Lupus Erythematosus. *Mod Treat.* Jan 1964;20:89-99.

[52] Felson DT, Anderson J. Evidence for the superiority of immunosuppressive drugs and prednisone over prednisone alone in lupus nephritis. Results of a pooled analysis. *N Engl J Med.* Dec 13 1984;311(24):1528-1533.

[53] Austin HA, 3rd, Klippel JH, Balow JE, et al. Therapy of lupus nephritis. Controlled trial of prednisone and cytotoxic drugs. *N Engl J Med.* Mar 6 1986;314(10):614-619.

[54] Boumpas DT, Austin HA, 3rd, Vaughn EM, et al. Controlled trial of pulse methylprednisolone versus two regimens of pulse cyclophosphamide in severe lupus nephritis. *Lancet.* Sep 26 1992;340(8822):741-745.

[55] Houssiau FA, Vasconcelos C, D'Cruz D, et al. Immunosuppressive therapy in lupus nephritis: the Euro-Lupus Nephritis Trial, a randomized trial of low-dose versus

high-dose intravenous cyclophosphamide. *Arthritis Rheum.* Aug 2002;46(8):2121-2131.

[56] Houssiau FA, Vasconcelos C, D'Cruz D, et al. The 10-year follow-up data of the Euro-Lupus Nephritis Trial comparing low-dose and high-dose intravenous cyclophosphamide. *Ann Rheum Dis.* Jan 2010;69(1):61-64.

[57] Zhu B, Chen N, Lin Y, et al. Mycophenolate mofetil in induction and maintenance therapy of severe lupus nephritis: a meta-analysis of randomized controlled trials. *Nephrol Dial Transplant.* Jul 2007;22(7):1933-1942.

[58] Walsh M, James M, Jayne D, Tonelli M, Manns BJ, Hemmelgarn BR. Mycophenolate mofetil for induction therapy of lupus nephritis: a systematic review and meta-analysis. *Clin J Am Soc Nephrol.* Sep 2007;2(5):968-975.

[59] Ginzler EM, Dooley MA, Aranow C, et al. Mycophenolate mofetil or intravenous cyclophosphamide for lupus nephritis. *N Engl J Med.* Nov 24 2005;353(21):2219-2228.

[60] Chan TM, Li FK, Tang CS, et al. Efficacy of mycophenolate mofetil in patients with diffuse proliferative lupus nephritis. Hong Kong-Guangzhou Nephrology Study Group. *N Engl J Med.* Oct 19 2000;343(16):1156-1162.

[61] Chan TM, Tse KC, Tang CS, Mok MY, Li FK. Long-term study of mycophenolate mofetil as continuous induction and maintenance treatment for diffuse proliferative lupus nephritis. *J Am Soc Nephrol.* Apr 2005;16(4):1076-1084.

[62] Appel GB, Contreras G, Dooley MA, et al. Mycophenolate mofetil versus cyclophosphamide for induction treatment of lupus nephritis. *J Am Soc Nephrol.* May 2009;20(5):1103-1112.

[63] Contreras G, Roth D, Pardo V, Striker LG, Schultz DR. Lupus nephritis: a clinical review for practicing nephrologists. *Clin Nephrol.* Feb 2002;57(2):95-107.

[64] Grootscholten C, Ligtenberg G, Hagen EC, et al. Azathioprine/methylprednisolone versus cyclophosphamide in proliferative lupus nephritis. A randomized controlled trial. *Kidney Int.* Aug 2006;70(4):732-742.

[65] Houssiau FA, D'Cruz D, Sangle S, et al. Azathioprine versus mycophenolate mofetil for long-term immunosuppression in lupus nephritis: results from the MAINTAIN Nephritis Trial. *Ann Rheum Dis.* Dec 2010;69(12):2083-2089.

[66] Diamanti AP, Rosado MM, Carsetti R, Valesini G. B cells in SLE: different biological drugs for different pathogenic mechanisms. *Autoimmun Rev.* Dec 2007;7(2):143-148.

[67] Terrier B, Amoura Z, Ravaud P, et al. Safety and efficacy of rituximab in systemic lupus erythematosus: results from 136 patients from the French AutoImmunity and Rituximab registry. *Arthritis Rheum.* Aug 2010;62(8):2458-2466.

[68] Ramos-Casals M, Soto MJ, Cuadrado MJ, Khamashta MA. Rituximab in systemic lupus erythematosus: A systematic review of off-label use in 188 cases. *Lupus.* Aug 2009;18(9):767-776.

[69] Looney RJ, Anolik JH, Campbell D, et al. B cell depletion as a novel treatment for systemic lupus erythematosus: a phase I/II dose-escalation trial of rituximab. *Arthritis Rheum.* Aug 2004;50(8):2580-2589.

[70] Ng KP, Cambridge G, Leandro MJ, Edwards JC, Ehrenstein M, Isenberg DA. B cell depletion therapy in systemic lupus erythematosus: long-term follow-up and predictors of response. *Ann. Rheum. Dis.* Sep 2007;66(9):1259-1262.

[71] Jonsdottir T, Gunnarsson I, Risselada A, Henriksson EW, Klareskog L, van Vollenhoven RF. Treatment of refractory SLE with rituximab plus cyclophosphamide: clinical effects, serological changes, and predictors of response. *Ann Rheum Dis.* Mar 2008;67(3):330-334.

[72] Tokunaga M, Saito K, Kawabata D, et al. Efficacy of rituximab (anti-CD20) for refractory systemic lupus erythematosus involving the central nervous system. *Ann Rheum Dis.* Apr 2007;66(4):470-475.

[73] Albert D, Dunham J, Khan S, et al. Variability in the biological response to anti-CD20 B cell depletion in systemic lupus erythaematosus. *Ann Rheum Dis.* Dec 2008;67(12):1724-1731.

[74] Gunnarsson I, Sundelin B, Jonsdottir T, Jacobson SH, Henriksson EW, van Vollenhoven RF. Histopathologic and clinical outcome of rituximab treatment in patients with cyclophosphamide-resistant proliferative lupus nephritis. *Arthritis Rheum.* Apr 2007;56(4):1263-1272.

[75] Merrill JT, Neuwelt CM, Wallace DJ, et al. Efficacy and safety of rituximab in moderately-to-severely active systemic lupus erythematosus: the randomized, double-blind, phase II/III systemic lupus erythematosus evaluation of rituximab trial. *Arthritis Rheum.* Jan 2010;62(1):222-233.

[76] Furie RA, Looney, R.J., Rovin, B., Latinis, K.M., Appel, G., Sanchez-Guerrero, J., et al. Efficacy and Safety of Rituximab in Subjects with Active Proliferative Lupus Nephritis (LN): Results From the Randomized, Double-Blind Phase III LUNAR Study [abstract]. *Arthritis Rheum.* 2009;60 Suppl(10):1149.

[77] Melander C, Sallee M, Trolliet P, et al. Rituximab in severe lupus nephritis: early B-cell depletion affects long-term renal outcome. *Clin J Am Soc Nephrol.* Mar 2009;4(3):579-587.

[78] Roccatello D, Sciascia S, Rossi D, et al. Intensive short-term treatment with rituximab, cyclophosphamide and methylprednisolone pulses induces remission in severe cases of SLE with nephritis and avoids further immunosuppressive maintenance therapy. *Nephrol. Dial. Transplant.* Mar 8 2011.

[79] Schwartz-Albiez R, Dorken B, Monner DA, Moldenhauer G. CD22 antigen: biosynthesis, glycosylation and surface expression of a B lymphocyte protein involved in B cell activation and adhesion. *Int. Immunol.* Jul 1991;3(7):623-633.

[80] Doody GM, Justement LB, Delibrias CC, et al. A role in B cell activation for CD22 and the protein tyrosine phosphatase SHP. *Science.* Jul 14 1995;269(5221):242-244.

[81] Nitschke L, Floyd H, Ferguson DJ, Crocker PR. Identification of CD22 ligands on bone marrow sinusoidal endothelium implicated in CD22-dependent homing of recirculating B cells. *J. Exp. Med.* May 3 1999;189(9):1513-1518.

[82] Dorner T, Kaufmann J, Wegener WA, Teoh N, Goldenberg DM, Burmester GR. Initial clinical trial of epratuzumab (humanized anti-CD22 antibody) for immunotherapy of systemic lupus erythematosus. *Arthrit. Res. Ther.* 2006;8(3):R74.

[83] Jacobi AM, Goldenberg DM, Hiepe F, Radbruch A, Burmester GR, Dorner T. Differential effects of epratuzumab on peripheral blood B cells of patients with systemic lupus erythematosus versus normal controls. *Ann. Rheum. Dis.* Apr 2008;67(4):450-457.

[84] Daridon C, Blassfeld D, Reiter K, et al. Epratuzumab targeting of CD22 affects adhesion molecule expression and migration of B-cells in systemic lupus erythematosus. *Arthritis Res Ther.* 2010;12(6):R204.
[85] Wallace DJ, Kalunian K.C., Petri, M.A., Strand, V., Kilgallen B., Kelley, L., Gordon C.P. Epretuzumab Demonstrates Clinically Meaningful Improvements in Patients with Moderate to Severe Systemic Lupus Erythematosus (SLE): Results from EMBLEM, a Phase IIb Study. *Arthritis Rheum.* 2010;62(Suppl 10):S605.
[86] www.clinicaltrials.gov.
[87] Mackay F, Schneider P. Cracking the BAFF code. *Nat Rev Immunol.* Jul 2009;9(7):491-502.
[88] Liu Z, Davidson A. BAFF and selection of autoreactive B cells. *Trends Immunol.* Aug 2011;32(8):388-394.
[89] Thanou-Stavraki A, Sawalha AH. An update on belimumab for the treatment of lupus. *Biologics.* 2011;5:33-43.
[90] Mackay F, Figgett WA, Saulep D, Lepage M, Hibbs ML. B-cell stage and context-dependent requirements for survival signals from BAFF and the B-cell receptor. *Immunol. Rev.* Sep 2010;237(1):205-225.
[91] Hoyer BF, Moser K, Hauser AE, et al. Short-lived plasmablasts and long-lived plasma cells contribute to chronic humoral autoimmunity in NZB/W mice. *J. Exp. Med.* Jun 7 2004;199(11):1577-1584.
[92] Ramanujam M, Davidson A. BAFF blockade for systemic lupus erythematosus: will the promise be fulfilled? *Immunol. Rev.* Jun 2008;223:156-174.
[93] Liu W, Szalai A, Zhao L, et al. Control of spontaneous B lymphocyte autoimmunity with adenovirus-encoded soluble TACI. *Arthritis Rheum.* Jun 2004;50(6):1884-1896.
[94] Cheema GS, Roschke V, Hilbert DM, Stohl W. Elevated serum B lymphocyte stimulator levels in patients with systemic immune-based rheumatic diseases. *Arthritis Rheum.* Jun 2001;44(6):1313-1319.
[95] Collins CE, Gavin AL, Migone TS, Hilbert DM, Nemazee D, Stohl W. B lymphocyte stimulator (BLyS) isoforms in systemic lupus erythematosus: disease activity correlates better with blood leukocyte BLyS mRNA levels than with plasma BLyS protein levels. *Arthritis Res Ther.* 2006;8(1):R6.
[96] Petri M, Stohl W, Chatham W, et al. Association of plasma B lymphocyte stimulator levels and disease activity in systemic lupus erythematosus. *Arthritis Rheum.* Aug 2008;58(8):2453-2459.
[97] Neusser MA, Lindenmeyer MT, Edenhofer I, et al. Intrarenal production of B-cell survival factors in human lupus nephritis. *Mod. Pathol.* Jan 2011;24(1):98-107.
[98] Wallace DJ, Stohl W, Furie RA, et al. A phase II, randomized, double-blind, placebo-controlled, dose-ranging study of belimumab in patients with active systemic lupus erythematosus. *Arthritis Rheum.* Sep 15 2009;61(9):1168-1178.
[99] Navarra SV, Guzman RM, Gallacher AE, et al. Efficacy and safety of belimumab in patients with active systemic lupus erythematosus: a randomised, placebo-controlled, phase 3 trial. *Lancet.* Feb 26 2011;377(9767):721-731.
[100] Petri M, Levy, R.A., Merrill, J. T., Navarra, S. C., Cervera, R., Van Vollenhoven, R.F., Manzi, S. Belimumab, a BlyS-Specific Inhibitor, Reduced Disease Activity, Flares and Prednisone Use in Patients with Seropositive SLE: Combined Efficacy results from the BLISS-52 and BLISS-76 Studies. *Arthritis Rheum.* 2010;62(Suppl 10).

[101] Manzi S, Sanchez-Guerrero, J., Merrill, J.T., Furie, R.A., Gladman, D., Navarra, S., Ginzler, E.M. Belimumab, A BLyS-Specific Inhibitor, Reduces Disease Activity Across Multiple Organ Domains: Combined Efficacy Results from the Phase 3 BLISS-52 and -76 Studies. *Arthritis Rheum.* 2010;62(Suppl 10).

[102] Munafo A, Priestley A, Nestorov I, Visich J, Rogge M. Safety, pharmacokinetics and pharmacodynamics of atacicept in healthy volunteers. *Eur. J. Clin. Pharmacol.* Jul 2007;63(7):647-656.

[103] Tak PP, Thurlings RM, Rossier C, et al. Atacicept in patients with rheumatoid arthritis: results of a multicenter, phase Ib, double-blind, placebo-controlled, dose-escalating, single- and repeated-dose study. *Arthritis Rheum.* Jan 2008;58(1):61-72.

[104] Ramanujam M, Wang X, Huang W, et al. Mechanism of action of transmembrane activator and calcium modulator ligand interactor-Ig in murine systemic lupus erythematosus. *J. Immunol.* Sep 1 2004;173(5):3524-3534.

[105] Dall'Era M, Chakravarty E, Wallace D, et al. Reduced B lymphocyte and immunoglobulin levels after atacicept treatment in patients with systemic lupus erythematosus: results of a multicenter, phase Ib, double-blind, placebo-controlled, dose-escalating trial. *Arthritis Rheum.* Dec 2007;56(12):4142-4150.

[106] Pena-Rossi C, Nasonov E, Stanislav M, et al. An exploratory dose-escalating study investigating the safety, tolerability, pharmacokinetics and pharmacodynamics of intravenous atacicept in patients with systemic lupus erythematosus. *Lupus.* May 2009;18(6):547-555.

[107] Bluestone JA. New perspectives of CD28-B7-mediated T cell costimulation. *Immunity.* Jun 1995;2(6):555-559.

[108] Finck BK, Linsley PS, Wofsy D. Treatment of murine lupus with CTLA4Ig. *Science.* Aug 26 1994;265(5176):1225-1227.

[109] Mihara M, Tan I, Chuzhin Y, et al. CTLA4Ig inhibits T cell-dependent B-cell maturation in murine systemic lupus erythematosus. *J Clin Invest.* Jul 2000;106(1):91-101.

[110] Schiffer L, Sinha J, Wang X, et al. Short term administration of costimulatory blockade and cyclophosphamide induces remission of systemic lupus erythematosus nephritis in NZB/W F1 mice by a mechanism downstream of renal immune complex deposition. *J Immunol.* Jul 1 2003;171(1):489-497.

[111] Merrill JT, Burgos-Vargas R, Westhovens R, et al. The efficacy and safety of abatacept in patients with non-life-threatening manifestations of systemic lupus erythematosus: results of a twelve-month, multicenter, exploratory, phase IIb, randomized, double-blind, placebo-controlled trial. *Arthritis Rheum.* Oct 2010;62(10):3077-3087.

[112] Lenert P. Nucleic acid sensing receptors in systemic lupus erythematosus: development of novel DNA- and/or RNA-like analogues for treating lupus. *Clin. Exp. Immunol.* Aug 2010;161(2):208-222.

[113] Anders HJ. A Toll for lupus. *Lupus.* 2005;14(6):417-422.

[114] Leadbetter EA, Rifkin IR, Hohlbaum AM, Beaudette BC, Shlomchik MJ, Marshak-Rothstein A. Chromatin-IgG complexes activate B cells by dual engagement of IgM and Toll-like receptors. *Nature.* Apr 11 2002;416(6881):603-607.

[115] Anders HJ, Vielhauer V, Eis V, et al. Activation of toll-like receptor-9 induces progression of renal disease in MRL-Fas(lpr) mice. *FASEB J.* Mar 2004;18(3):534-536.

[116] Pawar RD, Patole PS, Ellwart A, et al. Ligands to nucleic acid-specific toll-like receptors and the onset of lupus nephritis. *J. Am. Soc. Nephrol.* Dec 2006;17(12):3365-3373.

[117] Benigni A, Caroli C, Longaretti L, et al. Involvement of renal tubular Toll-like receptor 9 in the development of tubulointerstitial injury in systemic lupus. *Arthritis Rheum.* May 2007;56(5):1569-1578.

[118] Papadimitraki ED, Choulaki C, Koutala E, et al. Expansion of toll-like receptor 9-expressing B cells in active systemic lupus erythematosus: implications for the induction and maintenance of the autoimmune process. *Arthritis Rheum.* Nov 2006;54(11):3601-3611.

[119] Komatsuda A, Wakui H, Iwamoto K, et al. Up-regulated expression of Toll-like receptors mRNAs in peripheral blood mononuclear cells from patients with systemic lupus erythematosus. *Clin. Exp. Immunol.* Jun 2008;152(3):482-487.

[120] Ciferska H, Horak P, Konttinen YT, et al. Expression of nucleic acid binding Toll-like receptors in control, lupus and transplanted kidneys--a preliminary pilot study. *Lupus.* Jun 2008;17(6):580-585.

[121] Lau CM, Broughton C, Tabor AS, et al. RNA-associated autoantigens activate B cells by combined B cell antigen receptor/Toll-like receptor 7 engagement. *J. Exp. Med.* Nov 7 2005;202(9):1171-1177.

[122] Deane JA, Pisitkun P, Barrett RS, et al. Control of toll-like receptor 7 expression is essential to restrict autoimmunity and dendritic cell proliferation. *Immunity.* Nov 2007;27(5):801-810.

[123] Guiducci C, Gong M, Xu Z, et al. TLR recognition of self nucleic acids hampers glucocorticoid activity in lupus. *Nature.* Jun 17 2010;465(7300):937-941.

[124] Pisetsky DS, Reich CF. Inhibition of murine macrophage IL-12 production by natural and synthetic DNA. *Clin. Immunol.* Sep 2000;96(3):198-204.

[125] Krieg AM, Wu T, Weeratna R, et al. Sequence motifs in adenoviral DNA block immune activation by stimulatory CpG motifs. *Proc. Natl. Acad. Sci. U. S. A.* Oct 13 1998;95(21):12631-12636.

[126] Dong L, Ito S, Ishii KJ, Klinman DM. Suppressive oligodeoxynucleotides delay the onset of glomerulonephritis and prolong survival in lupus-prone NZB x NZW mice. *Arthritis Rheum.* Feb 2005;52(2):651-658.

[127] Graham KL, Lee LY, Higgins JP, Steinman L, Utz PJ, Ho PP. Treatment with a toll-like receptor inhibitory GpG oligonucleotide delays and attenuates lupus nephritis in NZB/W mice. *Autoimmunity.* Mar 2010;43(2):140-155.

[128] Barrat FJ, Meeker T, Gregorio J, et al. Nucleic acids of mammalian origin can act as endogenous ligands for Toll-like receptors and may promote systemic lupus erythematosus. *J. Exp. Med.* Oct 17 2005;202(8):1131-1139.

[129] Barrat FJ, Meeker T, Chan JH, Guiducci C, Coffman RL. Treatment of lupus-prone mice with a dual inhibitor of TLR7 and TLR9 leads to reduction of autoantibody production and amelioration of disease symptoms. *Eur. J. Immunol.* Dec 2007;37(12):3582-3586.

[130] Lenert P, Yasuda K, Busconi L, et al. DNA-like class R inhibitory oligonucleotides (INH-ODNs) preferentially block autoantigen-induced B-cell and dendritic cell activation in vitro and autoantibody production in lupus-prone MRL-Fas(lpr/lpr) mice in vivo. *Arthritis Res Ther*. 2009;11(3):R79.

Part 4

Diabetes and Kidney

11

Diabetic Nephropathy: Current and Novel Therapeutic Approaches to Prevent Its Development and Progression

Karly C. Sourris[1,2] and Josephine M. Forbes[1,2]
[1]*Glycation and Diabetes Complications*
Baker IDI Heart Research Institute, Melbourne, Victoria
[2]*Departments of Immunology and Medicine*
Monash University, Alfred Medical Research Education Precinct
Australia

1. Introduction

Diabetes is a metabolic disorder characterised by chronic hyperglycaemia, hypertension, dyslipidaemia, microalbuminuria and inflammation. Moreover, there are a number of vascular complications associated with this condition including retinopathy, neuropathy and nephropathy. Diabetic nephropathy is the major cause of end-stage renal disease in Western societies affecting a substantial proportion (25-40%) of patients with diabetes. Diabetic nephropathy is defined as a progressive decline in glomerular filtration rate, accompanied by proteinuria and other end-organ complications such as retinopathy.

It is widely accepted, that diabetic nephropathy is the product of hemodynamic and metabolic factors which act in concert and drive its development and progression. Metabolic factors include hyperglycaemia, hyperlipidaemia and advanced glycation. Hemodynamic factors include alterations in flow and pressure and the activation of the Renin-Angiotensin system (RAS). Together, the hemodynamic and metabolic factors activate common downstream signalling pathways, which potentiate the activation of target growth factors and signalling pathways which likely drive the development of DN. At present the most effective therapeutics for the treatment of DN target the renin-angiotensin system. Unfortunately, whilst they slow down the progression of DN they do not prevent it and thus novel therapeutics and potential targets required.

In recent times the downstream intracellular signalling pathways and their modulators have been central focus for the investigation of novel therapeutic targets for the treatment of DN. These targets include advanced glycation end products (AGEs) and their receptors, glucose transport molecules, NFκB, ROS, PKC, inflammatory molecules, including adipokines, chemokines, adhesion molecules and pro-inflammatory cytokines. Moreover, pro-fibrotic molecules , including EGF, VEGF, CTGF and arguably the most important, TGF-β, which are known to potentiate the morphological alterations associated with DN have also been targeted. Recently, epigenetic alterations, including histone, DNA methylation, metabolic memory and microRNA's have demonstrated their potential as novel therapeutic targets in the area of DN. Importantly a number of these potential therapies are the focus of clinical trials or are in pre-clinical investigations.

In summary this chapter will investigate the hemodynamic, metabolic and epigenetic factors which drive the development of diabetic nephropathy and their subsequent downstream signalling pathways. Importantly, we will discuss the limitations of current therapeutic strategies and development of novel therapeutic targets which are presently in either pre-clinical experimental investigations or clinical trials.

2. Diabetes

Today, it is estimated that approximately 180 million individuals worldwide have diabetes and WHO predicts that this is likely to double by the year 2030. The incidence of diabetes is increasing across the board, irrespective of age, sex or ethnicity (Sowers and Stump 2004). Diabetes is a metabolic disorder characterised by chronic hyperglycaemia, and often co-morbidities such as hypertension, dyslipidaemia and inflammation, with the major types being type 1 (insulin-dependant) or type 2 (commonly non-insulin dependant) (Sowers and Stump 2004; O'Connor and Schelling 2005). Both forms of diabetes are associated with micro- and macrovascular complications which include retinopathy, neuropathy, cardio/cerebrovascular disease and nephropathy which are the major cause of mortality and morbidity in diabetic patients (Cooper, Gilbert et al. 1998; Giacchetti, Sechi et al. 2005).

3. Diabetic nephropathy

Diabetic nephropathy is defined as a progressive decline in glomerular filtration rate, accompanied by proteinuria and other end-organ complications such as retinopathy (O'Connor and Schelling 2005). Diabetic nephropathy progresses to end-stage renal disease via a number of stages including normoalbuminuria, microalbuminuria/incipient diabetic nephropathy, macroalbuminuria and finally end-stage renal disease (Giacchetti, Sechi et al. 2005; O'Connor and Schelling 2005). Progression to end stage renal disease is enhanced by hyperglycaemia, hypertension and proteinuria, which are all common in diabetes (Cooper 1998; Mene, Festuccia et al. 2001; Marshall 2004; Wolf 2004).

Renal disease in diabetic patients is characterised by hemodynamic (hyperfiltration and hyperperfusion) as well as structural abnormalities (glomerulosclerosis, alterations in tubulointerstitium including interstitial fibrosis) and metabolic changes (Cooper 2001). More importantly, it appears that all renal cell types are affected by hyperglycaemic injury including glomerular podocytes, mesangial and endothelial cells, tubular epithelial cells, interstial fibroblasts, and vascular endothelia (Kanwar, Wada et al. 2008). Within glomeruli, there is thickening of basement membranes, mesangial expansion and hypertrophy and glomerular epithelial cell (podocyte) loss (Bohlender, Franke et al. 2005). In conjunction, disease progression is also seen in the tubulointerstitial compartment causing expansion of tubular basement membranes, tubular atrophy, interstitial fibrosis and arteriosclerosis (Marshall 2004).

To date, the most effective clinical treatments to prevent the progression of diabetic nephropathy are strict blood glucose control and anti-hypertensives (1998; 2002; 2003). Unfortunately, present therapies have failed to prevent new cases of diabetic nephropathy and progression as such novel therapeutic approaches are required. It is widely accepted that there metabolic, hemodynamic and genetic components of diabetic nephropathy. Novel therapeutics which are either in pre-clinical or clinical investigations target these factors in the hope of achieving the ultimate goal, prevention of diabetic nephropathy.

4. Potential therpeutic targets and approaches

4.1 Modulating hemodynamic pathways

Hyperfiltration, which presents as a marked increase in glomerular filtration rate, is widely recognised as being an early marker of diabetic nephropathy (Kanwar, Sun et al.; Anderson and Brenner 1988). Elevations in intra-renal pressure or glomerular capillary pressure are thought to induce the development of hyperfiltration thus highlighting the importance of the hemodynamic pathways in DN. Furthermore, the UK prospective diabetes study in type 2 diabetic patients, highlights the importance of hemodynamic influences in the development of DN. Diabetic subjects randomised to receive tighter blood pressure control, exhibited a concomitant reduction in microalbuminuria and clinical proteinuria (1998) To date the most effective treatments for both type 1 and type 2 diabetic patients to retard the progression of diabetic complications, are anti-hypertensives which target the renin-angiotensin system (Lewis, Hunsicker et al. 1993; Brenner, Cooper et al. 2001).

4.2 The Renin-Angiotensin System (RAS)

The renin-angiotensin system (RAS) is a co-ordinated hormonal cascade, which modulates vasoconstriction and facilitates renal-sodium absorption to maintain blood pressure control. The RAS cascade is initiated by the production of renin, which is released from renal juxtaglomerular cells, and converts angiotensinogen to angiotensin I. Angiotensin I, an inactive hormone, is subsequently cleaved into Angiotensin II by angiotensin converting enzyme (ACE). Angiotensin II drives the RAS and elicits its effects by binding to cellular receptors, the Angiotensin II type I receptor (AT1) or angiotensin type 2 receptor type II (AT2). It was originally postulated that AT1 was the primary receptor and modulator of the actions of Ang II, however in recent years it has been widely accepted that AT1 and AT2 elicit opposing actions upon ligand interaction with Ang II. The RAS is known to exist both systemically and locally in a number of different organs throughout the body including kidney, and vasculature (Wiecek, Chudek et al. 2003; Wolf 2004). Activation of the local renal RAS appears to be independent of the systemic RAS. In diabetes, the local RAS has been found to be up-regulated, in particular within the kidney, whilst the systemic RAS appears to be down-regulated (Gilbert, Krum et al. 2003; Wiecek, Chudek et al. 2003; Schrijvers, De Vriese et al. 2004; Forbes, Fukami et al. 2007).

To date the most effective treatments for diabetic nephropathy target the RAS. Whilst they slow down the progression of nephropathy, Clinical studies such as the RENAAL have demonstrated that these compounds do not prevent the relentless progression to end stage renal disease.

4.3 The endothelin pathway

The endothelin pathway has also been shown to be involved in the development and progression of diabetic nephropathy. There are three recognised endothelin proteins: ET-1, ET-2 and ET-3, all of which share a high level of homology and have demonstrated localisation in a variety of cell types. These vasoactive proteins bind to their receptors ET_A, ET_B, and ET_C. ET_A receptors have been shown to induce vasoconstriction and mitogenesis whilst ET_B receptors has been shown to induce vasoconstriction and vasodilatation (Seo,

Oemar et al. 1994; Roux, Breu et al. 1999; Candido and Allen 2002). Importantly, within the diabetic kidney, ET-1 has been found to be elevated and altered expression of the receptors has also been reported. In addition, modulation of this pathway through the employment of ET antagonists has been shown to reduce renal extracellular matrix (ECM) accumulation diabetic rats (Jandeleit-Dahm, Allen et al. 2000; Fukami, Cooper et al. 2005). Bosentan, an ET_A and ET_B receptor antagonist has demonstrated renoprotective benefits in the diabetic rat which was comparable to enalapril. Currently there are number of clinical trials examining the benefits of ET antagonists such as bosentan in diabetic nephropathy.

5. Modulation of metabolic pathways

5.1 Glycaemic control

A range of metabolic abnormalities in addition to hyperglycaemia, are seen in the diabetic milieu. However, it is obvious from studies in diabetic patients, that an elevation in circulating glucose is the predominant metabolic abnormality and strict glycaemic control, remains the ideal therapeutic approach to halt the progression of complications (1998; 2002). As well as promoting the formation of AGEs, chronic hyperglycaemia is also associated with increased inflammation and expression of associated inflammatory cytokines, such as MCP-1 (monocyte chemoattractant protein-1) (Dragomir, Tircol et al. 2006), and CTGF (connective tissue growth factor) (Makino, Mukoyama et al. 2003), elevated production of ROS (reactive oxygen species) and activation of a number of signalling pathways which are involved in diabetic nephropathy. At present glycaemic control is achieved through a number of approaches including improving insulin sensitivity via agents such as glitazones, increasing pancreatic insulin production with sulfonylureas and meglitinides, reducing hepatic glucose production with the administration of biguanides, limiting post-prandial glucose absorption with α-glucosidase inhibitors (Wagman and Nuss 2001; Fukami, Cooper et al. 2005).

A novel approach to modulate post-prandial glucose absorption is via targeting glucagon-like peptide-1 (GLP-1). GLP-1 is an incretin hormone which is known to stimulate insulin secretion, increase pro-insulin biosynthesis and improve pacreatic beta-cell viability. Recently it has been demonstrated that GLP-1 also posesses a number of extra pancreatic functions including anti-apoptotic and anti-inflammatory effects. The actions of GLP-1 are also modulated via an endogenous circulating enzyme DPP IV (dipeptidyl peptidase inhibitors). At present GLP-1 analogues and inhibitors of DPP-IV are under pre-clinical investigation for diabetic nephropathy. Specifically, administration of GLP-1 in an experimental model of type-1 diabetes exhibited renoprotective benefits independant of glucose control thus warrant further investigation (Kodera, Shikata et al.)

5.2 Modulation of glucose uptake

The initial step of glucose signalling it thought to be the translocation of glucose into the cells. Glucose uptake into renal cells is facilitated by various glucose transporters including SGLT2 (sodium-glucose transporter-2) , GLUT-1(glucose transporter -1) and GLUT-4 (glucose transporter-4). Hyperglycaemia is thought to induce an increase in expression and /or activity of these receptors which results in elevated intracellular glucose, which is one of the fundamental drivers for the development of diabetic nephropathy. One of the pathological outcomes of increased glucose transport is increased aldose reductase expression and up-regulation of PKC-MAPK (Protein kinase C- mitogen activated protein kinase) pathways which lead subsequent elevation in ECM (extracellular matrix) proteins such as collagen IV and fibronectin which are pivotal to the development of fibrotic lesions associated with DN (Kanwar, Sun et al.). Moreover, TGF-β (Transforming growth factor-β) is known to promote GLUT-1(glucose transporter-1) expression and facilitate elevations in intracellular glucose (Fukami, Yamagishi et al. 2007). Inhibitors of facilitative glucose transporter-2 (SGLT-2) (T-1095), have demonstrated potential as therapeutics for diabetic nephropathy in experimental models of type 1 diabetes. Administration of T-1095, a synthetic inhibitor of SGLT, reduced plasma glucose and urinary AER and a concomitant decrease in gene expression GLUT-2 (Fukami, Yamagishi et al. 2007). Thus targeting glucose transporters has exhibited renoprotective benefits and further investigation is warranted.

5.3 Advanced glycation end-products

AGEs are a heterogeneous and complex group of modifications, which play an important role in the development of diabetic nephropathy. They often present as a yellow-brown pigmentation, may be fluorescent and a number are primarily cross-links between proteins (Brownlee 1992; Brownlee 1995; Kalousova, Zima et al. 2004). AGEs are formed as a result of non-enzymatic biochemical reactions initiated as part of the Maillard Reaction. This reaction is a multi-step process, where a reactive carbonyl from glucose or its derivatives, are attached commonly to lysine and arginine residues on proteins, amino acids and nucleic acids (Njoroge and Monnier 1989; Ziyadeh, Cohen et al. 1997). Following further condensation, rearrangement and other reactions, the intermediate compounds of which some are "Schiff" bases and amadori products, are further irreversibly modified to become advanced glycation end products (AGEs) (Njoroge and Monnier 1989; Schrijvers, De Vriese et al. 2004). Physiologically, advanced glycation is thought to play an important role in the identification of senescent molecules, which are then subsequently cleaved and cleared, primarily via the kidneys (Jakus and Rietbrock 2004).

Within the body, AGEs accumulate from both endogenous and exogenous sources. Intracellularly, AGEs are formed as a by-product of a number of important biochemical reactions including oxidation of glucose to glyoxal, decomposition of amadori products and the fragmentation of glyceraldehydes. The reactive intracellular intermediates formed during these reactions, such as methylglyoxal, react with the amino groups of both intracellular and extracellular proteins to form AGEs (Brownlee 1992; Bierhaus, Hofmann et al. 1998).

AGEs may be broadly categorised on the basis of their action and function as either non-cross-linking adducts and cross-linking adducts such as hydroimidazoles (Bohlender, Franke et al. 2005). Some of the best characterised AGEs to date, include N-carboxymethyllysine (CML), N-carboxyethyllysine (CEL), pentosidine, imidazole, glyoxallysine dimer (GOLD) and pyrraline (Brownlee 1992; Schrijvers, De Vriese et al. 2004; Wolf 2004; Bohlender, Franke et al. 2005). In addition, there are a number of exogenous sources of AGEs identified in recent times, including food and tobacco smoke, which also contribute to the body's AGE pool (Cerami, Founds et al. 1997; Koschinsky, He et al. 1997).

Under normal physiological conditions, AGEs are cleared from the body via the kidney, following their degradation by reductase enzymes within cells such as macrophages. The kidney via a multi-step process, filters AGE modified-peptides and proteins. Following filtration via the glomeruli, they are subsequently reabsorbed by the proximal tubules where they are often further degraded and then excreted into the urine (Kalousova, Zima et al. 2004). In homeostasis, the rate of renal AGE removal is proportional to creatinine clearance, ensuring that there is no excess accumulation of tissue AGEs.

In metabolic disorders, such as diabetes, there is a marked increase in a number of factors which promote the formation and accumulation of AGEs within various susceptible organs, in particular, the kidney. As a direct result of the hyperglycaemia characteristic of diabetes, there is marked increase in both carbonyl and oxidative stress, which each promote in vivo AGE accumulation (Miyata, Haneda et al. 1996; Miyata and van Ypersele de Strihou 2003).

Excessive AGE accumulation can elicit a variety of deleterious effects on tissues and organs. These include altering the structure and function of both intracellular and extracellular molecules, increasing oxidative stress, modulation of cell activation, enhancement of signal transduction pathways and increasing the activation and expression of cytokines and growth factors. These actions have been shown to be mediated via both receptor dependant and independent mechanisms (Brownlee 1995; Schrijvers, De Vriese et al. 2004 Circulating levels of AGEs in diabetic patients are elevated with decreased renal function {Kubba, 2003 #916). Furthermore, AGE accumulation in tissues correlate with the severity of organ injury, particularly within glomerular lesions (Shimoike, Inoguchi et al. 2000; Kanauchi, Nishioka et al. 2001).

Dietary AGEs, are also thought to contribute to the development of diabetic nephropathy. Diets low in AGE content, when fed to non-obese diabetic mice (type 1) and db/db mice (type 2) reduced glomerular lesions, creatinine/albumin ratios and renal TGFβ1 expression when compared to their high AGE counterparts (Zheng, He et al. 2002). Moreover, diets high in AGE content are known to impair insulin sensitivity further confounding downstream complications (Hofmann, Dong et al. 2002). Harcourt et al, have recently demonstrated the benefits of low AGE diets on kidney function in pre-diabetic, obese individuals. Diets low in AGE content elicited improvements in renal function and reduction in inflammation (Harcourt, Sourris et al.). Various agents, including LR-90 (Figarola, Scott et al. 2003), aminoguanidine (Youssef, Nguyen et al. 1999), and ALT-711 (Forbes, Thallas et al. 2003) are potent in reducing AGE accumulation in renal tissues in experimental diabetic nephropathy, subsequently improving renal function. Many other agents have elicited similar benefits and have been extensively reviewed previously (Alderson, Chachich et al. 2004; Williams and Tuttle 2005; Williams 2006). In addition, pyridoxamine, an intermediate of vitamin B_6, attenuated the progression of human diabetic nephropathy and concurrently reduced AGE and urinary TGF-β(Williams, Bolton et al. 2007). Furthermore, benfotiamine (liposoluble vitamin B1 derivative), decreases AGE accumulation, inflammation and improves vascular function in type 2 diabetic patients consuming diets high in AGE content (Stirban, Negrean et al. 2006). To date there have been three clinical trials conducted which employed AGE-lowering therapies . Aminoguanidine and benfotiamine trials were stopped due to toxicity of the therapy. The third trial employed Alagaebrium in type 1 diabetic patients in addition to an ACE-inhibitor. This trial has now ended and results are pending.

5.4 AGE-receptors

The receptors for AGE are important modulators of the deleterious effects of these compounds. Receptors for AGEs may be loosely grouped as either inflammatory (RAGE, AGE-R2) or clearance type receptors (AGE-R1, AGE-R3, CD36, Scr-II, FEEL-1 and FEEL-2) (Vlassara and Bucala 1996; Vlassara 1997; Singh, Barden et al. 2001; Forbes, Yee et al. 2004; Schrijvers, De Vriese et al. 2004; Alikhani, Alikhani et al. 2005). Vascular, renal, neuronal and haematopoietic cells are all known to express receptors for AGEs (Goldin, Beckman et al. 2006; Sourris and Forbes 2009) AGEs contribute to the pathogenesis of diabetic nephropathy via receptor mediated mechanisms and indirectly via the generation of reactive oxygen species and by altering extracellular matrix (ECM) integrity.

Diabetes alters the expression of a number of AGE-receptors thought to drive the development and progression of diabetic nephropathy, in particular, the expression of RAGE on cells such as podocytes and tubular epithelial cells (Soulis, Thallas et al. 1997; Wendt, Tanji et al. 2003; Gu, Hagiwara et al. 2006; Li, Nakamura et al. 2006).

Another AGE receptor postulated to be involved in the development of diabetic nephropathy is AGE-R1, although converse to RAGE this is likely via a decrease in expression. In an experimental model of type 1 diabetes, renal AGE-R1 expression is reduced in association with a concurrent increase in AGE deposition and progression to diabetic nephropathy (He, Zheng et al. 2000; Vlassara 2001). In addition, we recently reported that in a small cohort of type 2 diabetic patients we found a positive correlation with AGE-R1 expression on the cell surface of peripheral blood mononuclear cells and renal function. We found that this was the most predictive biomarker for renal function and further investigation in a larger cohort is required {Sourris, #9145}.

The contribution of AGE-R3 to the development and progression of diabetic nephropathy has not been extensively researched. However, AGE-induced increases in the expression of AGE-R3 has been demonstrated in cultured endothelial cells and within renal tissues in the diabetic milieu (Iacobini, Oddi et al. 2005; Kumar, Narang et al. 2006). This however, may indicate a protective role for AGE-R3 given that AGE-R3 deficient mice develop more severe renal disease and have marked increases in renal AGE deposition (Iacobini, Oddi et al. 2005). Furthermore, AGE-R3 deficient mice develop albuminuria, mesangial expansion and fibrosis within the kidney cortex which is more pronounced with diabetes. Importantly, the deletion of AGE-R3 was also associated with a decrease in AGE-R1 and increased expression of RAGE demonstrating the existence of AGE-receptor cross talk. This study highlights that the role of AGE-R3 in the clearance of AGEs (Pugliese, Pricci et al. 2000) is likely more important in diabetic nephropathy than its ability to modulate immune function. The modulation of AGEs and their receptors have been extensively reviewed previously (Sourris and Forbes 2009).

6. Hyperlipidaemia

Hyperlipidaemia is a comorbidity often seen in diabetic patients and is thought to be an important contributor to progressive micro and macrovascular complications. This is most clearly demonstrated by the renoprotection which is seemingly afforded with HMG CoA reductase inhibitors (Tonolo, Ciccarese et al. 1997; Fujii, Inoguchi et al. 2007; Matsumoto, Tanimoto et al. 2008). Obesity is one the leading factors which drive the development of type 2 diabetes and its complications such as nephropathy. Moreover, it has also been shown to lead to kidney disease in the absence of diabetes. As one of the leading causes of chronic kidney disease, the WHO has recommended that lifestyle changes such as dietary and exercise are the most cost-effective approaches to combating this epidemic. We have recently reported the benefits of dietary intervention and renal function in a obese, non-diabetic population (Harcourt, Sourris et al.).

7. Reactive oxygen species

Reactive oxygen species are important intermediates in the formation of AGEs and are often excessively generated in the kidney in diabetes (Forbes, Coughlan et al. 2008). In addition, concomitant dysregulation of anti-oxidant enzymes in diabetes, leads to a state of oxidative stress (Forbes, Coughlan et al. 2008). To date, it is unclear as to why exogenous administration of antioxidants *per se* has demonstrated such poor renoprotection in humans, despite exciting positive preclinical research findings. However, it seems evident that therapies such as vitamins may not be the ideal antioxidant strategy in human DN. Vitamin B6 derivatives (Hammes, Du et al. 2003; Endo, Nishiyama et al. 2007), metformin (Rahbar, Natarajan et al. 2000), OPB-9195 (Wada, Nishizawa et al. 2001; Mizutani, Ikeda et al. 2002), ACEi (Miyata, van Ypersele de Strihou et al. 2002; Coughlan, Thallas-Bonke et al. 2007), AT1 antagonists (Miyata, van Ypersele de Strihou et al. 2002), ALA (Coughlan, Thallas-Bonke et al. 2007) and sRAGE (Wautier, Zoukourian et al. 1996) have exhibited beneficial effects on excess superoxide generation within tissues, associated with improvements in the development and/or progression of diabetic complications.

Vitamin B-related therapeutics are effective scavengers of ROS intermediates. Pyridoxamine, inhibits superoxide radical generation, as well as preventing the progression of neuropathy and retinopathy (Jain and Lim 2001). In addition benfotiamine and thiamine, Vitamin B1 derivatives, have shown beneficial effects in normalising ROS production and reducing the activity of aldose reductase (Berrone, Beltramo et al. 2006). Paradoxically, thiamine administered to human with diabetic renal disease actually worsened renal function (Rabbani, Alam et al. 2009). The role of ROS in diabetic kidney disease has been extensively reviewed previously (Forbes, Coughlan et al. 2008).

8. Inhibition of protein kinase C (PKC) activity

There has been a growing body of evidence suggesting the central role of PKC, which is broadly involved in signal transduction from the plasma membrane to the nucleus, in diabetes induced vascular dysfunction (Inoguchi, Battan et al. 1992; Xia, Inoguchi et al. 1994). PKC has 11 different isoforms, many of which have been shown to be involved in diabetic complications, in particular nephropathy. (Koya, Jirousek et al. 1997; Koya, Haneda et al. 2000; Meier, Park et al. 2003). Of the 11 isoforms, PKC-α, -β, -δ, -ε, -ξ are expressed within the kidney (Kanwar, Sun et al.) PKC pathway is known to be activated by many factors including: Elevations in diacylglycerol, hydrogen peroxide, increased activity of polyol pathway, mitochondrial superoxide activity (Geraldes and King) and following AGE-RAGE interactions (Kanwar, Sun et al.). PKC isoforms have been associated with many cellular and vascular alterations and processes including: endothelial dysfunction, angiogenesis, vascular permeability, cell growth and apoptosis, basement membrane thickening, extracellular matrix (ECM) expansion. PKC pathway is known to be activation of numerous cellular pathways including NADH, ROS, Na^+/K^+ ATPase , Endothelin (ET-1), Ang II, MAPK and phospolipase A2 and VEGF (Geraldes and King; Kanwar, Sun et al.).

We have recently reported the attenuation of PKC-α phosphorylation and translocation with ALA in both *in vivo* models of DN and *in vitro* studies (Thallas-Bonke, Lindschau et al. 2004). It remains to be determined if this action of alagebrium on PKCα phosphorylation partly explains its renoprotective actions. Modulation of PKC activity within the diabetic kidney has also been exhibited by various vitamin B derivatives (Babaei-Jadidi, Karachalias et al.

2003; Hammes, Du et al. 2003). Interestingly, both ACEi and aminoguanidine prevent diabetes associated increases in PKC β activation in renal glomeruli (Osicka, Yu et al. 2000). The effects of aminoguanidine and ACEi on PKC β activity were also observed at other sites of vascular injury including the retina and mesenteric vascular bed (Osicka, Kiriazis et al. 2001; Miyata, van Ypersele de Strihou et al. 2002). In addition, AT-1 receptor antagonists, also attenuate diabetes induced increases in PKC -epsilon activity within the diabetic heart (Malhotra, Reich et al. 1997). Furthermore, modulation of PKC has been demonstrated in vascular endothelial cells with the insulin sensitizing agent metformin (Isoda, Young et al. 2006) and the anti-thrombotic therapeutic, aspirin (Dragomir, Manduteanu et al. 2004). We have demonstrated that in our experimental models of diabetes translocation of PKC α to the membrane is associated with parallel increases in superoxide production and elevated urinary VEGF thus highlighting the importance of this pathway in DN. In the clinical setting, roboxistaurin, is a PKC inhibitor which Tuttle et al, demonstrated that 32mg/day in addition to an ACEi for 12 months reduced urinary ACR (Geraldes and King). Moreover, renal biopsies from diabetic patients exhibited almost 10-fold increase in PKC β gene expression compared to their control (Geraldes and King; Langham, Kelly et al. 2008). In addition, the importance of PCK isoforms has been demonstrated in experimental models of diabetic nephropathy. PCK-α and β knockout mice exhibited a high level of resistance to the development of diabetic renal disease (Meier, Park et al. 2007; Meier, Menne et al. 2009; Tossidou, Starker et al. 2009).

9. Nuclear transcription factor kappa-B (NF-κB)

NF-κB is a transcription factor composed of two subunits, the most common of which are the p50 and p65 subunits (Barnes and Larin 1997) which are thought to be important modulators of diabetic complications. The active p65 subunit in particular, is thought to be central in the activation of numerous genes including cytokines, adhesion molecules, NO synthase, angiotensinogen and many other inflammatory and proliferative proteins implicated in the process of diabetic nephropathy (Barnes and Larin 1997; Bierhaus, Schiekofer et al. 2001). NF-κB is activated by a range of stimuli including glucose (Pieper and Riazulhaq 1997) and ROS (Nishikawa, Edelstein et al. 2000). AGEs are also involved in activation of NF-κB via a RAGE-dependent pathway leading to its translocation to the nucleus where it induces transcription of target genes such as IL-6 and TNF-α (Yan, Schmidt et al. 1994). The diverse actions of NF-κB and the capacity of various factors such as AII and AGEs to activate this transcription factor (Ruiz-Ortega, Lorenzo et al. 2000; Ruiz-Ortega, Lorenzo et al. 2000), are consistent with NF-κB playing a pivotal role in the pathogenesis of diabetic complications.

Pyrrolidine dithiocarbamate (PDTC) is a NF-κB inhibitor which has been used in both diabetic (Lee, Cao et al. 2004) and non-diabetic animal models of renal disease where it is renoprotective (Rangan, Wang et al. 1999), although its toxicity does not allow for direct translation to the clinical setting. Indeed, our group has demonstrated the importance of NF-κB in the pathogenesis of early renal macrophage infiltration in experimental diabetes, which could be modulated by interruption of the RAS (Lee, Cao et al. 2004; Liu, Wei et al. 2006). Moreover, diabetes-induced increases in NF-κB activation are prevented by numerous therapeutics including Metformin (Isoda, Young et al. 2006) aspirin (Zheng, Howell et al. 2007) Vitamin B derivatives (Hammes, Du et al. 2003) carnosine (Odashima,

Otaka et al. 2006) and thiazolidinediones (Marx, Walcher et al. 2004). It is possible that NF-κB, like PKC, is a central mediator which drives the downstream pathogenic consequences of interactions between hemodynamic and glucose dependent pathways in diabetic vascular complications. However, approaches to inhibit NF-κB have not been explored fully in DN, most likely due to the intimate involvement of this transcription factor in a number of essential cellular processes including apoptosis.

10. Inflammatory cytokines and growth factors

Diabetic nephropathy was not traditionally considered to be an inflammatory condition, however, there is a growing body of evidence in recent times highlighting the central role of inflammation in its development and progression (Wu, Huang et al. 2002; Forbes, Cooper et al. 2003; Chow, Ozols et al. 2004; Chow, Nikolic-Paterson et al. 2004; Chow, Nikolic-Paterson et al. 2006; Nguyen, Ping et al. 2006; Chow, Nikolic-Paterson et al. 2007; Ninichuk, Khandoga et al. 2007; Giunti, Tesch et al. 2008; Hohenstein, Hugo et al. 2008). Indeed, both hemodynamic and metabolic factors involved in the development of diabetic complications such as nephropathy activate common downstream targets, including cytokines and growth factors (Cooper, Gilbert et al. 1998). In particular, Monocyte Chemoattractant Protein (MCP-1), Transforming Growth Factor-β1 (TGF-β1), Connective Tissue Growth Factor (cTGF) and Vascular Endothelial Growth Factor (VEGF) have all been implicated in both experimental and human studies to be involved in the development and progression of diabetic nephropathy.

10.1 Monoctye chemoattractant protein -1 (MCP-1)

MCP-1 is a potent chemokine which encourages monocyte/macrophage infiltration into the kidney, which likely contributes to the progression of DN. MCP-1 production and secretion from damaged renal cells in diabetes are postulated to be a response to hyperglycaemia subsequently activating a number of signalling pathways including those mediated by PKC and NF-κB (Tesch 2008). In an experimental model of type 2 diabetic nephropathy, a deficiency in MCP-1 resulted in a significant reduction in renal inflammatory infiltration and renoprotection, Furthermore administration of propagermanium, an antagonist of the MCP-1 receptor, in model of diabetic nephropathy, resulted in reduced renal hypertrophy and macrophage infiltration in renal glomeruli (Kanamori, Matsubara et al. 2007). Indeed, it has been demonstrated that elevations in urinary excretion of MCP-1 may be a valid diagnostic marker of diabetic nephropathy in type 2 diabetic patients (Wang and Chen 2009). These studies suggest that MCP-1 is a central mediator of diabetic renal disease, although its utility as a therapeutic target remains to be determined (Chow, Nikolic-Paterson et al. 2007).

10.2 Modulation of growth factors

Growth factors such as transforming growth factor-β (TGF-β), a fibrogenic cytokine, and connective tissue growth factor (CTGF), which is primarily induced by TGF- β1, have been implicated as key effector molecules which promote diabetic renal disease. Transforming growth factor beta is a superfamily with three mammalian isoforms. The major isoform, TGF-β1 is synthesised as an inactive or latent form, which subsequently is subjected to proteolytic cleavage leading to the generation of the active form. TGF-β1 binds to the type II receptor and subsequently binds to the type I receptor (Wrana, Attisano et al. 1994) inducing phosphorylation and intracellular signalling involving the SMAD proteins (Massague 1998). In vitro studies have shown that a range of stimuli increase TGF-β1 expression including hyperglycaemia, AGEs, stretch, AII, endothelin, lipids and various products of oxidative stress such as F_2 isoprostanes, all factors relevant to DN (Rocco, Neilson et al. 1992; Wolf, Ziyadeh et al. 1995; Herman, Emancipator et al. 1998; Gruden, Thomas et al. 1999; Jandeleit-Dahm, Cao et al. 1999; Montero, Munger et al. 2000). Ziyadeh *et al* have previously examined the effects of long-term administration of a neutralizing TGF-β1 antibody on renal function and structure in diabetic *db/db* mice (Ziyadeh, Hoffman et al. 2000) and STZ diabetic mice (Sharma, Jin et al. 1996). Although most of the benefits have been attributed to TGF-β1, Hill *et al.* have suggested that another isoform, TGF-β2, is closely linked to fibrogenesis in diabetic nephropathy (Hill, Flyvbjerg et al. 2000). The utility of TGF-β1 as a target for therapeutic intervention in DN, however, is impeded by its essential role in inflammatory and immune processes. Therefore it may be preferable to modulate renal TGF-β1 levels by an alternative approach such as therapies which focus on upstream advanced glycation pathways. A clinical trial in type 2 diabetic patients has recently ended and reports have been released. In this study by Sharma et al, they employed the anti-fibrotic therapeutic, Pirfenidone at two different doses to investigate the benefits on renal function. Administration of Perfenidone at the lower dose of 1200mg resulted in a concurrent improvement in renal function and reduction in TGF-β thus demonstrating its benefits as a potential therapeutic for diabetic nephropathy (Sharma, Ix et al.).

10.3 Connective tissue growth factor

Another pro-sclerotic cytokine, connective tissue growth factor (CTGF) has increased renal (Riser, Denichilo et al. 2000; Twigg, Cao et al. 2002) and in particular, glomerular expression in diabetes (Murphy, Godson et al. 1999; Riser, Denichilo et al. 2000) and elevated in both early and late diabetic nephropathy in humans (Ito, Aten et al. 1998). Currently a Phase II study of FG-3019, a humanised anti-CTGF antibody, has been completed in patients with diabetic nephropathy (microalbuminuria) which was well tolerated and improved albuminuria. Subsequent, studies are planned in diabetic patients with macroalbuminuria (http://www.fibrogen.com/trials).

CTGF expression is thought to be mediated by a number of factors common in diabetic nephropathy including TGF-β1, hyperglycaemia or mechanical stretch (Riser, Denichilo et al. 2000). Interestingly, AGEs have been reported to specifically increase CTGF expression, initially in fibroblasts (Twigg, Chen et al. 2001) but subsequently in mesangial cells (Twigg, Chen et al. 2001). Moreover, aspirin has also been shown to prevent the diabetes-mediated increase in CTGF and mesangial expansion in experimental models of DN (Makino, Mukoyama et al. 2003).

10.4 Vascular endothelial growth factor (VEGF)

Vascular endothelial growth factor (VEGF) is a cytokine whose major role in diabetes was initially considered to be central for the pathogenesis of diabetic retinopathy and in particular retinal neovascularisation. Recent findings, however, have demonstrated the importance of VEGF within the diabetic kidney (De Vriese, Tilton et al. 2001; Wada, Nishizawa et al. 2001; Rizkalla, Forbes et al. 2003; Wendt, Tanji et al. 2003; Thallas-Bonke, Lindschau et al. 2004)]. We and others have previously shown both in vivo and in vitro decreases in VEGF expression with a number of therapies including alagebrium (Thallas-

Bonke, Lindschau et al. 2004), ACE inhibitors (Thallas-Bonke, Lindschau et al. 2004), sRAGE (Wendt, Tanji et al. 2003) and OPB-9195 (Wada, Nishizawa et al. 2001). Despite this suppression of VEGF as a result of current therapeutics, the benefits of VEGF suppression remain controversial with some studies suggesting that VEGF blockade is renoprotective (De Vriese, Tilton et al. 2001), whereas recent studies, albeit in a non-diabetic context, suggest that VEGF is a critical renal survival factor and that blockade may in fact promote renal damage (Advani, Kelly et al. 2007). This is perhaps best demonstrated by the differential effects seen with anti-VEGF antibodies (192,193). Studies on the renal effects of blockade of VEGF receptor (VEGFR) signalling are currently being performed. Indeed, a recent preliminary report has shown that SU5416, a VEGFR tyrosine kinase inhibitor, reduces albuminuria in *db/db* mice (Sung 2004). In experimental models of DN, VEGF expression is also decreased by an inhibitor of AGE formation (Tsuchida, Makita et al. 1999) and with the AGE cross-link breaker, ALA (Thallas-Bonke, Lindschau et al. 2004) further confirming the link between AGEs and VEGF expression.

11. Targeting genetic mediators of diabetic nephropathy

Whilst, genetic factors and gene mutations have been implicated in the development and pathogenesis of diabetes for some time, recent evidence has implicated the involvement of , microRNA's, histone methylation and metabolic memory in diabetes and specifically its complications.

11.1 MicroRNAs (miRNAs)

MiRNAs are regulatory RNAs that act as post-transcriptional repressors by binding to the 3'untranslated region of target genes (Akkina and Becker; Guay, Roggli et al.). The mammalian genome encodes for several hundred miRNAs, and within the kidney, the miRNA profile differs from that of other tissues and indeed within different compartments of the kidney (Akkina and Becker; Guay, Roggli et al.). Initially miRNAs are transcribed as long pre-miRNA molecules which are subsequently modified to become their mature miRNA form, approximately 19-25 nucleotides in length, via a number of different processes. A strand of mature miRNA enters the RNA-inducing silencing complex (RISC) where it binds to the 3' untranslated region of its target mRNA thus resulting in reduced expression of the targeted gene (Akkina and Becker) The miRNA which are in greatest abundance within the kidney include: miR-192, 194, 204, 215 and 216. Kantharidis et al have demonstrated in-vitro and ex-vivo potential of miRNA as therapeutic targets in diabetic nephropathy. Specifically, they have demonstrated the role of microRNA's in the fibrosis associated with diabetic nephropathy. MicroRNA-192/215 was found to regulate the pro-fibrotic protein e-cadherin whilst miRNA-200a was found to repress the expression of TGF-ß2 (Wang, Herman-Edelstein et al.; Wang, Koh et al.) Natarajan et al have alos extensively investigated microRNA in diabetic renal disease in experimental models (Kato, Arce et al.; Kato, Arce et al. 2009; Kato and Natarajan 2009; Kato, Putta et al. 2009). This therefore highlights the potential of microRNA's as therapeutic targets for diabetic nephropathy and further pre-clinical work is warranted.

11.2 Metabolic memory

A number of pre-clinical and clinical trials have implicated the involvement of metabolic memory and the development of diabetic complications. Metabolic memory refers to an earlier hyperglycaemic or erratic metabolic controlled state which is then followed by "normoglycaemia" or good glycaemia control. This phenomenon is poorly understood, however it suggests that despite improved glycemic control, the original exposure to hyperglycaemia is enough to sustain prolonged deleterious effects and outcomes. Metabolic memory has been demonstrated in both experimental and cell culture models of diabetes. In addition, numerous clinical trials, including the United Kingdom Prospective Diabetes Study (UKPDS) and The Action in Diabetes and Vascular Disease: Preterax and Diamicron Modified Release Controlled Evaluation (ADVANCE) demonstrated that intensive glycaemia control may help decrease micro and macrovasuclar complications thus suggesting the existence of metabolic memory (Villeneuve and Natarajan). Brassacchio et al have demonstrated the existence of "hyperglycaemic memory" in an in-vitro model of diabetes (Brasacchio, Okabe et al. 2009) however further investigation into this phenomenon is warranted and would undoubtedly reduce the onset and progression of diabetic complications, including nephropathy.

11.3 Histone modifications

Post-translational modifications that occur at the histone tails including: acetylation, methylation, and phosphorylation, one of the many methods through which regulation of gene transcription is achieved. Traditionally, post-translational modifications, such as DNA methylation have been extensively studied in the area of cancer. Recent reports have demonstrated the importance of histone modifications in diabetic complications. Pre-clinical studies in white blood cells including monocytes from diabetic patients have exhibited epigenetic modifications including increases in H3K9me2 AND H3K4me2 which are associated with immune and inflammatory pathways (Villeneuve and Natarajan). In addition, TGF- ß treatment of renal mesangial cells were found to induce an increase in HMT SET7/9 which was associated with a profibrotic phenotype (Villeneuve and Natarajan). Histone modifications therefore demonstrate great potential as therapeutic targets.

12. Clinical trials: The current state of affairs

It is clearly evident that there is an abundance of potential therapeutic targets for the treatment of diabetic nephropathy. So why are we failing to translate these into positive outcomes in patients? We investigated the NIH database for clinical trials (completed and running) which targeted diabetic nephropathy. Of the 200 trials listed in the database, we categorised the interventions into their broad subject groups (Table 1). Our search found that 35% of all trials, employed interventional therapies which targeted the renin-aldosterone-angiotensin system, which to date have proven to be the most beneficial therapeutic approach (Table 1). Approximately 13.5% of all clinical trials were investigating therapies which target glycaemic control (including insulin). Dietary intervention is a more cost effective therapeutic approach for the treatment of diabetic nephropathy constituted some 20% of all clinical trials registered within the NIH data base. It is evident that the wider research community is actively investigating novel therapeutic targets other than those which target the RAAS, demonstrated by the variety of interventions and categories. Of particular interest, is that of all of these trials, almost 10% of these targeted ROS whilst 5% employed anti-inflammatories. In addition, 1.5% of all trials targeted AGEs and/or their receptors (Table 1). The remainder of the trials targeted thrombosis, fibrosis, erythropoiesis, heparin, PKC, calcium transport, endothelin and genetics (Table 1). A recent search into the diabetic nephropathy patent database has identified that other new novel therapeutics including vasohibin (20100113354), myostatin (20110008357), Oligotide (20100291098), modulators of prostacyclin (20110053872), inhibitors of galectin-3 (20080219973) and inhibitors of fatty acid oxidation (20110048980) are being considered for the treatment of diabetic renal disease. Moreover, novel biomarkers for the development and progression of diabetic nephropathy are also under investigation including urinary: precursor α-2-HS-glycoprotein, α-1-antitrypsin, α-1-acid glycoprotein and osteopontin.

TARGET	PERCENTAGE
Glycaemic Control (including insulin and glucose transport)	14.5%
Advanced Glycation End-Products	1.5%
Reactive Oxygen Species	9%
Inflammation	5%
Renin-aldosterone-angiotensin system	35%
Endothelin	2.5%
Dietary Interventions	17.5%
Pro-fibrotic molecules	2%
Anti-Thrombotic	1.5%
Genetics	1%
Protein Kinase C- inhibitors	1%
Anti-Lipidaemic	4.5%
Calcium Blockers	1.5%
Others - diuretics, hormones, apoptosis,	5%

Table 1. Therapeutics in clinical trials for treatment of diabetic nephropathy Representative table of Clinical Trials run to treat diabetic nephropathy and registered on NIH webpage.

13. Conclusion

Diabetic nephropathy is a multifaceted disease which encompasses hemodynamic, metabolic and genetic factors which are central to its development and progression. At present therapeutics which target the hemodynamic factors, specifically the renin-aldosterone-angiotensin system are the most effective treatments. Unfortunately, their benefits are limited and as such additional novel therapeutics are required. In this chapter we have described an number of potential therapeutic targets which have been identified and which are either in clinical or pre-clinical investigation. In the future, it is hoped that current clinical trials will show benefits of some of these novel agents and that there will be significant advanced in our management of individuals with diabetic renal disease.

14. References

(1998). "Tight blood pressure control and risk of macrovascular and microvascular complications in type 2 diabetes: UKPDS 38. UK Prospective Diabetes Study Group." *Bmj* 317(7160): 703-13.

(2002). "Effect of intensive therapy on the microvascular complications of type 1 diabetes mellitus." *Jama* 287(19): 2563-9.

(2003). "Sustained effect of intensive treatment of type 1 diabetes mellitus on development and progression of diabetic nephropathy: the Epidemiology of Diabetes Interventions and Complications (EDIC) study." *Jama* 290(16): 2159-67.

Advani, A., D. J. Kelly, et al. (2007). "Role of VEGF in maintaining renal structure and function under normotensive and hypertensive conditions." *Proc Natl Acad Sci U S A* 104(36): 14448-53.

Akkina, S. and B. N. Becker "MicroRNAs in kidney function and disease." *Transl Res* 157(4): 236-40.

Alderson, N. L., M. E. Chachich, et al. (2004). "Effect of antioxidants and ACE inhibition on chemical modification of proteins and progression of nephropathy in the streptozotocin diabetic rat." *Diabetologia* 47(8): 1385-95.

Alikhani, Z., M. Alikhani, et al. (2005). "Advanced glycation end products enhance expression of pro-apoptotic genes and stimulate fibroblast apoptosis through cytoplasmic and mitochondrial pathways." *J Biol Chem* 280(13): 12087-95.

Anderson, S. and B. M. Brenner (1988). "Pathogenesis of diabetic glomerulopathy: hemodynamic considerations." *Diabetes Metab Rev* 4(2): 163-77.

Babaei-Jadidi, R., N. Karachalias, et al. (2003). "Prevention of incipient diabetic nephropathy by high-dose thiamine and benfotiamine." *Diabetes* 52(8): 2110-20.

Barnes, P. J. and M. Larin (1997). "MECHANISMS OF DISEASE - NUCLEAR FACTOR-KAPPA-B - A PIVOTAL TRANSCRIPTION FACTOR IN CHRONIC INFLAMMATORY DISEASES [Review]." *New England Journal of Medicine* 336(15): 1066-1071.

Berrone, E., E. Beltramo, et al. (2006). "Regulation of intracellular glucose and polyol pathway by thiamine and benfotiamine in vascular cells cultured in high glucose." *J Biol Chem* 281(14): 9307-13.

Bierhaus, A., M. A. Hofmann, et al. (1998). "AGEs and their interaction with AGE-receptors in vascular disease and diabetes mellitus. I. The AGE concept." *Cardiovasc Res* 37(3): 586-600.

Bierhaus, A., S. Schiekofer, et al. (2001). "Diabetes-associated sustained activation of the transcription factor nuclear factor-kappaB." *Diabetes* 50(12): 2792-808.

Bohlender, J., S. Franke, et al. (2005). "Advanced glycation end products: a possible link to angiotensin in an animal model." *Ann N Y Acad Sci* 1043: 681-4.

Bohlender, J. M., S. Franke, et al. (2005). "Advanced glycation end products and the kidney." *Am J Physiol Renal Physiol* 289(4): F645-59.

Brasacchio, D., J. Okabe, et al. (2009). "Hyperglycemia induces a Dynamic Cooperativity of Histone Methylase and Demethylase Enzymes associated with Gene-Activating Epigenetic Marks that co-exist on the Lysine Tail." *Diabetes*.

Brenner, B. M., M. E. Cooper, et al. (2001). "Effects of losartan on renal and cardiovascular outcomes in patients with type 2 diabetes and nephropathy." *N Engl J Med* 345(12): 861-9.

Brownlee, M. (1992). "Glycation products and the pathogenesis of diabetic complications." *Diabetes Care* 15(12): 1835-43.

Brownlee, M. (1995). "Advanced protein glycosylation in diabetes and aging." *Annu Rev Med* 46: 223-34.

Brownlee, M. (1995). "The pathological implications of protein glycation." *Clin Invest Med* 18(4): 275-81.

Candido, R. and T. J. Allen (2002). "Haemodynamics in microvascular complications in type 1 diabetes." *Diabetes Metab Res Rev* 18(4): 286-304.

Cerami, C., H. Founds, et al. (1997). "Tobacco smoke is a source of toxic reactive glycation products." *Proc Natl Acad Sci U S A* 94(25): 13915-20.

Chow, F., E. Ozols, et al. (2004). "Macrophages in mouse type 2 diabetic nephropathy: correlation with diabetic state and progressive renal injury." *Kidney Int* 65(1): 116-28.

Chow, F. Y., D. J. Nikolic-Paterson, et al. (2004). "Macrophages in streptozotocin-induced diabetic nephropathy: potential role in renal fibrosis." *Nephrol Dial Transplant* 19(12): 2987-96.

Chow, F. Y., D. J. Nikolic-Paterson, et al. (2007). "Monocyte chemoattractant protein-1-induced tissue inflammation is critical for the development of renal injury but not type 2 diabetes in obese db/db mice." *Diabetologia* 50(2): 471-80.

Chow, F. Y., D. J. Nikolic-Paterson, et al. (2006). "Monocyte chemoattractant protein-1 promotes the development of diabetic renal injury in streptozotocin-treated mice." *Kidney Int* 69(1): 73-80.

Cooper, M. E. (1998). "Pathogenesis, prevention, and treatment of diabetic nephropathy." *Lancet* 352(9123): 213-9.

Cooper, M. E. (2001). "Interaction of metabolic and haemodynamic factors in mediating experimental diabetic nephropathy." *Diabetologia* 44(11): 1957-72.

Cooper, M. E., R. E. Gilbert, et al. (1998). "Pathophysiology of diabetic nephropathy." *Metabolism* 47(12 Suppl 1): 3-6.

Coughlan, M. T., V. Thallas-Bonke, et al. (2007). "Combination therapy with the advanced glycation end product cross-link breaker, alagebrium, and angiotensin converting enzyme inhibitors in diabetes: synergy or redundancy?" *Endocrinology* 148(2): 886-95.

De Vriese, A. S., R. G. Tilton, et al. (2001). "Vascular endothelial growth factor is essential for hyperglycemia-induced structural and functional alterations of the peritoneal membrane." *J Am Soc Nephrol* 12(8): 1734-41.

Dragomir, E., I. Manduteanu, et al. (2004). "Aspirin rectifies calcium homeostasis, decreases reactive oxygen species, and increases NO production in high glucose-exposed human endothelial cells." *J Diabetes Complications* 18(5): 289-99.

Dragomir, E., M. Tircol, et al. (2006). "Aspirin and PPAR-alpha activators inhibit monocyte chemoattractant protein-1 expression induced by high glucose concentration in human endothelial cells." *Vascul Pharmacol* 44(6): 440-9.

Endo, N., K. Nishiyama, et al. (2007). "Vitamin B6 suppresses apoptosis of NM-1 bovine endothelial cells induced by homocysteine and copper." *Biochim Biophys Acta* 1770(4): 571-7.

Figarola, J. L., S. Scott, et al. (2003). "LR-90 a new advanced glycation endproduct inhibitor prevents progression of diabetic nephropathy in streptozotocin-diabetic rats." *Diabetologia* 46(8): 1140-52.

Forbes, J. M., M. E. Cooper, et al. (2003). "Role of advanced glycation end products in diabetic nephropathy." *J Am Soc Nephrol* 14(8 Suppl 3): S254-8.

Forbes, J. M., M. T. Coughlan, et al. (2008). "Oxidative stress as a major culprit in kidney disease in diabetes." *Diabetes* 57(6): 1446-54.

Forbes, J. M., K. Fukami, et al. (2007). "Diabetic nephropathy: where hemodynamics meets metabolism." *Exp Clin Endocrinol Diabetes* 115(2): 69-84.

Forbes, J. M., V. Thallas, et al. (2003). "The breakdown of preexisting advanced glycation end products is associated with reduced renal fibrosis in experimental diabetes." *Faseb J* 17(12): 1762-4.

Forbes, J. M., L. T. Yee, et al. (2004). "Advanced glycation end product interventions reduce diabetes-accelerated atherosclerosis." *Diabetes* 53(7): 1813-23.

Fujii, M., T. Inoguchi, et al. (2007). "Pitavastatin ameliorates albuminuria and renal mesangial expansion by downregulating NOX4 in db/db mice." *Kidney Int* 72(4): 473-80.

Fukami, K., M. E. Cooper, et al. (2005). "Agents in development for the treatment of diabetic nephropathy." *Expert Opin Investig Drugs* 14(3): 279-94.

Fukami, K., S. Yamagishi, et al. (2007). "Novel therapeutic targets for diabetic nephropathy." *Endocr Metab Immune Disord Drug Targets* 7(2): 83-92.

Geraldes, P. and G. L. King "Activation of protein kinase C isoforms and its impact on diabetic complications." *Circ Res* 106(8): 1319-31.

Giacchetti, G., L. A. Sechi, et al. (2005). "The renin-angiotensin-aldosterone system, glucose metabolism and diabetes." *Trends Endocrinol Metab* 16(3): 120-6.

Gilbert, R. E., H. Krum, et al. (2003). "The renin-angiotensin system and the long-term complications of diabetes: pathophysiological and therapeutic considerations." *Diabet Med* 20(8): 607-21.

Giunti, S., G. H. Tesch, et al. (2008). "Monocyte chemoattractant protein-1 has prosclerotic effects both in a mouse model of experimental diabetes and in vitro in human mesangial cells." *Diabetologia* 51(1): 198-207.

Goldin, A., J. A. Beckman, et al. (2006). "Advanced glycation end products: sparking the development of diabetic vascular injury." *Circulation* 114(6): 597-605.

Gruden, G., S. Thomas, et al. (1999). "Interaction of angiotensin II and mechanical stretch on vascular endothelial growth factor production by human mesangial cells." *J Am Soc Nephrol* 10(4): 730-7.

Gu, L., S. Hagiwara, et al. (2006). "Role of receptor for advanced glycation end-products and signalling events in advanced glycation end-product-induced monocyte chemoattractant protein-1 expression in differentiated mouse podocytes." *Nephrol Dial Transplant* 21(2): 299-313.

Guay, C., E. Roggli, et al. "Diabetes mellitus, a microRNA-related disease?" *Transl Res* 157(4): 253-64.

Hammes, H. P., X. Du, et al. (2003). "Benfotiamine blocks three major pathways of hyperglycemic damage and prevents experimental diabetic retinopathy." *Nat Med* 9(3): 294-9.

Harcourt, B. E., K. C. Sourris, et al. "Targeted reduction of advanced glycation improves renal function in obesity." *Kidney Int.*

He, C. J., F. Zheng, et al. (2000). "Differential expression of renal AGE-receptor genes in NOD mice: possible role in nonobese diabetic renal disease." *Kidney Int* 58(5): 1931-40.

Herman, W. H., S. N. Emancipator, et al. (1998). "Vascular and glomerular expression of endothelin-1 in normal human kidney." *Am J Physiol* 275(1 Pt 2): F8-17.

Hill, C., A. Flyvbjerg, et al. (2000). "The renal expression of transforming growth factor-beta isoforms and their receptors in acute and chronic experimental diabetes in rats." *Endocrinology* 141(3): 1196-208.

Hofmann, S. M., H. J. Dong, et al. (2002). "Improved insulin sensitivity is associated with restricted intake of dietary glycoxidation products in the db/db mouse." *Diabetes* 51(7): 2082-9.

Hohenstein, B., C. P. Hugo, et al. (2008). "Analysis of NO-synthase expression and clinical risk factors in human diabetic nephropathy." *Nephrol Dial Transplant* 23(4): 1346-54.

Iacobini, C., G. Oddi, et al. (2005). "Development of age-dependent glomerular lesions in galectin-3/AGE-receptor-3 knockout mice." *Am J Physiol Renal Physiol* 289(3): F611-21.

Inoguchi, T., R. Battan, et al. (1992). "Preferential elevation of protein kinase C isoform beta II and diacylglycerol levels in the aorta and heart of diabetic rats: differential reversibility to glycemic control by islet cell transplantation." *Proc Natl Acad Sci U S A* 89(22): 11059-63.

Isoda, K., J. L. Young, et al. (2006). "Metformin inhibits proinflammatory responses and nuclear factor-kappaB in human vascular wall cells." *Arterioscler Thromb Vasc Biol* 26(3): 611-7.

Ito, Y., J. Aten, et al. (1998). "Expression of connective tissue growth factor in human renal fibrosis." *Kidney Int* 53(4): 853-61.

Jain, S. K. and G. Lim (2001). "Pyridoxine and pyridoxamine inhibits superoxide radicals and prevents lipid peroxidation, protein glycosylation, and (Na+ + K+)-ATPase activity reduction in high glucose-treated human erythrocytes." *Free Radic Biol Med* 30(3): 232-7.

Jakus, V. and N. Rietbrock (2004). "Advanced glycation end-products and the progress of diabetic vascular complications." *Physiol Res* 53(2): 131-42.

Jandeleit-Dahm, K., T. J. Allen, et al. (2000). "Is there a role for endothelin antagonists in diabetic renal disease?" *Diabetes Obes Metab* 2(1): 15-24.

Jandeleit-Dahm, K., Z. Cao, et al. (1999). "Role of hyperlipidemia in progressive renal disease: focus on diabetic nephropathy." *Kidney Int Suppl* 71: S31-6.

Kalousova, M., T. Zima, et al. (2004). "Advanced glycation end products in clinical nephrology." *Kidney Blood Press Res* 27(1): 18-28.

Kanamori, H., T. Matsubara, et al. (2007). "Inhibition of MCP-1/CCR2 pathway ameliorates the development of diabetic nephropathy." *Biochem Biophys Res Commun* 360(4): 772-7.

Kanauchi, M., H. Nishioka, et al. (2001). "Serum levels of advanced glycosylation end products in diabetic nephropathy." *Nephron* 89(2): 228-30.

Kanwar, Y. S., L. Sun, et al. "A glimpse of various pathogenetic mechanisms of diabetic nephropathy." *Annu Rev Pathol* 6: 395-423.

Kanwar, Y. S., J. Wada, et al. (2008). "Diabetic nephropathy: mechanisms of renal disease progression." *Exp Biol Med (Maywood)* 233(1): 4-11.

Kato, M., L. Arce, et al. (2009). "MicroRNAs and their role in progressive kidney diseases." *Clin J Am Soc Nephrol* 4(7): 1255-66.

Kato, M., L. Arce, et al. "A microRNA circuit mediates transforming growth factor-beta1 autoregulation in renal glomerular mesangial cells." *Kidney Int.*

Kato, M. and R. Natarajan (2009). "microRNA cascade in diabetic kidney disease: Big impact initiated by a small RNA." *Cell Cycle* 8(22): 3613-4.

Kato, M., S. Putta, et al. (2009). "TGF-beta activates Akt kinase through a microRNA-dependent amplifying circuit targeting PTEN." *Nat Cell Biol* 11(7): 881-9.

Kodera, R., K. Shikata, et al. "Glucagon-like peptide-1 receptor agonist ameliorates renal injury through its anti-inflammatory action without lowering blood glucose level in a rat model of type 1 diabetes." *Diabetologia* 54(4): 965-78.

Koschinsky, T., C. J. He, et al. (1997). "Orally absorbed reactive glycation products (glycotoxins): an environmental risk factor in diabetic nephropathy." *Proc Natl Acad Sci U S A* 94(12): 6474-9.

Koya, D., M. Haneda, et al. (2000). "Amelioration of accelerated diabetic mesangial expansion by treatment with a PKC beta inhibitor in diabetic db/db mice, a rodent model for type 2 diabetes." *FASEB J* 14(3): 439-47.

Koya, D., M. R. Jirousek, et al. (1997). "Characterization of protein kinase C beta isoform activation on the gene expression of transforming growth factor-beta, extracellular matrix components, and prostanoids in the glomeruli of diabetic rats." *J Clin Invest* 100(1): 115-26.

Kumar, B., T. Narang, et al. (2006). "A clinico-aetiological and ultrasonographic study of Peyronie's disease." *Sex Health* 3(2): 113-8.

Langham, R. G., D. J. Kelly, et al. (2008). "Increased renal gene transcription of protein kinase C-beta in human diabetic nephropathy: relationship to long-term glycaemic control." *Diabetologia* 51(4): 668-74.

Lee, F. T., Z. Cao, et al. (2004). "Interactions between angiotensin II and NF-kappaB-dependent pathways in modulating macrophage infiltration in experimental diabetic nephropathy." *J Am Soc Nephrol* 15(8): 2139-51.

Lewis, E. J., L. G. Hunsicker, et al. (1993). "The effect of angiotensin-converting-enzyme inhibition on diabetic nephropathy. The Collaborative Study Group." *N Engl J Med* 329(20): 1456-62.

Li, H., S. Nakamura, et al. (2006). "N2-carboxyethyl-2'-deoxyguanosine, a DNA glycation marker, in kidneys and aortas of diabetic and uremic patients." *Kidney Int* 69(2): 388-92.

Liu, H. Q., X. B. Wei, et al. (2006). "Angiotensin II stimulates intercellular adhesion molecule-1 via an AT1 receptor/nuclear factor-kappaB pathway in brain microvascular endothelial cells." *Life Sci* 78(12): 1293-8.

Makino, H., M. Mukoyama, et al. (2003). "Roles of connective tissue growth factor and prostanoids in early streptozotocin-induced diabetic rat kidney: the effect of aspirin treatment." *Clin Exp Nephrol* 7(1): 33-40.

Malhotra, A., D. Reich, et al. (1997). "Experimental diabetes is associated with functional activation of protein kinase C epsilon and phosphorylation of troponin I in the heart, which are prevented by angiotensin II receptor blockade." *Circ Res* 81(6): 1027-33.

Marshall, S. M. (2004). "Recent advances in diabetic nephropathy." *Postgrad Med J* 80(949): 624-33.

Marx, N., D. Walcher, et al. (2004). "Thiazolidinediones reduce endothelial expression of receptors for advanced glycation end products." *Diabetes* 53(10): 2662-8.

Massague, J. (1998). "TGF-beta signal transduction." *Annu Rev Biochem* 67: 753-91.

Matsumoto, M., M. Tanimoto, et al. (2008). "Effect of pitavastatin on type 2 diabetes mellitus nephropathy in KK-Ay/Ta mice." *Metabolism* 57(5): 691-7.

Meier, M., J. Menne, et al. (2009). "Targeting the protein kinase C family in the diabetic kidney: lessons from analysis of mutant mice." *Diabetologia* 52(5): 765-75.

Meier, M., J. K. Park, et al. (2003). "Knockout of protein kinase C alpha protect against the development of albuminuria but not renal hypertrophy." *Diabetes* In Press, Accepted 10th December, 2003.

Meier, M., J. K. Park, et al. (2007). "Deletion of protein kinase C-beta isoform in vivo reduces renal hypertrophy but not albuminuria in the streptozotocin-induced diabetic mouse model." *Diabetes* 56(2): 346-54.

Mene, P., F. Festuccia, et al. (2001). "Diabetic nephropathy and advanced glycation end products." *Contrib Nephrol*(131): 22-32.

Miyata, S., T. Haneda, et al. (1996). "Renin-angiotensin system in stretch-induced hypertrophy of cultured neonatal rat heart cells." *Eur J Pharmacol* 307(1): 81-8.

Miyata, T. and C. van Ypersele de Strihou (2003). "Angiotensin II receptor blockers and angiotensin converting enzyme inhibitors: implication of radical scavenging and transition metal chelation in inhibition of advanced glycation end product formation." *Arch Biochem Biophys* 419(1): 50-4.

Miyata, T., C. van Ypersele de Strihou, et al. (2002). "Angiotensin II receptor antagonists and angiotensin-converting enzyme inhibitors lower in vitro the formation of advanced glycation end products: biochemical mechanisms." *J Am Soc Nephrol* 13(10): 2478-87.

Mizutani, K., K. Ikeda, et al. (2002). "Inhibitor for advanced glycation end products formation attenuates hypertension and oxidative damage in genetic hypertensive rats." *J Hypertens* 20(8): 1607-14.

Montero, A., K. A. Munger, et al. (2000). "F(2)-isoprostanes mediate high glucose-induced TGF-beta synthesis and glomerular proteinuria in experimental type I diabetes." *Kidney Int* 58(5): 1963-72.

Murphy, M., C. Godson, et al. (1999). "Suppression subtractive hybridization identifies high glucose levels as a stimulus for expression of connective tissue growth factor and other genes in human mesangial cells." *J Biol Chem* 274(9): 5830-4.

Nguyen, D., F. Ping, et al. (2006). "Macrophage accumulation in human progressive diabetic nephropathy." *Nephrology (Carlton)* 11(3): 226-31.

Ninichuk, V., A. G. Khandoga, et al. (2007). "The role of interstitial macrophages in nephropathy of type 2 diabetic db/db mice." *Am J Pathol* 170(4): 1267-76.

Nishikawa, T., D. Edelstein, et al. (2000). "Normalizing mitochondrial superoxide production blocks three pathways of hyperglycaemic damage." *Nature* 404(6779): 787-90.

Njoroge, F. G. and V. M. Monnier (1989). "The chemistry of the Maillard reaction under physiological conditions: a review." *Prog Clin Biol Res* 304: 85-107.

O'Connor, A. S. and J. R. Schelling (2005). "Diabetes and the kidney." *Am J Kidney Dis* 46(4): 766-73.

Odashima, M., M. Otaka, et al. (2006). "Zinc L-carnosine protects colonic mucosal injury through induction of heat shock protein 72 and suppression of NF-kappaB activation." *Life Sci* 79(24): 2245-50.

Osicka, T. M., Z. Kiriazis, et al. (2001). "Ramipril and aminoguanidine restore renal lysosomal processing in streptozotocin diabetic rats." *Diabetologia* 44(2): 230-236.

Osicka, T. M., Y. X. Yu, et al. (2000). "Prevention of albuminuria by aminoguanidine or ramipril in streptozotocin-induced diabetic rats is associated with the normalization of glomerular protein kinase C." *Diabetes* 49(1): 87-93.

Pieper, G. M. and Riazulhaq (1997). "Activation of Nuclear Factor-Kappa-B in Cultured Endothelial Cells by Increased Glucose Concentration - Prevention by Calphostin C." *Journal of Cardiovascular Pharmacology* 30(4): 528-532.

Pugliese, G., F. Pricci, et al. (2000). "The diabetic milieu modulates the advanced glycation end product-receptor complex in the mesangium by inducing or upregulating galectin-3 expression." *Diabetes* 49(7): 1249-57.

Rabbani, N., S. S. Alam, et al. (2009). "High-dose thiamine therapy for patients with type 2 diabetes and microalbuminuria: a randomised, double-blind placebo-controlled pilot study." *Diabetologia* 52(2): 208-12.

Rahbar, S., R. Natarajan, et al. (2000). "Evidence that pioglitazone, metformin and pentoxifylline are inhibitors of glycation." *Clin Chim Acta* 301(1-2): 65-77.

Rangan, G. K., Y. P. Wang, et al. (1999). "Inhibition of nuclear factor-kappa B activation reduces cortical tubulointerstitial injury in proteinuric rats." *Kidney International* 56(1): 118-134.

Riser, B. L., M. Denichilo, et al. (2000). "Regulation of connective tissue growth factor activity in cultured rat mesangial cells and its expression in experimental diabetic glomerulosclerosis." *J Am Soc Nephrol* 11(1): 25-38.

Rizkalla, B., J. M. Forbes, et al. (2003). "Increased renal vascular endothelial growth factor and angiopoietins by angiotensin II infusion is mediated by both AT1 and AT2 receptors." *J Am Soc Nephrol* 14(12): 3061-71.

Rocco, M. V., E. G. Neilson, et al. (1992). "Attenuated expression of epithelial cell adhesion molecules in murine polycystic kidney disease." *Am J Physiol* 262(4 Pt 2): F679-86.

Roux, S., V. Breu, et al. (1999). "Endothelin antagonism with bosentan: a review of potential applications." *J Mol Med* 77(4): 364-76.

Ruiz-Ortega, M., O. Lorenzo, et al. (2000). "Angiotensin III increases MCP-1 and activates NF-kappaB and AP-1 in cultured mesangial and mononuclear cells." *Kidney Int* 57(6): 2285-98.

Ruiz-Ortega, M., O. Lorenzo, et al. (2000). "Angiotensin II activates nuclear transcription factor kappaB through AT(1) and AT(2) in vascular smooth muscle cells: molecular mechanisms." *Circ Res* 86(12): 1266-72.

Schrijvers, B. F., A. S. De Vriese, et al. (2004). "From hyperglycemia to diabetic kidney disease: the role of metabolic, hemodynamic, intracellular factors and growth factors/cytokines." *Endocr Rev* 25(6): 971-1010.

Seo, B., B. S. Oemar, et al. (1994). "Both ETA and ETB receptors mediate contraction to endothelin-1 in human blood vessels." *Circulation* 89(3): 1203-8.

Sharma, K., J. H. Ix, et al. "Pirfenidone for diabetic nephropathy." *J Am Soc Nephrol* 22(6): 1144-51.

Sharma, K., Y. Jin, et al. (1996). "Neutralization of TGF-beta by anti-TGF-beta antibody attenuates kidney hypertrophy and the enhanced extracellular matrix gene expression in STZ-induced diabetic mice." *Diabetes* 45(4): 522-30.
Shimoike, T., T. Inoguchi, et al. (2000). "The meaning of serum levels of advanced glycosylation end products in diabetic nephropathy." *Metabolism* 49(8): 1030-5.
Singh, R., A. Barden, et al. (2001). "Advanced glycation end-products: a review." *Diabetologia* 44(2): 129-46.
Soulis, T., V. Thallas, et al. (1997). "Advanced glycation end products and their receptors co-localise in rat organs susceptible to diabetic microvascular injury." *Diabetologia* 40(6): 619-28.
Sourris, K. C. and J. M. Forbes (2009). "Interactions between advanced glycation end-products (AGE) and their receptors in the development and progression of diabetic nephropathy - are these receptors valid therapeutic targets." *Curr Drug Targets* 10(1): 42-50.
Sowers, J. R. and C. S. Stump (2004). "Insights into the biology of diabetic vascular disease: what's new?" *Am J Hypertens* 17(11 Pt 2): 2S-6S; quiz A2-4.
Stirban, A., M. Negrean, et al. (2006). "Benfotiamine prevents macro- and microvascular endothelial dysfunction and oxidative stress following a meal rich in advanced glycation end products in individuals with type 2 diabetes." *Diabetes Care* 29(9): 2064-71.
Sung, e. a. (2004). *J Am Soc Nephrol* 15: 720A.
Tesch, G. H. (2008). "MCP-1/CCL2: a new diagnostic marker and therapeutic target for progressive renal injury in diabetic nephropathy." *Am J Physiol Renal Physiol* 294(4): F697-701.
Thallas-Bonke, V., C. Lindschau, et al. (2004). "Attenuation of extracellular matrix accumulation in diabetic nephropathy by the advanced glycation end product cross-link breaker ALT-711 via a protein kinase C-alpha-dependent pathway." *Diabetes* 53(11): 2921-30.
Tonolo, G., M. Ciccarese, et al. (1997). "Reduction of albumin excretion rate in normotensive microalbuminuric type 2 diabetic patients during long-term simvastatin treatment." *Diabetes Care* 20(12): 1891-5.
Tossidou, I., G. Starker, et al. (2009). "PKC-alpha modulates TGF-beta signaling and impairs podocyte survival." *Cell Physiol Biochem* 24(5-6): 627-34.
Tsuchida, K., Z. Makita, et al. (1999). "Suppression of transforming growth factor beta and vascular endothelial growth factor in diabetic nephropathy in rats by a novel advanced glycation end product inhibitor, OPB-9195." *Diabetologia* 42(5): 579-88.
Twigg, S. M., Z. Cao, et al. (2002). "Renal Connective Tissue Growth Factor Induction in Experimental Diabetes is prevented by aminoguanidine." *Endocrinology* 143(12): 4907-4915.
Twigg, S. M., M. M. Chen, et al. (2001). "Advanced glycosylation end products up-regulate connective tissue growth factor (insulin-like growth factor-binding protein-related protein 2) in human fibroblasts: A potential mechanism for expansion of extracellular matrix in diabetes mellitus." *Endocrinology* 142(5): 1760-1769.
Villeneuve, L. M. and R. Natarajan "The role of epigenetics in the pathology of diabetic complications." *Am J Physiol Renal Physiol* 299(1): F14-25.

Vlassara, H. (1997). "Recent progress in advanced glycation end products and diabetic complications." *Diabetes* 46 Suppl 2: S19-25.

Vlassara, H. (2001). "The AGE-receptor in the pathogenesis of diabetic complications." *Diabetes Metab Res Rev* 17(6): 436-43.

Vlassara, H. and R. Bucala (1996). "Recent progress in advanced glycation and diabetic vascular disease: role of advanced glycation end product receptors." *Diabetes* 45 Suppl 3: S65-6.

Wada, R., Y. Nishizawa, et al. (2001). "Effects of OPB-9195, anti-glycation agent, on experimental diabetic neuropathy." *Eur J Clin Invest* 31(6): 513-20.

Wagman, A. S. and J. M. Nuss (2001). "Current therapies and emerging targets for the treatment of diabetes." *Curr Pharm Des* 7(6): 417-50.

Wang, B., M. Herman-Edelstein, et al. "E-cadherin expression is regulated by miR-192/215 by a mechanism that is independent of the profibrotic effects of transforming growth factor-beta." *Diabetes* 59(7): 1794-802.

Wang, B., P. Koh, et al. "miR-200a Prevents renal fibrogenesis through repression of TGF-beta2 expression." *Diabetes* 60(1): 280-7.

Wang, Q. Y. and F. Q. Chen (2009). "Clinical significance and different levels of urinary monocyte chemoattractant protein-1 in type 2 diabetes mellitus." *Diabetes Res Clin Pract* 83(2): 215-9.

Wautier, J. L., C. Zoukourian, et al. (1996). "Receptor-mediated endothelial cell dysfunction in diabetic vasculopathy. Soluble receptor for advanced glycation end products blocks hyperpermeability in diabetic rats." *J Clin Invest* 97(1): 238-43.

Wendt, T., N. Tanji, et al. (2003). "Glucose, glycation, and RAGE: implications for amplification of cellular dysfunction in diabetic nephropathy." *J Am Soc Nephrol* 14(5): 1383-95.

Wendt, T. M., N. Tanji, et al. (2003). "RAGE drives the development of glomerulosclerosis and implicates podocyte activation in the pathogenesis of diabetic nephropathy." *Am J Pathol* 162(4): 1123-37.

Wiecek, A., J. Chudek, et al. (2003). "Role of angiotensin II in the progression of diabetic nephropathy-therapeutic implications." *Nephrol Dial Transplant* 18 Suppl 5: v16-20.

Williams, M. E. (2006). "New potential agents in treating diabetic kidney disease: the fourth act." *Drugs* 66(18): 2287-98.

Williams, M. E., W. K. Bolton, et al. (2007). "Effects of pyridoxamine in combined phase 2 studies of patients with type 1 and type 2 diabetes and overt nephropathy." *Am J Nephrol* 27(6): 605-14.

Williams, M. E. and K. R. Tuttle (2005). "The next generation of diabetic nephropathy therapies: an update." *Adv Chronic Kidney Dis* 12(2): 212-22.

Wolf, G. (2004). "New insights into the pathophysiology of diabetic nephropathy: from haemodynamics to molecular pathology." *Eur J Clin Invest* 34(12): 785-96.

Wolf, G., F. N. Ziyadeh, et al. (1995). "Angiotensin II-stimulated expression of transforming growth factor beta in renal proximal tubular cells: attenuation after stable transfection with the c-mas oncogene." *Kidney Int* 48(6): 1818-27.

Wrana, J. L., L. Attisano, et al. (1994). "Mechanism of activation of the TGF-beta receptor." *Nature* 370(6488): 341-7.

Wu, C. H., C. M. Huang, et al. (2002). "Advanced glycosylation end products induce NF-kappaB dependent iNOS expression in RAW 264.7 cells." *Mol Cell Endocrinol* 194(1-2): 9-17.

Xia, P., T. Inoguchi, et al. (1994). "Characterization of the Mechanism for the Chronic Activation of Diacylglycerol-Protein Kinase C Pathway in Diabetes and Hypergalactosemia." *Diabetes* 43(9): 1122-1129.

Yan, S. D., A. M. Schmidt, et al. (1994). "Enhanced cellular oxidant stress by the interaction of advanced glycation end products with their receptors/binding proteins." *J Biol Chem* 269(13): 9889-97.

Youssef, S., D. T. Nguyen, et al. (1999). "Effect of diabetes and aminoguanidine therapy on renal advanced glycation end-product binding." *Kidney Int* 55(3): 907-16.

Zheng, F., C. He, et al. (2002). "Prevention of diabetic nephropathy in mice by a diet low in glycoxidation products." *Diabetes Metab Res Rev* 18(3): 224-37.

Zheng, L., S. J. Howell, et al. (2007). "Salicylate-based anti-inflammatory drugs inhibit the early lesion of diabetic retinopathy." *Diabetes* 56(2): 337-45.

Ziyadeh, F. N., M. P. Cohen, et al. (1997). "RAGE mRNA expression in the diabetic mouse kidney." *Mol Cell Biochem* 170(1-2): 147-52.

Ziyadeh, F. N., B. B. Hoffman, et al. (2000). "Long-term prevention of renal insufficiency, excess matrix gene expression, and glomerular mesangial matrix expansion by treatment with monoclonal antitransforming growth factor-beta antibody in db/db diabetic mice." *Proc Natl Acad Sci U S A* 97(14): 8015-20.

12

Antioxidant Therapy for Diabetic Kidney Disease

Alina Livshits[1] and Axel Pflueger[2]
[1]*Department of Molecular Pharmacology and Experimental Therapeutics Mayo Clinic College of Medicine, Rochester, MN*
[2]*Division of Nephrology and Hypertension, College of Medicine Mayo Clinic, Rochester, MN USA*

1. Introduction

Diabetic kidney disease (DKD) is the single most common cause of end stage renal disease (ESRD) with the annual costs of caring for patients with DKD exceeding more than $9 billion in the United States (Centers of Disease Control and Prevention, 2005). Every diabetic patient has up to a 40% lifetime risk to develop DKD, if the patient does not die prematurely of cardiovascular disease (CVD) (Parving, Osterby, & Ritz, 2000). DKD can present as different phenotypes, progressive and nonprogressive (Figure 1 and 2).

Stages of CKD	GFR (mL/min/ 1.73m²)	Proteinuria/Albuminuria and/or Hematuria
1	≥90	+
2	60-89	+
3	30-59	±
4	15-29	±
5	<15	±

Stages of DKD	GFR (mL/min/ 1.73m²)	Albuminuria (mg/g)
1	≥90	-
2	60-89	30-300
3	30-59	>300
4	15-29	>3000 NS
5	<15	±

NS= Nephrotic Range Proteinuria

Fig. 1. A-B. The stages of CKD (A) and DKD (B).

Approximately, a third of patients can have progressive DKD which presents with progressive proteinuria, mainly albuminuria, a subsequent decline in glomerular filtration rate (GFR), and in some patients, progression to ESRD. Clinical studies show that renal vascular dysfunction can precede the onset of proteinuria in diabetes. Ishimura et al. demonstrated that patients with stage 1 DKD have increased resistive indices in the renal vasculature, indicating a diminished renal vasodilatory blood flow reserve (Ishimura et al., 1997). Furthermore, Frauchiger et al. validated that patients with early DKD have a diminished renal blood flow response to nitroglycerin compared to healthy controls (Frauchiger, Nussbaumer, Hugentobler, & Staub, 2000). In addition, Epstein et al. elegantly demonstrated that renal blood flow oxygenation, as quantified by blood oxygenation level-dependent magnet resonance imaging, is diminished in response to a water load in patients with stage 1 DKD compared to healthy controls, suggesting that oxygen delivery may be impaired in early stages of DKD, at least in part, due to vascular and/or endothelial dysfunction (Epstein, Veves, & Prasad, 2002). The cause for these observations is incompletely understood, but several studies suggest that inactivation of Nitric Oxide (NO) by increased reactive oxygen species (ROS) generation in diabetes may be an underlying mechanism. It has been suggested that increased generation of ROS in diabetes mellitus, namely of superoxide anion (O_2-), reduces vascular endothelial function. This endothelial dysfunction is characterized by a decreased NO-dependent vasodilation which has been demonstrated in the renal vasculature of early DKD and may also contribute to the increased cardiovascular mortality in these patients (Dai, Diederich, Skopec, & Diederich, 1993; Diederich, 1997; Kanwar et al., 2008). Any form of DKD is associated with a markedly increased cardiovascular mortality and in recent years, even low levels of albuminuria, which were previously thought to be normal, have been shown to be associated with up to 10-fold increased cardiovascular mortality (Rachmani et al., 2000).

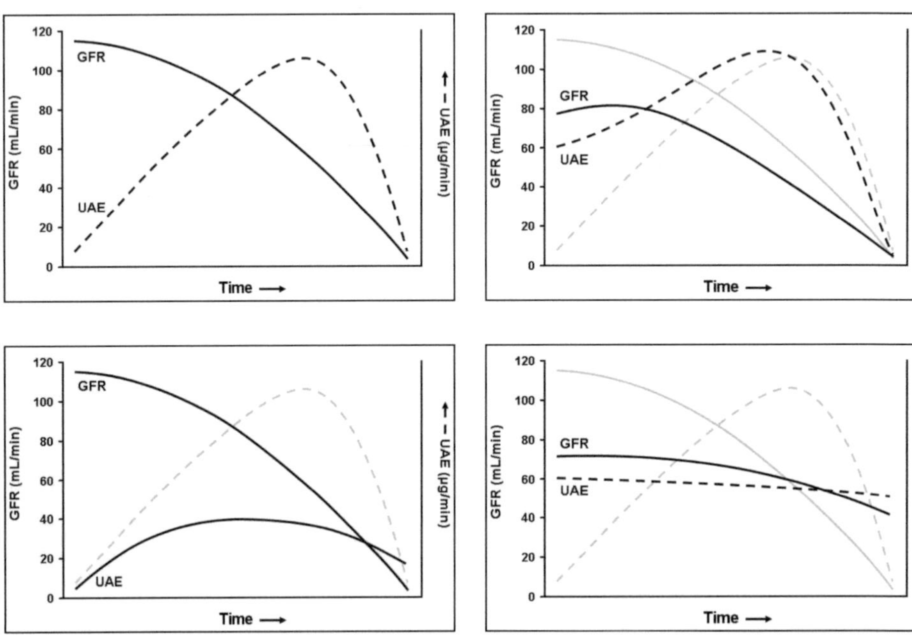

Fig. 2. A-D. Different phenotypes of DKD including progressive (A-C) and non-progressive or slowly progressive DKD (D), GFR, glomerular filtration rate; UAE, Urine albumin excretion.

The therapeutic strategies for DKD are limited due to several factors: (1) Lack of screening for DKD, (2) Lack of implementation of optimal standard therapy for DKD, and (3) Current therapies primarily slow down, but do not halt the progression of DKD. These therapies include: blood pressure, lipid, glycemic, and weight control; diet and lifestyle modifications; antiplatelet aggregation therapy; and initiation of therapy with inhibition of the renin angiotensin system (RAS) by angiotensin converting enzyme inhibitors (ACEIs), angiotensin receptor blockers (ARBs), and renin inhibitors.

A major role of DKD pathogenesis has been attributed to the increased generation of ROS in diabetes.(Figure 3)

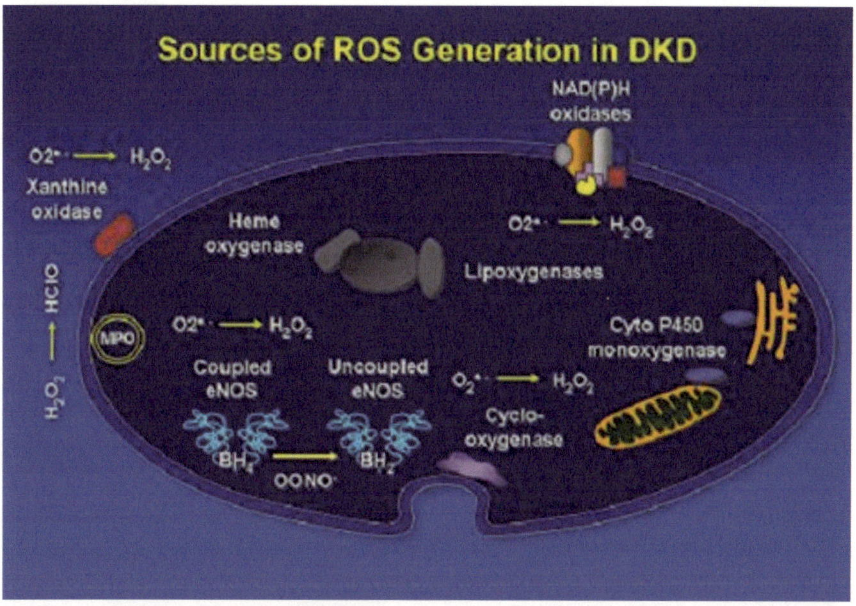

Fig. 3. Sources of ROS Generation in DKD

ROS are natural by-products of oxygen metabolism that are generated during oxidative phosphorylation and play an important role in cell signalizing, aging, cancer prevention and degenerative diseases. Oxidative radicals are highly reactive ROS capable of changing the form and function of many cellular components. Under normal conditions, common ROS, including superoxide anion (O_2-), hydrogen peroxide (H_2O_2), hydroxyl radical (OH-) and hypochlorous acid (HClO) are detoxified via electron transfer by cellular antioxidant enzyme systems (superoxide dismutase, catalase, and glutathione peroxidase). However, during periods of stress, including environmental, physical (e.g. radiation, ultraviolet light), and chemical (e.g. hyperglycemia), these free radicals are produced in excess, overwhelming the detoxification capacity of cellular antioxidant enzymes and causing cell damage. This damage is mediated directly by electron shifts or due to cytokine-mediated signal transduction and amplification, DNA damage and structural changes of lipids and proteins.

The overproduction of ROS in the kidney has been demonstrated in both animals (Koya et al., 2003) and humans with DKD (Brezniceanu et al., 2007). In addition, the products of increased ROS generation, such as 13-hydroxyoctadecadienoic acid, dimethylarginine,

8-hydroxyguanosine, and oxidized glutathione are increased in DKD (Aslam, Santha, Leone, & Wilcox, 2006). Vascular endothelium is especially prone to ROS-mediated damage (Inoguchi et al., 2003; H. B. Lee, Ha, & King, 2003; H. B. Lee, Yu, Yang, Jiang, & Ha, 2003; Li & Shah, 2003). Superoxide anion generation has been shown to inactivate NO-dependent vasodilation, likely by scavenging NO and generating the very potent ROS peroxynitrite: $NO\cdot + O_2^- \rightarrow ONOO$ (Figure 5A) (Hogg & Griffith, 1997).

The challenges antioxidant therapy faces in the clinic are two-fold: (1) prevention of further ROS generation and, (2) achieving an appropriate and constant antioxidant level at the site of injury (mitochondria). Many antioxidant molecules get converted to oxidant radicals during the redox reaction involved in scavenging ROS. Moreover, the mitochondria are the major site of ROS generation and it is questionable if most antioxidants currently in clinical use (e.g. N-acetylcysteine, vitamin C, vitamin E) are reaching their target and acting within the mitochondria in order to effectively decrease ROS generation. Some newer antioxidants, such as ubiquinones, may be more mitochondria-specific and will be discussed later (James, Cocheme, Smith, & Murphy, 2005; James et al., 2007). (Figure 3 & 4)

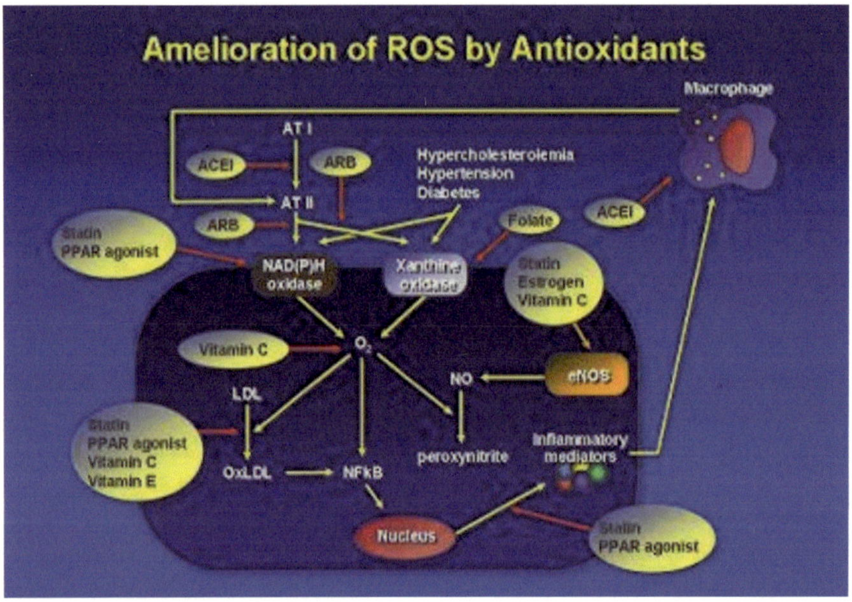

Fig. 4. Amelioration of ROS by Antioxidants

Both enzymatic (NADPH oxidase, G6PDH, xanthine oxidase, NO synthase and glycolysis pathway enzymes) and non-enzymatic reactions (glucose auto-oxidation and advanced glycation) are involved in hyperglycemia-induced overproduction of ROS. Glucose-induced protein kinase C (PKC), advanced glycosylation end-products (AGE), polyol pathways, and nuclear factor kappa B (NF-kB) activation are the 4 critical pathways involved in DKD. Agents with potential antioxidant effects currently investigated in animals and humans which will be discussed below include renin angiotensin inhibitors, protein kinase C inhibitors, TGF-B inhibitors, pentoxifylline, selective mitochondrial antioxidants, statins, vitamins C and E, sodium bicarbonate, N-acetylcysteine, bardoxolone methyl, omega-3 fatty acids, coenzyme Q10, and tempol.

2. Antioxidant therapy: ROS inhibition for the treatment of DKD

Several studies have demonstrated that inhibition of ROS generation by various therapeutic strategies and targeting different pathways are beneficial in the prevention and/or progression of DKD. An ideal antioxidant agent would be one that targets several ROS-generating pathways, in particular, mitochondrial-derived ROS. Such agents studied for the treatment of DKD are yet to be identified. Potential novel treatment strategies may include the following (see also Figure 5).

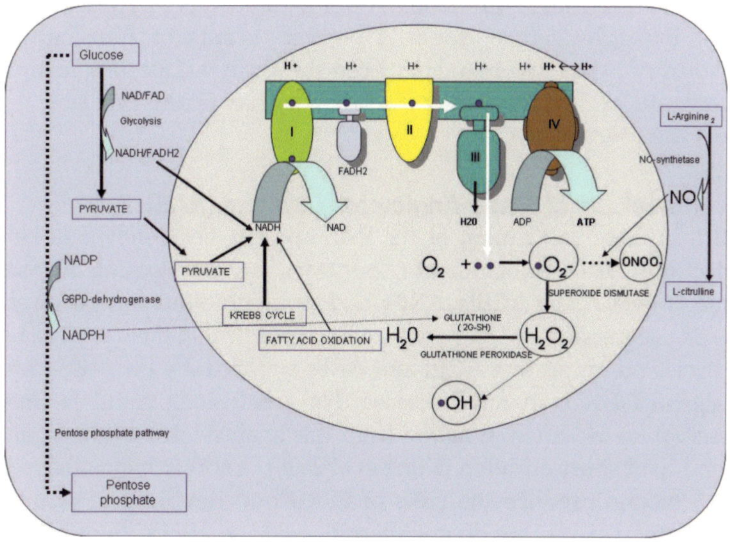

(A)

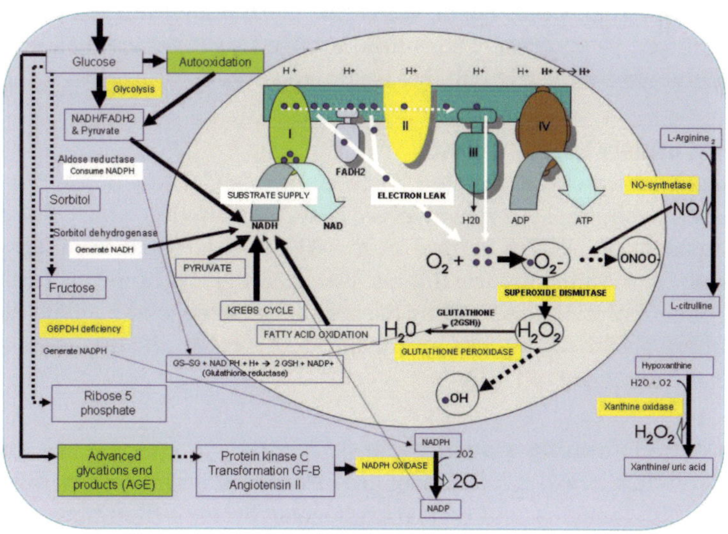

(B)

Fig. 5. A-B. Mitochondrial pathways of ROS generation in non-diabetic (A) and diabetic conditions (B).

2.1 Glycemic control

In hyperglycemia, excess glucose undergoes auto-oxidation and glycolysis to produce large amounts of NADH and FADH2 which feed into and overwhelm the electron transport chain, causing electron leaks and ROS overproduction in renal and other cells (El-Osta et al., 2008). Currently, standard therapy for DKD includes tight glycemic control, directed by glycosylated hemoglobin A1c (HbA1c) levels to prevent hyperglycemia-induced, ROS-related DKD. Target HbA1c levels of less than 7.0% have been recommended to improve DKD and/or prevent its progression in several trials (National Kidney Foundation, 2010).

Generally, elevated HbA1c levels are indicative of chronic hyperglycemia, but insensitive to detect transient hyperglycemic episodes. However, events of transient hyperglycemia (as short as 6 hours of hyperglycemia) have been shown to induce long-lasting activation of NF-kB (El-Osta et al., 2008) and are now considered a risk factor for diabetic complications independent of HbA1c levels.

2.2 Inhibition or blockade of Renin-Angiotensin System (RAS)

Angiotensin II is a major constituent of the RAS and has been shown to be an important pathogenetic factor in DKD development (Andersen, Tarnow, Rossing, Hansen, & Parving, 2000). Inhibition of the RAS by ACEIs, ARBs, and renin inhibitors have been shown to delay the onset and/or progression of DKD in numerous studies. A meta-analysis by Kunz et al analyzed 110 trials and found that ACEI and ARBs significantly decreased proteinuria, one of the early signs of DKD, in renal disease. No conclusions could be made, however, regarding preservation of kidney function from this analysis due to the variable quality of these studies and their short duration (Kunz et al 2008). Another meta-analysis of 24 studies found that RAS blockers reduce the risks of ESRD and doubling of serum creatinine in diabetic nephropathy patients, but do not affect all-cause mortality (Sarafidis et al 2008). The beneficial effects of RAS inhibitors in DKD may in part be due to their antioxidant properties (Onozato, Tojo, Goto, Fujita, & Wilcox, 2002). However, the use and benefit of these agents is limited by potentially harmful side effects such as hyperkalemia, reduction in the GFR, and failure to completely halt disease progression.

2.3 Inhibition of protein kinase C (PKC)

Hyperglycemia-mediated overexpression of protein kinase C (PKC)-β results in activation of NADPH oxidase, a lysosomal enzyme involved in ROS generation which is also increased in experimental models of DKD (Onozato et al., 2002). Ruboxistaurin, a PKC-β inhibitor, reduced proteinuria in animal models (Inoguchi et al., 2003) and humans (Tuttle et al., 2005). However, larger clinical trials are pending to confirm the safety and validate the prospective benefits of ruboxistaurin. Other PKC-β inhibitors are currently under investigation for possible use in the treatment of DKD.

2.4 Inhibitors of transforming growth factor-β (TGF-β)

Transforming growth factor-β is a family of growth and differentiation factors that includes TGF-β1, β-2, and β-3 , activins, and bone morphogenic proteins (Bottinger, 2007). TGF-β1 is a pleotrophic cytokine with complex biological activities that depend on cell type and cell context. Cell cycle control, regulation of early development, cell differentiation, angiogenesis, and immune system regulation are all activities ascribed to TGF-β1 (Schmidt-Weber & Blaser, 2004{Ghosh, 2005 #132). TGF-β is also a major regulator of the extracellular

matrix and tissue repair. A highly validated deleterious action of TGF-β is its contribution to the progressive fibrosis of CKD (Bottinger & Bitzer, 2002) and DKD (Chen et al., 2001). TGF-β1 appears to be the predominant isotype mediating disease progression. Experimental evidence indcates that TGF-β1 is the most abundant isoform expressed in the kidney. The TGF-β2 and-β3 isoforms have been shown to mediate part of their effect through upregulation of β1 expression (Chen et al., 2001). In addition, it has been demonstrated in the *db/db* mouse model of DKD that a neutralizing monoclonical antibody (mAb) specific for TGF-β-1 was as effective in reducing renal damage as an mAb against all 3 TGF-β isoforms (Ziyadeh et al., 2000). Thus, modulation of TGF-β1 activity would be expected to retard DKD progression without interfering with either important regulatory roles of TGF-β2 and -β3. Humanized IgG4 mAb that has potent and selective neralizing activity against active TGF-β1 (known as CAT-192) is being tested for DKD therapy. Monoclonal antibodies against TGF-β are currently under clinical investigation for DKD.
TGF-β is not only fibrogenic and causes glomerulosclerosis(Sharma, Jin, Guo, & Ziyadeh, 1996) but can also generate ROS by inducting NADPH oxidase (Misra & Rabideau, 2000). Pirfenidone is an inhibitor of fibroblast growth factor, platelet derived growth factor, and TGF-β. Pirfenidone has antioxidant properities, and has been shown to slow the progression of glomerulosclerosis (Misra & Rabideau, 2000; RamachandraRao et al., 2009). Pirfenidone has been clinically used for the treatement of interstitial lung disease, and recently been shown to have beneficial effects for DKD (Sharma et al., 2011).

2.5 Inhibition of non-enzymatic glycation

Advance glycation end-product (AGE) are endogenous proteins which are non-enzymatically glycated following auto-oxidation of glucose, primarily in diabetes. The interaction between AGE and their receptors (RAGE) in the kidney has been shown to activate expression of NF-kB which stimulates ROS production, contributing to DKD (Schmidt et al., 1995). Pyridoxamine inhibits glycation of proteins and decreases AGE deposition in animal models of DKD (Degenhardt et al., 2002). One clinical trial in DKD patients who were treated with pyridoxamine demonstrated a reduced progression of DKD defined as the improvement of the serum creatinine; however, a reduction of urinary albumin excretion was not observed (Williams et al., 2007). A multi-center, randomized controlled trial studying the effects of pyridoxamine in DKD is currently being conducted.

2.6 Removal of catalytic iron

Hyperglycemia-induced glycation of proteins increases their affinity for iron, forming glycochelates. Glycochelates, as well as catalytic iron, have also been implicated in DKD (Swaminathan, Fonseca, Alam, & Shah, 2007). Desferoxamine, a commonly used iron chelator(Miller, M.J., 1989), restores endothelial function mediated by inhibition of ROS (Koo, Casper, Otto, Gira, & Swerlick, 2003). The drug has the ability to penetrate cell membranes and chelate intracellular iron species. The role of iron chelators in decreasing ROS in DKD warrants evaluation in randomized controlled clinical trials.

2.7 Role of pentoxifylline

Pentoxifylline has numerous pharmacological roles, including antioxidant and platelet aggregation inhibitor. For example, tissue necrosis factor α (TNF-α) promotes the local generation of ROS in the glomerular capillary wall, increasing albuminuria in DKD (McCarthy et al., 1998). Pentoxifylline decreases TNF-α expression and reduces proteinuria in DKD (Navarro et al., 1999). Clinical trials have demonstrated that pentoxifylline has additional mild benefits in reducing albuminuria in DKD patients who are already on ACEI or ARB therapy (Harmankaya, Seber, & Yilmaz, 2003; Navarro, Mora, Muros, & Garcia, 2005). However, pentoxifylline has anti-platelet aggregating properties and as such, may increase the risk for bleeding in patients who are already on aspirin therapy (unpublished observations by the authors).

2.8 Selective mitochondrial antioxidants

Some of the newer developed antioxidants are the ubiquinones, and in particular, MitoQ10 has been characterized as an effective mitochondrial antioxidant (Green, Brand, & Murphy, 2004). Furthermore, MitoQ10 is not itself converted to a ROS after it scavenges ROS, making it a safer antioxidant (James et al., 2005; James et al., 2007). Thus, MitoQ10 might be a promising new agent for the treatment of DKD. Idebenone (Hausse et al., 2002), is another safe mitochondrial antioxidant which has a high mitochondrial uptake. Neither the role of Idebenone nor MitoQ10 have been studied yet in the treatment of DKD and remain to be elucidated.

2.9 Statins

Statins have been shown to have multiple antioxidant properties and improve vascular remodeling (Briones et al., 2009). Statins have also been shown to reduce proteinuria (Nakamura et al., 2005) and the progression of DKD (Agarwal, 2007). Therefore, patients with DKD may benefit from intensified statin therapy, even in the setting of an already controlled LDL cholesterol level. In our practice, we have observed a significant reduction in urinary albumin excretion in patients with progressive DKD who are taking statins and are either intolerable for ACEI/ARB therapy or who are already on maximal ACEI/ARB therapy (unpublished findings). Whether these benefits for the treatment of DKD are due to the antioxidant properties of statins, still needs to be determined. Furthermore, the recently published results of the Study of Heart and Renal Protection (SHARP trial) demonstrated the safety of statins in patients with DKD, however, no significant benefits with regard to improved kidney function have been demonstrated (Baigent, C. et al. 2011). However, a population based cohort study demonstrated possible renal toxic effects of statin therapy, in that all statins were associated with acute renal failure over five years, however, the risk of that was extremely low (Hippisley-Cox and Coupland, 2010). For example, in women, the number needed to harm (NNH) for an additional case of acute kidney injury over years was 434 (ranging from 284-783).

2.10 Vitamin C and E

Vitamin C activates vitamin E and each exhibits multiple antioxidant effects, including inhibition of monocyte adhesion. Their effects have been shown in animal models of experimental diabetes mellitus (E. Y. Lee, Lee, Hong, Chung, & Hong, 2007; Nakano et al., 2008; Simsek, Naziroglu, & Erdinc, 2005). Furthermore, vitamin E protected against ROS-induced DKD in diabetic mice with the haptoglobin (Hp) 2-2 genotype (Nakhoul et al., 2009). A small randomized clinical trial of 69, type 2, diabetic patients with DKD, demonstrated a benefit with the administration of vitamin C (200 mg) and E (100 IU) in reducing urinary albumin excretion (Farvid, Jalali, Siassi, & Hosseini, 2005). Larger trials are warranted to further validate these findings.

2.11 Sodium bicarbonate

The administration of sodium bicarbonate for patients with DKD has primarily been utilized for the prevention of contrast-induced acute kidney injury (CIAKI) (Brar et al., 2008; Maioli et al., 2008; Merten et al., 2004). The pathogenesis of CIAKI involves renal ischemia and ROS generation. Therefore, the use of sodium bicarbonate, a pro-oxidant, to countervail an ROS mediated and generated process such as CIAKI, would seem questionable and counter-intuitive. Consistent with these biochemical observations (From et al., 2008), a retrospective cohort study of 7,977 patients undergoing contrast media (CM) procedures found that the administration of sodium bicarbonate for CIAKI prevention was associated with a 3-fold higher risk to develop CIAKI, compared to N-acetylcysteine alone. However, a recent study found a decrease in the progression of chronic kidney disease (CKD) and DKD in patients taking sodium bicarbonate for 2 years (de Brito-Ashurst, Varagunam, Raftery, & Yaqoob, 2009). However, sodium bicarbonate did not change proteinuria in these patients. Further studies are needed to validate these findings and the underlying mechanism.

2.12 N-acetylcysteine (NAC)

NAC has several antioxidant properties, including induction of synthesis of glutathione, which is used by glutathione peroxidase to reduce H_2O_2. Furthermore, NAC has been successfully utilized for the prevention of CIAKI in patients with DKD, since both DKD and CIAKI are associated with increased ROS generation (A. Pflueger, Abramowitz, & Calvin, 2009).

The first study of NAC for CIAKI prevention was conducted by Tepel and colleagues (Tepel et al., 2000). The investigators used 600 mg orally, twice daily, on the day before and the day of iodine CM administration and 0.45% saline intravenous hydration in comparison to 0.45% saline hydration alone. Forty-eight hours after CM administration, CIAKI tended to occur and the serum creatinine tended to increase from 2.4 to 2.6 mg/dL (P=0.18) in the control group, whereas in the NAC group, serum creatinine decreased significantly from 2.5 to 2.1 mg/dL (P=0.01). Several studies followed with conflicting results (Fishbane, 2008; Sterling, Tehrani, & Rudnick, 2008). Several factors have been postulated to contribute to these varying results, including different formulations of NAC.

Dose and treatment duration are the most decisive factors in NAC's prevention of CIAKI. NAC is commonly given for only two days (Tepel et al., 2000), and treatment duration may be too brief to effectively countervail CIAKI-induced ROS production. This treatment duration was chosen because ROS production was thought to occur only shortly after CM induction. However, this concept may need to be revised since the effects of ROS-induction may last much longer than previously assumed, particularly in diabetes. Recently, Michael Brownlee and his group (El-Osta et al., 2008) demonstrated that short-term exposure (1 hour) of high glucose induces ROS-mediated, long-lasting activation of NF-kB subunit p65 in aortic endothelial cells, both in vitro and in vivo. Interestingly, the effects of this short-term ROS-mediated induction on transcription factor activation could be observed for at least six days after the initial induction. Therefore, CIAKI prevention strategies may need to be applied for longer than two days in order to countervail ROS production and induction of other cell signaling mechanisms. In our practice, we have given NAC as long as six days after CM administration with good tolerability and outcome (unpublished observation).

Furthermore, like many antioxidants, NAC has a very short plasma half-life and plasma target levels are difficult to assess. Dosing twice daily may be insufficient to achieve consistent renoprotective effects. Moreover, the bioavailability of NAC by oral administration is limited by extensive first-pass metabolism, perhaps explaining why studies of intravenous NAC have tended to show greater efficacy in CIAKI prevention (Fishbane, 2008; Sterling et al., 2008).

NAC has been successfully used for the treatment of acetaminophen-induced ROS liver toxicity, typically utilizing 40-fold higher doses than the current recommended dose of NAC (MW: 163.19) for CIAKI prevention, which is 1200 mg daily or 7 x 10^{-3} moles. The daily physiological production of superoxide anion (MW: 31.99) has been estimated to be 1.75 kg, or 5.5 x 10^{4} moles (Frei, 1994). Furthermore, ROS production is increased in patients with diabetes and CIAKI. Therefore, it may be presumptuous to assume that 7 x 10^{-3} moles NAC would cause a meaningful reduction in a daily ROS generation of more than 5.5 x 10^{4} moles of superoxide anion, which is a greater than 7 million-fold difference. Marenzi et al. have demonstrated that doubling the dose of NAC (1200 mg twice daily) improves CIAKI prevention rates (Marenzi et al., 2006). Thus, it would seem that higher doses of NAC and longer treatment periods are necessary for more efficacious CIAKI prevention. No clinical trials studying the long-term effects of NAC on DKD have been conducted, though given its low cost and good side-effect profile, they may well be worthwhile.

2.13 Induction of transcription factor Nrf2: Bardoxolone methyl

Bardoxolyne methyl, an inducer of transcription factor Nrf2, can induce the generation of over 250 antioxidant enzymes (Dinkova-Kostova et al., 2005). Recently, Bardoxolone methyl has been shown to significantly improve the creatinine GFR and cystatin C GFR in patients with DKD after only 4 weeks (Schwartz, Denham, Hurwitz, Meyer, & Pergola, 2009). However, Bardoxolone methyl did not improve urinary albumin excretion. Moreover, a recent landmark phase 2 trial of 227 adults with CKD and type 2 DM demonstrated that bardoxolone methyl improved GFR by at least 8.2 +/-1.5 ml/min over placebo after 24 weeks of treatment and that this effect was maintained after a year of therapy. (Pergola, et al., 2011). Even though bardoxolone did not effect proteinuria in this trial.

2.14 Role of haptoglobin (Hp) genotype

Hp is a hemoglobin-binding protein that has a major role in protecting against heme-induced ROS (Levy et al., 2010; Nakhoul, Miller-Lotan, Awaad, Asleh, & Levy, 2007). There are three common Hp genotypes: Hp 1-1, Hp 2-1, and Hp 2-2. The antioxidant protection provided by Hp in DKD has been shown to be genotype-dependent in animals (Miller-Lotan et al., 2005) and humans (Burbea et al., 2004), with Hp 1-1 providing superior antioxidant protection compared with Hp 2-2. Diabetic patients with the genotype Hp 2-2 are more likely to develop DKD than those with the Hp 2-1 or Hp 1-1 genotypes (Burbea et al., 2004; Levy et al., 2010; Nakhoul et al., 2007). However, no clinical therapeutic application has been studied in connection with Hp for DKD.

2.15 Plant-derived omega-3 fatty acids: Alpha linolenic acid

Omega-3 fatty acids are incorporated into cell membrane lipids, making them less susceptible to a free radical attack. Additionally, omega-3 fatty acids up-regulate the gene expression of antioxidant enzymes and down-regulate the gene expression of genes associated with ROS production (Takahashi et al., 2002). One of the most important plant-derived omega-3 fatty acids is alpha linolenic acid, found in rapeseed (canola), chia, kiwifruit seed, soybean oil and in especially high content in flaxseed oil (Kris-Etherton, Harris, & Appel, 2003). Alpha linolenic acid has been shown to prevent the progression of DKD including reduction of proteinuria, glomerular sclerosis, and tubular abnormalities in streptozotocin (STZ)-induced diabetic rats (Barcelli, Weiss, Beach, Motz, & Thompson, 1990).

2.16 Animal-derived omega-3 fatty acids: Fish oil

Important animal-derived fatty acids include eicosapentaenoic acid (EPA) and docosahexaenoic acid (DHA) found primarily in fish oil. Among their many antioxidant effects, EPA has been shown to inhibit the production of phospholipase A2, an important pro-oxidant enzyme (von Schacky, Siess, Fischer, & Weber, 1985; Zhang et al., 2006), and DHA has been shown to decrease NADPH oxidase activity (Diep et al., 2002). However, these fatty acids are also susceptible to auto-oxidation and may, theoretically, increase ROS and lead to progression of DKD (Nenseter & Drevon, 1996).

The antioxidant effects of fish oil-derived omega-3 fatty acids have also shown promising results in animal models of DKD. Several studies have noted a decrease in albuminuria (Garman, Mulroney, Manigrasso, Flynn, & Maric, 2009; Hagiwara et al., 2006; Zhang et al., 2006) and general proteinuria (Velasquez et al., 2003) in rat and mouse models of diabetes mellitus. The percentage of glomerular abnormalities, defined as either mesangial expansion (Velasquez et al., 2003; Zhang et al., 2006) or glomerulosclerosis (Garman et al., 2009), was less in rodent diabetic models fed omega-3 fatty acids, versus placebo. The extent of tubulointerstitial fibrosis was also less in these animals (Garman et al., 2009; Velasquez et al., 2003; Zhang et al., 2006).

Fish oil-derived omega-3 fatty acid effects on human DKD subjects have been less impressive. Two double-blind, randomized controlled studies, each involving 29 type 1 diabetic patients at a tertiary center, were performed comparing fish oil (4.6 g fish oil/d) with olive oil placebo (Myrup et al., 2001; Rossing et al., 1996). In one of these studies, although triglyceride and VLDL levels were lower in the fish oil group, total and LDL cholesterol were increased in that group, when compared to placebo (Rossing et al., 1996). There was no significant change in albuminuria,(Myrup et al., 2001; Rossing et al., 1996) nor in GFR (Rossing et al., 1996) between the fish oil and control groups in type 1 diabetic patients. Currently, the data in vivo concerning the antioxidant effect of omega-3 fatty acids is inconclusive.

2.17 Red wine polyphenols

The antioxidant renoprotective effects of red wine have largely been attributed to their polyphenol constituents, which include resveratrol, quercetin, anthocyanins, gallic acid, catechin, tannic acid and myercetin. Many other alcoholic beverages as well as tea, garlic, and other plants also are known to contain increased amounts of polyphenols (Rodrigo & Bosco, 2006). Among their antioxidant mechanisms, polyphenols have been shown to increase the activity of glutathione peroxidase and prevent deactivation of endothelial nitric oxide synthase (eNOS). eNOS is an isoenzyme of nitric oxide synthase (NOS) which uses NADPH to generate NO during oxidation of L-arginine and leads to vasodilation. Low starting reagent levels result in uncoupling of NOS and generation of superoxide via NADPH oxidase instead. Decreased NO-dependent renal vasodilation has been demonstrated in early DKD in both animals (Matsumoto, Koshiishi, Inoguchi, Nawata, &

Utsumi, 2003; A. C. Pflueger, Larson, Hagl, & Knox, 1999; A. C. Pflueger, Osswald, & Knox, 1999; A. C. Pflueger, Schenk, & Osswald, 1995) and humans (Frauchiger et al., 2000), also suggesting an uncoupling of the NO signal transduction pathway.

Several studies have also been carried out on rodent DKD models. For example, direct quercetin administration resulted in reduced levels of oxidative stress and attenuation of diabetic proteinuria, polyuria, serum creatinine, and blood urea nitrogen in STZ-induced diabetic rats when compared to STZ diabetic controls (Anjaneyulu & Chopra, 2004). Green tea polyphenol with partially hydrolyzed gaur gum has also been shown to reduce oxidative stress and improve kidney weight, blood urea nitrogen levels, serum creatinine, and creatinine clearance in partially nephrectasized and STZ-induced diabetic rats (Yokozawa, Nakagawa, Oya, Okubo, & Juneja, 2005). Another study on STZ rats led by the Montilla group included administration of red wine four weeks after, as well as two weeks prior to STZ injection. Treatment with red wine significantly prevented changes induced by STZ, including decreased albuminuria, proteinuria, glucosuria, triglycerides, and total cholesterol, when compared with the control STZ rat group (Montilla et al., 2005).

Several studies in humans suggest that chronic exposure to moderate amounts of red wine improve DKD. A large cross sectional study involving 157 type 1 diabetes patients with macroalbuminuria found that those who consume moderate amounts (30-70 g/week) of alcoholic beverages including red wine and beer, had a significantly lower incidence of macroalbuminuria than those who did not (Beulens et al., 2008). A randomized, controlled study involving moderate red wine versus white wine consumption (4 oz/day, for 6 months) in type 2 diabetes patients with DKD showed a statistically significant decrease in proteinuria, as well as in excretion of 8-hydroxydeoxyguanosine and liver type fatty acid-binding protein (markers of tubulointerstitial damage and of CKD, respectively) only in the red wine group (Nakamura, Fujiwara, Sugaya, Ueda, & Koide, 2009). Red wine has a higher content of polyphenols than white wine. Another randomized, controlled trial in diabetic patients showed that the administration of moderate amounts of red wine with a polyphenol-enriched, low-iron-available, carbohydrate-restricted diet was 40-50% more effective in improving renal and overall survival rates than the standard protein restriction diet (Facchini & Saylor, 2003). Further studies need to be conducted in order to investigate the full benefit of these compounds in patients with DKD.

2.18 Berry polyphenols

An important subgroup of polyphenol-containing foods are berries, such as acai berries, bilberries, raspberries, black currants, strawberries, blueberries, lingonberry extracts, and grapes (Pacheco-Palencia, Talcott, Safe, & Mertens-Talcott, 2008; Schauss et al., 2006; Seeram et al., 2008; Spada, de Souza, Bortolini, Henriques, & Salvador, 2008; Sun et al., 2010).

The most beneficial antioxidant molecules in berries are polyphenolic acids, including gallic acid, hydroxybenzoic acids, and flavanoids, including flavan-3-ols along with cyaniding 3-*O*- rutinoside and cyaniding 3-*O*-glucoside. One example is the acai fruit berry. Acai is a palm fruit from South America, and the pulp and oil extracts have been studied and shown to inhibit cell proliferation and demonstrate antioxidant properties (Mertens-Talcott et al., 2008; Pacheco-Palencia et al., 2008). Acai extract has been shown to improve endothelium-dependent vasodilatation in the mesenteric vascular bed of rats (Rocha et al., 2007). Furthermore, acai juice and pulp have been shown to increase plasma antioxidant capacity in humans up to threefold, albeit without an elevation in urinary antioxidants (Mertens-

Talcott et al., 2008). The benefits of the acai berry from pulp and oil in vitro have been demonstrated in humans with a dual effect on ROS generation, in that lower concentrations of acai extract may increase ROS generation, whereas higher concentrations have antioxidant properties (Pacheco-Palencia et al., 2008).

The antioxidant capacity of polyphenolics has further been demonstrated in freeze-dried acai extract (Schauss et al., 2006) and in other frozen fruits (Spada et al., 2008), suggesting that processed food items still retain antioxidant properties (Mertens-Talcott et al., 2008).

In one study, the antioxidant property of acai extract, assessed by SOD-induced scavenging of superoxide anion, was remarkably higher than in other reported fruit and vegetables. Seeram and colleagues also compared the antioxidant properties of several polyphenol-rich beverages, including acai juice. Their analyses revealed that the highest antioxidant index and gallic acid equivalence occur in the following order, from highest to lowest antioxidant properties: pomegranate juice, red wine, grape juice, blueberry juice, blackberry juice, acai juice, cranberry juice, orange juice, apple juice, green tea, and black tea (Seeram et al., 2008).

2.19 Role of heme oxygenase (HO)

HO is a heme degradation enzyme which is expressed in several organs, including liver and kidney. It is involved in the production of several molecules known to have antioxidant properties including, carbon monoxide, biliverdin/bilirubin, and iron/ferritin (Stocker, Yamamoto, McDonagh, Glazer, & Ames, 1987). HO-2 is constituitively expressed, while the inducible isoform, HO-1 is generated in response to oxidative stress. HO's specific functions in the kidney include maintaining renal blood flow, vasotonic equilibrium, and sodium and fluid absorption in the Loop of Henle (Abraham, Cao, Sacerdoti, Li, & Drummond, 2009). HO-1 has also been shown to enhance renal mitochondrial transport carriers and cytochrome c oxidase activity (Di Noia et al., 2006). CO, one of the products of heme degradation, has been shown to have both pro-oxidant (via vasoconstriction) and antioxidant (via vasodilation) effects (Abraham et al., 2009; Lamon et al., 2009).

The antioxidant effects of HO-1 have also been demonstrated in rodent DKD models. Goodman, et al. examined the differences between HO-2 (-/-) knockout and HO-2 (+/+) wildtype mice. When diabetes was induced by STZ in both groups, HO-2 (-/-) mice demonstrated increased plasma creatinine levels, acute tubular damage and microvascular pathology when compared to their wildype HO-2 counterparts. An inverse relationship was demonstrated between HO and superoxide levels. These results clearly indicate that HO activity is essential in preserving renal function and morphology in STZ-induced diabetic mice (Abraham et al., 2009; Goodman et al., 2006).

Although there are studies showing the causative role of pro-oxidants, including endothelin-1, TGF-β and platelet-derived growth factor (PDGF) in DKD patients (Gilbert, Akdeniz, Allen, & Jerums, 2001; Jandeleit-Dahm, Allen, Youssef, Gilbert, & Cooper, 2000; Langham et al., 2003) and HO-1 has been shown to inhibit these pro-oxidants (Abraham et al., 2009; A. Pflueger et al., 2005), no human studies have been performed demonstrating the direct effect of HO on alleviating DKD.

2.20 Role of bilirubin

As noted above, bilirubin is a degradation product of HO and is long known to have antioxidant properties (Stocker, Glazer, & Ames, 1987; Stocker, Yamamoto, et al., 1987). The ROS scavenging properties of bilirubin have been demonstrated in rat tissue samples. In rat liver tissue exposed to oxidative stresses including UVA radiation, menadione bisulfite, or copper sulfate, the addition of low doses of bilirubin prevented lipid peroxidation and attenuation of glutathione reductase antioxidant enzyme (Ossola, Groppa, & Tomaro, 1997; Ossola, Kristoff, & Tomaro, 2000; Ossola & Tomaro, 1995, 1998). Bilirubin and biliverdin (bilirubin's immediate precursor) inhibit CO-induced superoxide generation in rat renal arteries (Lamon et al., 2009). Bilirubin also demonstrated important effects on angiotensin II (AII) activity: in vitro, AII administration results in vascular smooth muscle contraction and generation of superoxide anion, a powerful ROS. Administration of bilirubin was shown to normalize the pressor and pro-oxidant effects of AII (A. Pflueger et al., 2005).

Despite the aforementioned beneficial properties, high levels of bilirubin have also been associated with adverse effects in cells. In our own experiments, higher bilirubin concentrations (≥100 μM, ≥5.8 mg/dL) were associated with apoptosis (unpublished observations by the authors). Bilirubin has also been shown to inhibit mitochondrial enzymes, cause DNA damage, and inhibit protein synthesis (Chuniaud et al., 1996). Moreover, bilirubin has been shown to have inhibitory effects on ion exchange and water transport in the kidney (Sellinger, Haag, Burckhardt, Gerok, & Knauf, 1990).

A few studies involving bilirubin and renal damage that may mimic DKD have been carried out in animal models. Recently, Adin and colleagues demonstrated that micromolar doses of bilirubin improved renal vascular resistance, urine output, GFR, tubular function, and mitochondrial integrity in rats exposed to ischemia/reperfusion renal injury (which can occur in DKD) (Abraham et al., 2009; Adin, Croker, & Agarwal, 2005). The attenuating effect of bilirubin on AII has also been shown in animal models although AII administration caused a significant decrease in GFR and impairment of both endothelium-dependent and endothelium-independent vasodilators in control rats, hyperbilirubinemic Gunn rats were resistant to such effects (A. Pflueger et al., 2005). Another study by Fujii et al. suggests a protective effect of bilirubin in diabetic animal models via downregulation of NADPH oxidase. Diabetic, hyperbilirubinemic Gunn j/j rats and biliverdin-treated diabetic db/db mice were found to have a lack of progression of mesangial expansion and less albuminuria than the control diabetic, j/+ Gunn rats and non-biliverdin-treated db/db mice, respectively, suggesting a bilirubin- and biliverdin-induced resistance to the development of DKD. In vascular endothelial and mesangial cells cultured from these animals, bilirubin and biliverdin were found to significantly inhibit NADPH-dependent superoxide production, as well as hyperglycemic- and AII-induced production of ROS, suggesting that this bilirubin- and biliverdin-induced protection is mediated by an antioxidant mechanism (Fujii et al., 2010).

Several human studies have recently been conducted studying the antioxidant effects of bilirubin on DKD. A cross-sectional, population-based study of 93,909 Korean subjects found that CKD due to diabetes mellitus was significantly lower in women with higher bilirubin levels, but not in men (Han et al., 2010). However, another cross-sectional study using demographic data from 13,184 US patients found higher serum bilirubin levels to be associated with lower estimated GFR and higher albuminuria, but found no significant associations in diabetic patients (Targher et al., 2009). A recent case control study compared bilirubin levels of 32 type 2 diabetic patients with DKD to those of 32 likewise diabetic patients without DKD, matched for gender, age, and diabetes duration. Bilirubin was 5.5 +/-2.3 umol/l in cases versus 7.3+/- 3.3 umol/l in controls ($P = 0.02$), suggesting a protective effect of bilirubin on DKD in humans (Zelle, Deetman, Alkhalaf, Navis, & Bakker, 2011).

2.21 Role of coenzyme Q10

Coenzyme Q10 (also known as ubiquinone, or "Q10") is a lipid-soluble component of the electron transport chain. In its reduced form (ubiquinol-10), coenzyme Q10 acts as an antioxidant, inhibiting lipid peroxidation and free radical oxidative damage.

Studies involving Q10's renal effects have thus far been sparse. No rodent studies focusing on DKD have been performed. However, the effects of Q10 on renal function in human diabetics are beginning to be conducted. A 1998 study by Suzuki (Suzuki et al., 1998) and colleagues studied the effect of Q10 on 28 subjects with a rare form of diabetes called maternally inherited diabetes mellitus and deafness (MIDD), caused by a mutation of one of the tRNA genes in the mitochondrial DNA. The subjects were given daily doses of 150mg of Q10 over a period of three years. Results showed that Q10 improved insulin secretory response, post-exercise lactate levels, and progression of hearing loss in these patients. However, Q10 was not shown to improve diabetic complications in these patients, including DKD.

A recent randomized, controlled 8-week trial involving 74 subjects by Mori and colleagues showed that when taken in conjunction with omega-3 fatty acids (4g/d), Q10 (200mg/d) improves systolic and especially diastolic blood pressure in (non-diabetic) moderate-to-severe CKD patients. This effect on diastolic blood pressure using combination therapy was only marginally better than the results of omega-3 fatty acids being used alone (3.4 mm Hg decrease for combination therapy versus 2.9 mm Hg decrease for omega-3 alone), and thus, the effects of Q10 alone on blood pressure need confirmation. When Q10 was used alone on such patients, no benefit on blood pressure was observed; in fact, Q10 demonstrated a slight tachycardic effect. Since hypertension is an important prognostic factor in the progression of CKD, the authors of this study suggested that Q10 may slow down CKD progression when used in conjunction with omega-3 fatty acids (Mori et al., 2009). However, more studies involving Q10 used alone and in combination with omega-3 fatty acids would have to be performed in order to elucidate its effect on CKD. Studies involving Coenzyme Q10 and diabetes-induced CKD and other manifestations of DKD would also need to be performed in order to investigate Q10's effect on this aspect of diabetes.

2.22 Tempol

Nitroxides, also known as superoxide dismutase mimetics, are a class of potent, synthetic antioxidants. One of the nitroxides, tempol, has been studied extensively for its antioxidant properties. Tempol metabolizes superoxide anion to by a catalase-like action. Furthermore, nitroxides metabolize, detoxify, or prevent the formation or action of a wide range of other ROS (Wilcox & Pearlman, 2008).

In animals, tempol has been shown to prevent the development of hypertension, proteinuria, oxidative ROS, podocyte damage, and upregulation of the aldosterone effector kinase-1 in glomerular podocytes of uni-nephrectomized rats (Ebenezer, Mariappan, Elks, Haque, & Francis, 2009). The authors have suggested that the beneficial effects of tempol on the reduction of proteinuria and glomerular damage are due to its antioxidant properties (Wilcox & Pearlman, 2008). Interestingly, tempol has been shown to improve renal oxygenation in rats and thereby may improve bioavailability of NO. Numerous studies have demonstrated blood pressure-reducing effects of tempol which are outlined in a detailed review article published by Wilcox and Pearlman (Wilcox & Pearlman, 2008). Tempol has also been demonstrated to reduce SOD activity in the renal cortical tissue of diabetic Zucker rats, thereby reducing the expression of numerous pro-

oxidant factors such as TNF, NF-kB and NADPH oxidase (Ebenezer et al., 2009). Furthermore, the reduction of renal SOD reduced the progression of DKD in the C57 BL\6 Akita diabetic mouse model (Fujita et al., 2009).
However, to date, tempol has never been studied in clinical trials for the treatment of DKD. Although tempol has potential properties to be effective in clinical trials, it can act as a pro-oxidant when used in high doses. Therefore, appropriate dosing regimens have to be determined clinically (Wilcox & Pearlman, 2008).

2.23 Other potential antioxidants for the treatment of DKD

Other potential antioxidant agents for the treatment of DKD include the following, with the potential antioxidant mechanism in parenthesis: selenium (cofactor for glutathione peroxidase), reduced glutathione (reducing agent by virtue of an SH-group), ceruloplasmin (binding iron), transferrin (binding iron), albumin (binding iron and copper), uric acid (binding iron and copper), amino-steroids (e.g. methylprednisolone; inhibit lipid peroxidation by non-glucocorticoid action), metformin (inhibits lipid peroxidation, increases SOD and glutathione levels), thiazolidinediones (inhibit lipid peroxidation, decrease inflammatory mediators, decrease $p47^{phox}$ expression), folate (decreases eNOS and xanthine oxidase-mediated O_2^- production), estrogen (decreases eNOS transcription), NOS inhibitors (decrease NO and potentially $ONOO^-$), endothelin receptor antagonists, and vitamin B. However, these agents have not been studied systematically to determine their clinical effects in the treatment of DKD and warrant further evaluation.

3. Conclusions

The increased generation of ROS production in diabetes plays a critical role in the pathogenesis of DKD. Appropriate and successful antioxidant therapy for the treatment of DKD will vitally depend on several factors, including: mechanism of action, site of action, auto-oxidation and conversion to ROS while serving as an antioxidant, plasma half-life, mode of delivery, safety, and tolerability. In the past, the benefits of antioxidant therapy have been limited by ineffective targeting of ROS pathways and ROS production at the site of injury or disease process. Antioxidant agents acting directly at the mitochondrial site may promise higher efficacy than non-specific antioxidant agents. However, clinical trials and the development of further appropriate and more effective antioxidant agents are warranted.

4. Acknowledgements

The authors gratefully acknowledge the editorial assistance of Jody Clikeman and Dawn Bergen. Furthermore, the authors appreciate the valuable support of Elana Pflueger.

5. References

Abraham, N. G., Cao, J., Sacerdoti, D., Li, X., & Drummond, G. (2009). Heme oxygenase: the key to renal function regulation. *Am J Physiol Renal Physiol, 297*(5), F1137-1152. doi: 10.1152/ajprenal.90449.2008

Adin, C. A., Croker, B. P., & Agarwal, A. (2005). Protective effects of exogenous bilirubin on ischemia-reperfusion injury in the isolated, perfused rat kidney. *Am J Physiol Renal Physiol, 288*(4), F778-784. doi: 10.1152/ajprenal.00215.2004

Agarwal, R. (2007). Effects of statins on renal function. *Mayo Clin Proc, 82*(11), 1381-1390.

Andersen, S., Tarnow, L., Rossing, P., Hansen, B. V., & Parving, H. H. (2000). Renoprotective effects of angiotensin II receptor blockade in type 1 diabetic patients with diabetic nephropathy. *Kidney Int, 57*(2), 601-606. doi: 10.1046/j.1523-1755.2000.00880.x

Anjaneyulu, M., & Chopra, K. (2004). Quercetin, an anti-oxidant bioflavonoid, attenuates diabetic nephropathy in rats. *Clin Exp Pharmacol Physiol, 31*(4), 244-248. doi: 10.1111/j.1440-1681.2004.03982.x

Aslam, S., Santha, T., Leone, A., & Wilcox, C. (2006). Effects of amlodipine and valsartan on oxidative stress and plasma methylarginines in end-stage renal disease patients on hemodialysis. *Kidney Int, 70*(12), 2109-2115. doi: 10.1038/sj.ki.5001983

Baignet, C., Landray, M., Reith, C., Emberson, J., Wheeler, D.C., Tomson, C ...Collins, R. (2011). The effect of lowering LDL cholesterol with simvastatin plus ezetimibe in patients with chronic kidney disease (Study of Heart and Renal Protection): a randomised placebo-controlled trial. The Lancet, 377:2181-2192. doi:10:1016/S0140-6736(11)60739-3.

Barcelli, U. O., Weiss, M., Beach, D., Motz, A., & Thompson, B. (1990). High linoleic acid diets ameliorate diabetic nephropathy in rats. *Am J Kidney Dis, 16*(3), 244-251.

Beulens, J. W., Kruidhof, J. S., Grobbee, D. E., Chaturvedi, N., Fuller, J. H., & Soedamah-Muthu, S. S. (2008). Alcohol consumption and risk of microvascular complications in type 1 diabetes patients: the EURODIAB Prospective Complications Study. *Diabetologia, 51*(9), 1631-1638. doi: 10.1007/s00125-008-1091-z

Bottinger, E. P. (2007). TGF-beta in renal injury and disease. *Semin Nephrol, 27*(3), 309-320. doi: 10.1016/j.semnephrol.2007.02.009

Bottinger, E. P., & Bitzer, M. (2002). TGF-beta signaling in renal disease. *J Am Soc Nephrol, 13*(10), 2600-2610.

Brar, S. S., Shen, A. Y., Jorgensen, M. B., Kotlewski, A., Aharonian, V. J., Desai, N., . . . Burchette, R. J. (2008). Sodium bicarbonate vs sodium chloride for the prevention of contrast medium-induced nephropathy in patients undergoing coronary angiography: a randomized trial. *JAMA, 300*(9), 1038-1046. doi: 10.1001/jama.300.9.1038

Brezniceanu, M. L., Liu, F., Wei, C. C., Tran, S., Sachetelli, S., Zhang, S. L., . . . Chan, J. S. (2007). Catalase overexpression attenuates angiotensinogen expression and apoptosis in diabetic mice. *Kidney Int, 71*(9), 912-923. doi: 10.1038/sj.ki.5002188

Briones, A. M., Rodriguez-Criado, N., Hernanz, R., Garcia-Redondo, A. B., Rodrigues-Diez, R. R., Alonso, M. J., . . . Salaices, M. (2009). Atorvastatin prevents angiotensin II-induced vascular remodeling and oxidative stress. *Hypertension, 54*(1), 142-149. doi: 10.1161/hypertensionaha.109.133710

Burbea, Z., Nakhoul, F., Zoabi, R., Hochberg, I., Levy, N. S., Benchetrit, S., . . . Levy, A. P. (2004). Haptoglobin phenotype as a predictive factor of mortality in diabetic haemodialysis patients. *Ann Clin Biochem, 41*(Pt 6), 469-473. doi: 10.1258/0004563042466758

Centers of Disease Control and Prevention. (2005). National Diabetes Fact Sheet, 2005. Retrieved July 5, 2011, from http://www.cdc.gov/diabetes/pubs/factsheet05.htm

Chen, S., Hong, S. W., Iglesias-de la Cruz, M. C., Isono, M., Casaretto, A., & Ziyadeh, F. N. (2001). The key role of the transforming growth factor-beta system in the pathogenesis of diabetic nephropathy. *Ren Fail, 23*(3-4), 471-481.

Chuniaud, L., Dessante, M., Chantoux, F., Blondeau, J. P., Francon, J., & Trivin, F. (1996). Cytotoxicity of bilirubin for human fibroblasts and rat astrocytes in culture. Effect of the ratio of bilirubin to serum albumin. *Clin Chim Acta, 256*(2), 103-114.

Dai, F. X., Diederich, A., Skopec, J., & Diederich, D. (1993). Diabetes-induced endothelial dysfunction in streptozotocin-treated rats: role of prostaglandin endoperoxides and free radicals. *J Am Soc Nephrol, 4*(6), 1327-1336.

de Brito-Ashurst, I., Varagunam, M., Raftery, M. J., & Yaqoob, M. M. (2009). Bicarbonate supplementation slows progression of CKD and improves nutritional status. *J Am Soc Nephrol, 20*(9), 2075-2084. doi: 10.1681/asn.2008111205

Degenhardt, T. P., Alderson, N. L., Arrington, D. D., Beattie, R. J., Basgen, J. M., Steffes, M. W., . . . Baynes, J. W. (2002). Pyridoxamine inhibits early renal disease and dyslipidemia in the streptozotocin-diabetic rat. *Kidney Int, 61*(3), 939-950. doi: 10.1046/j.1523-1755.2002.00207.x

Di Noia, M. A., Van Driesche, S., Palmieri, F., Yang, L. M., Quan, S., Goodman, A. I., & Abraham, N. G. (2006). Heme oxygenase-1 enhances renal mitochondrial transport carriers and cytochrome C oxidase activity in experimental diabetes. *J Biol Chem, 281*(23), 15687-15693. doi: 10.1074/jbc.M510595200

Diederich, D. (1997). Nitric oxide in diabetic nephropathy. In M. Golligorsky, Gorss, S. (Ed.), *Nitric Oxide and the Kidney: Physiology and Pathophysiology* (pp. 349-367). New York, : Chapman & Hall.

Diep, Q. N., Amiri, F., Touyz, R. M., Cohn, J. S., Endemann, D., Neves, M. F., & Schiffrin, E. L. (2002). PPARalpha activator effects on Ang II-induced vascular oxidative stress and inflammation. *Hypertension, 40*(6), 866-871.

Dinkova-Kostova, A. T., Liby, K. T., Stephenson, K. K., Holtzclaw, W. D., Gao, X., Suh, N., . . . Talalay, P. (2005). Extremely potent triterpenoid inducers of the phase 2 response: correlations of protection against oxidant and inflammatory stress. *Proc Natl Acad Sci U S A, 102*(12), 4584-4589. doi: 10.1073/pnas.0500815102

Ebenezer, P. J., Mariappan, N., Elks, C. M., Haque, M., & Francis, J. (2009). Diet-induced renal changes in Zucker rats are ameliorated by the superoxide dismutase mimetic TEMPOL. *Obesity (Silver Spring), 17*(11), 1994-2002. doi: 10.1038/oby.2009.137

El-Osta, A., Brasacchio, D., Yao, D., Pocai, A., Jones, P. L., Roeder, R. G., . . . Brownlee, M. (2008). Transient high glucose causes persistent epigenetic changes and altered gene expression during subsequent normoglycemia. *J Exp Med, 205*(10), 2409-2417. doi: 10.1084/jem.20081188

Epstein, F. H., Veves, A., & Prasad, P. V. (2002). Effect of diabetes on renal medullary oxygenation during water diuresis. *Diabetes Care, 25*(3), 575-578.

Facchini, F. S., & Saylor, K. L. (2003). A low-iron-available, polyphenol-enriched, carbohydrate-restricted diet to slow progression of diabetic nephropathy. *Diabetes, 52*(5), 1204-1209.

Farvid, M. S., Jalali, M., Siassi, F., & Hosseini, M. (2005). Comparison of the effects of vitamins and/or mineral supplementation on glomerular and tubular dysfunction in type 2 diabetes. *Diabetes Care, 28*(10), 2458-2464.

Fishbane, S. (2008). N-acetylcysteine in the prevention of contrast-induced nephropathy. *Clin J Am Soc Nephrol, 3*(1), 281-287. doi: 10.2215/cjn.02590607

Frauchiger, B., Nussbaumer, P., Hugentobler, M., & Staub, D. (2000). Duplex sonographic registration of age and diabetes-related loss of renal vasodilatory response to nitroglycerine. *Nephrol Dial Transplant, 15*(6), 827-832.

Frei, B. (1994). Reactive oxygen species and antioxidant vitamins: mechanisms of action. *Am J Med, 97*(3A), 5S-13S; discussion 22S-28S.

From, A. M., Bartholmai, B. J., Williams, A. W., Cha, S. S., Pflueger, A., & McDonald, F. S. (2008). Sodium bicarbonate is associated with an increased incidence of contrast nephropathy: a retrospective cohort study of 7977 patients at mayo clinic. *Clin J Am Soc Nephrol, 3*(1), 10-18. doi: 10.2215/cjn.03100707

Fujii, M., Inoguchi, T., Sasaki, S., Maeda, Y., Zheng, J., Kobayashi, K., & Takayanagi, R. (2010). Bilirubin and biliverdin protect rodents against diabetic nephropathy by downregulating NAD(P)H oxidase. *Kidney Int, 78*(9), 905-919. doi: 10.1038/ki.2010.265

Fujita, H., Fujishima, H., Chida, S., Takahashi, K., Qi, Z., Kanetsuna, Y., . . . Takahashi, T. (2009). Reduction of renal superoxide dismutase in progressive diabetic nephropathy. *J Am Soc Nephrol, 20*(6), 1303-1313. doi: 10.1681/asn.2008080844

Garman, J. H., Mulroney, S., Manigrasso, M., Flynn, E., & Maric, C. (2009). Omega-3 fatty acid rich diet prevents diabetic renal disease. *Am J Physiol Renal Physiol, 296*(2), F306-316. doi: 10.1152/ajprenal.90326.2008

Gilbert, R. E., Akdeniz, A., Allen, T. J., & Jerums, G. (2001). Urinary transforming growth factor-beta in patients with diabetic nephropathy: implications for the pathogenesis of tubulointerstitial pathology. *Nephrol Dial Transplant, 16*(12), 2442-2443.

Goodman, A. I., Chander, P. N., Rezzani, R., Schwartzman, M. L., Regan, R. F., Rodella, L., . . . Abraham, N. G. (2006). Heme oxygenase-2 deficiency contributes to diabetes-mediated increase in superoxide anion and renal dysfunction. *J Am Soc Nephrol, 17*(4), 1073-1081. doi: 10.1681/asn.2004121082

Green, K., Brand, M. D., & Murphy, M. P. (2004). Prevention of mitochondrial oxidative damage as a therapeutic strategy in diabetes. *Diabetes, 53 Suppl 1*, S110-118.

Hagiwara, S., Makita, Y., Gu, L., Tanimoto, M., Zhang, M., Nakamura, S., . . . Tomino, Y. (2006). Eicosapentaenoic acid ameliorates diabetic nephropathy of type 2 diabetic KKAy/Ta mice: involvement of MCP-1 suppression and decreased ERK1/2 and p38 phosphorylation. *Nephrol Dial Transplant, 21*(3), 605-615. doi: 10.1093/ndt/gfi208

Han, S. S., Na, K. Y., Chae, D. W., Kim, Y. S., Kim, S., & Chin, H. J. (2010). High serum bilirubin is associated with the reduced risk of diabetes mellitus and diabetic nephropathy. *Tohoku J Exp Med, 221*(2), 133-140.

Harmankaya, O., Seber, S., & Yilmaz, M. (2003). Combination of pentoxifylline with angiotensin converting enzyme inhibitors produces an additional reduction in microalbuminuria in hypertensive type 2 diabetic patients. *Ren Fail, 25*(3), 465-470.

Hausse, A. O., Aggoun, Y., Bonnet, D., Sidi, D., Munnich, A., Rotig, A., & Rustin, P. (2002). Idebenone and reduced cardiac hypertrophy in Friedreich's ataxia. *Heart, 87*(4), 346-349.

Hippisley-Cox, J. & Coupland, C. (2010). Unintended effects of statins: population based cohort study. British Medical Journal 340:c2197.

Hogg, N., & Griffith, O. (1997). The biological chemistry of NO. *Nitric Oxide and the Kidney, MS Goligorsky and SS Gross*, 3-21.

Inoguchi, T., Sonta, T., Tsubouchi, H., Etoh, T., Kakimoto, M., Sonoda, N., . . . Nawata, H. (2003). Protein kinase C-dependent increase in reactive oxygen species (ROS) production in vascular tissues of diabetes: role of vascular NAD(P)H oxidase. *J Am Soc Nephrol, 14*(8 Suppl 3), S227-232.

Ishimura, E., Nishizawa, Y., Kawagishi, T., Okuno, Y., Kogawa, K., Fukumoto, S., . . . Morii, H. (1997). Intrarenal hemodynamic abnormalities in diabetic nephropathy measured by duplex Doppler sonography. *Kidney Int, 51*(6), 1920-1927.

James, A. M., Cocheme, H. M., Smith, R. A., & Murphy, M. P. (2005). Interactions of mitochondria-targeted and untargeted ubiquinones with the mitochondrial respiratory chain and reactive oxygen species. Implications for the use of exogenous ubiquinones as therapies and experimental tools. *J Biol Chem, 280*(22), 21295-21312. doi: 10.1074/jbc.M501527200

James, A. M., Sharpley, M. S., Manas, A. R., Frerman, F. E., Hirst, J., Smith, R. A., & Murphy, M. P. (2007). Interaction of the mitochondria-targeted antioxidant MitoQ with phospholipid bilayers and ubiquinone oxidoreductases. *J Biol Chem, 282*(20), 14708-14718. doi: 10.1074/jbc.M611463200

Jandeleit-Dahm, K., Allen, T. J., Youssef, S., Gilbert, R. E., & Cooper, M. E. (2000). Is there a role for endothelin antagonists in diabetic renal disease? *Diabetes Obes Metab, 2*(1), 15-24.

Kanwar, Y. S., Wada, J., Sun, L., Xie, P., Wallner, E. I., Chen, S., . . . Danesh, F. R. (2008). Diabetic nephropathy: mechanisms of renal disease progression. *Exp Biol Med (Maywood), 233*(1), 4-11. doi: 10.3181/0705-mr-134

Koo, S. W., Casper, K. A., Otto, K. B., Gira, A. K., & Swerlick, R. A. (2003). Iron chelators inhibit VCAM-1 expression in human dermal microvascular endothelial cells. *J Invest Dermatol, 120*(5), 871-879. doi: 10.1046/j.1523-1747.2003.12144.x

Koya, D., Hayashi, K., Kitada, M., Kashiwagi, A., Kikkawa, R., & Haneda, M. (2003). Effects of antioxidants in diabetes-induced oxidative stress in the glomeruli of diabetic rats. *J Am Soc Nephrol, 14*(8 Suppl 3), S250-253.

Kris-Etherton, P. M., Harris, W. S., & Appel, L. J. (2003). Fish consumption, fish oil, omega-3 fatty acids, and cardiovascular disease. *Arterioscler Thromb Vasc Biol, 23*(2), e20-30.

Kunz, R., Friedrich, C., Wolbers, M., Mann, J.F. (2008). Meta-analysis: effect of monotherapy and combination therapy with inhibitors of the renin angiotensin system on proteinuria in renal disease. Ann Intern Med 148:30-48.

Lamon, B. D., Zhang, F. F., Puri, N., Brodsky, S. V., Goligorsky, M. S., & Nasjletti, A. (2009). Dual pathways of carbon monoxide-mediated vasoregulation: modulation by redox mechanisms. *Circ Res, 105*(8), 775-783. doi: 10.1161/circresaha.109.197434

Langham, R. G., Kelly, D. J., Maguire, J., Dowling, J. P., Gilbert, R. E., & Thomson, N. M. (2003). Over-expression of platelet-derived growth factor in human diabetic nephropathy. *Nephrol Dial Transplant, 18*(7), 1392-1396.

Lee, E. Y., Lee, M. Y., Hong, S. W., Chung, C. H., & Hong, S. Y. (2007). Blockade of oxidative stress by vitamin C ameliorates albuminuria and renal sclerosis in experimental diabetic rats. *Yonsei Med J, 48*(5), 847-855. doi: 10.3349/ymj.2007.48.5.847

Lee, H. B., Ha, H., & King, G. (2003). Reactive Oxygen Species and Diabetic Nephropathy. *J Am Soc Nephrol, 14*, S209-S210.

Lee, H. B., Yu, M. R., Yang, Y., Jiang, Z., & Ha, H. (2003). Reactive oxygen species-regulated signaling pathways in diabetic nephropathy. *J Am Soc Nephrol, 14*(8 Suppl 3), S241-245.

Levy, A. P., Asleh, R., Blum, S., Levy, N. S., Miller-Lotan, R., Kalet-Litman, S., . . . Goldenstein, H. (2010). Haptoglobin: basic and clinical aspects. *Antioxid Redox Signal, 12*(2), 293-304. doi: 10.1089/ars.2009.2793

Li, J. M., & Shah, A. M. (2003). ROS generation by nonphagocytic NADPH oxidase: potential relevance in diabetic nephropathy. *J Am Soc Nephrol, 14*(8 Suppl 3), S221-226.

Maioli, M., Toso, A., Leoncini, M., Gallopin, M., Tedeschi, D., Micheletti, C., & Bellandi, F. (2008). Sodium bicarbonate versus saline for the prevention of contrast-induced nephropathy in patients with renal dysfunction undergoing coronary angiography or intervention. *J Am Coll Cardiol, 52*(8), 599-604. doi: 10.1016/j.jacc.2008.05.026

Marenzi, G., Assanelli, E., Marana, I., Lauri, G., Campodonico, J., Grazi, M., . . . Bartorelli, A. L. (2006). N-acetylcysteine and contrast-induced nephropathy in primary angioplasty. *N Engl J Med, 354*(26), 2773-2782. doi: 10.1056/NEJMoa054209

Matsumoto, S., Koshiishi, I., Inoguchi, T., Nawata, H., & Utsumi, H. (2003). Confirmation of superoxide generation via xanthine oxidase in streptozotocin-induced diabetic mice. *Free Radic Res, 37*(7), 767-772.

McCarthy, E. T., Sharma, R., Sharma, M., Li, J. Z., Ge, X. L., Dileepan, K. N., & Savin, V. J. (1998). TNF-alpha increases albumin permeability of isolated rat glomeruli through the generation of superoxide. *J Am Soc Nephrol, 9*(3), 433-438.

Merten, G. J., Burgess, W. P., Gray, L. V., Holleman, J. H., Roush, T. S., Kowalchuk, G. J., . . . Kennedy, T. P. (2004). Prevention of contrast-induced nephropathy with sodium bicarbonate: a randomized controlled trial. *JAMA, 291*(19), 2328-2334. doi: 10.1001/jama.291.19.2328

Mertens-Talcott, S. U., Rios, J., Jilma-Stohlawetz, P., Pacheco-Palencia, L. A., Meibohm, B., Talcott, S. T., & Derendorf, H. (2008). Pharmacokinetics of anthocyanins and antioxidant effects after the consumption of anthocyanin-rich acai juice and pulp (Euterpe oleracea Mart.) in human healthy volunteers. *J Agric Food Chem, 56*(17), 7796-7802. doi: 10.1021/jf8007037

Miller, M.J. (1989). Syntheses and therapeutic potential of hydroxamic acid based siderophores and analogs. Chem Rev 89:1563-1579.

Miller-Lotan, R., Herskowitz, Y., Kalet-Litman, S., Nakhoul, F., Aronson, D., Zoabi, R., . . . Levy, A. P. (2005). Increased renal hypertrophy in diabetic mice genetically modified at the haptoglobin locus. *Diabetes Metab Res Rev, 21*(4), 332-337. doi: 10.1002/dmrr.556

Misra, H. P., & Rabideau, C. (2000). Pirfenidone inhibits NADPH-dependent microsomal lipid peroxidation and scavenges hydroxyl radicals. *Mol Cell Biochem, 204*(1-2), 119-126.

Montilla, P., Barcos, M., Munoz, M. C., Bujalance, I., Munoz-Castaneda, J. R., & Tunez, I. (2005). Red wine prevents brain oxidative stress and nephropathy in streptozotocin-induced diabetic rats. *J Biochem Mol Biol, 38*(5), 539-544.

Mori, T. A., Burke, V., Puddey, I., Irish, A., Cowpland, C. A., Beilin, L., . . . Watts, G. F. (2009). The effects of [omega]3 fatty acids and coenzyme Q10 on blood pressure and heart rate in chronic kidney disease: a randomized controlled trial. *J Hypertens, 27*(9), 1863-1872.

Myrup, B., Rossing, P., Jensen, T., Parving, H. H., Holmer, G., Gram, J., . . . Jespersen, J. (2001). Lack of effect of fish oil supplementation on coagulation and transcapillary escape rate of albumin in insulin-dependent diabetic patients with diabetic nephropathy. *Scand J Clin Lab Invest, 61*(5), 349-356.

Nakamura, T., Fujiwara, N., Sugaya, T., Ueda, Y., & Koide, H. (2009). Effect of red wine on urinary protein, 8-hydroxydeoxyguanosine, and liver-type fatty acid-binding protein excretion in patients with diabetic nephropathy. *Metabolism, 58*(8), 1185-1190. doi: 10.1016/j.metabol.2009.03.019

Nakamura, T., Sugaya, T., Kawagoe, Y., Ueda, Y., Osada, S., & Koide, H. (2005). Effect of pitavastatin on urinary liver-type fatty acid-binding protein levels in patients with early diabetic nephropathy. *Diabetes Care, 28*(11), 2728-2732.

Nakano, M., Onodera, A., Saito, E., Tanabe, M., Yajima, K., Takahashi, J., & Nguyen, V. C. (2008). Effect of astaxanthin in combination with alpha-tocopherol or ascorbic acid against oxidative damage in diabetic ODS rats. *J Nutr Sci Vitaminol (Tokyo), 54*(4), 329-334.

Nakhoul, F. M., Miller-Lotan, R., Awaad, H., Asleh, R., & Levy, A. P. (2007). Hypothesis--haptoglobin genotype and diabetic nephropathy. *Nat Clin Pract Nephrol, 3*(6), 339-344. doi: 10.1038/ncpneph0467

Nakhoul, F. M., Miller-Lotan, R., Awad, H., Asleh, R., Jad, K., Nakhoul, N., . . . Levy, A. P. (2009). Pharmacogenomic effect of vitamin E on kidney structure and function in transgenic mice with the haptoglobin 2-2 genotype and diabetes mellitus. *Am J Physiol Renal Physiol, 296*(4), F830-838. doi: 10.1152/ajprenal.90655.2008

National Kidney Foundation. (2010). *Clinical practice guidelines and clinical practice recommendations for diabetes and chornic kidney disease- guidline 2: management of hyperglycemia and general diabetes care in chronic kidney disease*. New York.

Navarro, J. F., Mora, C., Muros, M., & Garcia, J. (2005). Additive antiproteinuric effect of pentoxifylline in patients with type 2 diabetes under angiotensin II receptor blockade: a short-term, randomized, controlled trial. *J Am Soc Nephrol, 16*(7), 2119-2126. doi: 10.1681/asn.2005010001

Navarro, J. F., Mora, C., Rivero, A., Gallego, E., Chahin, J., Macia, M., . . . Garcia, J. (1999). Urinary protein excretion and serum tumor necrosis factor in diabetic patients with advanced renal failure: effects of pentoxifylline administration. *Am J Kidney Dis, 33*(3), 458-463.

Nenseter, M. S., & Drevon, C. A. (1996). Dietary polyunsaturates and peroxidation of low density lipoprotein. *Curr Opin Lipidol, 7*(1), 8-13.

Onozato, M. L., Tojo, A., Goto, A., Fujita, T., & Wilcox, C. S. (2002). Oxidative stress and nitric oxide synthase in rat diabetic nephropathy: effects of ACEI and ARB. *Kidney Int, 61*(1), 186-194. doi: 10.1046/j.1523-1755.2002.00123.x

Ossola, J. O., Groppa, M. D., & Tomaro, M. L. (1997). Relationship between oxidative stress and heme oxygenase induction by copper sulfate. *Arch Biochem Biophys, 337*(2), 332-337.

Ossola, J. O., Kristoff, G., & Tomaro, M. L. (2000). Heme oxygenase induction by menadione bisulfite adduct-generated oxidative stress in rat liver. *Comp Biochem Physiol C Toxicol Pharmacol, 127*(1), 91-99.

Ossola, J. O., & Tomaro, M. L. (1995). Heme oxygenase induction by cadmium chloride: evidence for oxidative stress involvement. *Toxicology, 104*(1-3), 141-147.

Ossola, J. O., & Tomaro, M. L. (1998). Heme oxygenase induction by UVA radiation. A response to oxidative stress in rat liver. *Int J Biochem Cell Biol, 30*(2), 285-292.

Pacheco-Palencia, L. A., Talcott, S. T., Safe, S., & Mertens-Talcott, S. (2008). Absorption and biological activity of phytochemical-rich extracts from acai (Euterpe oleracea Mart.) pulp and oil in vitro. *J Agric Food Chem, 56*(10), 3593-3600. doi: 10.1021/jf8001608

Parving, H., Osterby, R., & Ritz, E. (2000). Diabetic Nephropathy. In B. Brenner (Ed.), *Brenner & Rector's The Kidney* (6 ed., pp. 1731-1773). Philadelphia: WB Saunders Co.

Pergola, P.E., Raskin, P., Toto, R.D., Meyer, C.J., Huff, J.W., Grossman, E.B., Krauth, M., Ruiz, S., Audhya, P., Christ-Schmidt, H., Wittes, J., Warnock, D.G., BEAM Study Investigators. (2011). Bardoxolone methyl and kidney function in CKD with type 2 -diabetes. N Engl J Med 365(4):327-336.

Pflueger, A., Abramowitz, D., & Calvin, A. D. (2009). Role of oxidative stress in contrast-induced acute kidney injury in diabetes mellitus. *Med Sci Monit, 15*(6), RA125-136.

Pflueger, A., Croatt, A. J., Peterson, T. E., Smith, L. A., d'Uscio, L. V., Katusic, Z. S., & Nath, K. A. (2005). The hyperbilirubinemic Gunn rat is resistant to the pressor effects of angiotensin II. *Am J Physiol Renal Physiol, 288*(3), F552-558. doi: 10.1152/ajprenal.00278.2004

Pflueger, A. C., Larson, T. S., Hagl, S., & Knox, F. G. (1999). Role of nitric oxide in intrarenal hemodynamics in experimental diabetes mellitus in rats. *Am J Physiol, 277*(3 Pt 2), R725-733.

Pflueger, A. C., Osswald, H., & Knox, F. G. (1999). Adenosine-induced renal vasoconstriction in diabetes mellitus rats: role of nitric oxide. *Am J Physiol, 276*(3 Pt 2), F340-346.

Pflueger, A. C., Schenk, F., & Osswald, H. (1995). Increased sensitivity of the renal vasculature to adenosine in streptozotocin-induced diabetes mellitus rats. *Am J Physiol, 269*(4 Pt 2), F529-535.

Rachmani, R., Levi, Z., Lidar, M., Slavachevski, I., Half-Onn, E., & Ravid, M. (2000). Considerations about the threshold value of microalbuminuria in patients with diabetes mellitus: lessons from an 8-year follow-up study of 599 patients. *Diabetes Res Clin Pract, 49*(2-3), 187-194.

RamachandraRao, S. P., Zhu, Y., Ravasi, T., McGowan, T. A., Toh, I., Dunn, S. R., . . . Sharma, K. (2009). Pirfenidone is renoprotective in diabetic kidney disease. *J Am Soc Nephrol, 20*(8), 1765-1775. doi: 10.1681/asn.2008090931

Rocha, A. P., Carvalho, L. C., Sousa, M. A., Madeira, S. V., Sousa, P. J., Tano, T., . . . Soares de Moura, R. (2007). Endothelium-dependent vasodilator effect of Euterpe oleracea Mart. (Acai) extracts in mesenteric vascular bed of the rat. *Vascul Pharmacol, 46*(2), 97-104. doi: 10.1016/j.vph.2006.08.411

Rodrigo, R., & Bosco, C. (2006). Oxidative stress and protective effects of polyphenols: comparative studies in human and rodent kidney. A review. *Comp Biochem Physiol C Toxicol Pharmacol, 142*(3-4), 317-327. doi: 10.1016/j.cbpc.2005.11.002

Rossing, P., Hansen, B. V., Nielsen, F. S., Myrup, B., Holmer, G., & Parving, H. H. (1996). Fish oil in diabetic nephropathy. *Diabetes Care, 19*(11), 1214-1219.

Sarafidis, P.A., Stafylas, P.C., Kanaki, A.I., Lasaridis, A.N. (2008). Effects of renin-angiotensin system blockers on renal outcomes and all-cause mortality in patients with diabetic nephropathy: an updated meta-analysis. Am J Mypertens. 21(8):922-929.

Schauss, A. G., Wu, X., Prior, R. L., Ou, B., Huang, D., Owens, J., . . . Shanbrom, E. (2006). Antioxidant capacity and other bioactivities of the freeze-dried Amazonian palm berry, Euterpe oleraceae mart. (acai). *J Agric Food Chem, 54*(22), 8604-8610. doi: 10.1021/jf0609779

Schmidt-Weber, C. B., & Blaser, K. (2004). Regulation and role of transforming growth factor-beta in immune tolerance induction and inflammation. *Curr Opin Immunol, 16*(6), 709-716. doi: 10.1016/j.coi.2004.09.008

Schmidt, A. M., Hori, O., Chen, J. X., Li, J. F., Crandall, J., Zhang, J., . . . Stern, D. (1995). Advanced glycation endproducts interacting with their endothelial receptor induce expression of vascular cell adhesion molecule-1 (VCAM-1) in cultured human endothelial cells and in mice. A potential mechanism for the accelerated vasculopathy of diabetes. *J Clin Invest, 96*(3), 1395-1403. doi: 10.1172/jci118175

Schrijvers, B.F., De Vriese, A.S., Flyvbjerg, A. (2004). From hyperglycemia to diabetic kidney disease: the role of metabolic, hemodynamic, intracellular factors and growth factors/cytokines. Endocr Rev. 25(6):971-1010.

Schwartz, S., Denham, D., Hurwitz, C., Meyer, C., & Pergola, P. (2009). Bardoxolone, a novel oral antioxidant-inflammation modulator improves renal function in patients with diabetes and CKD. *Am J Kidney Dis, 53*, B61.

Seeram, N. P., Aviram, M., Zhang, Y., Henning, S. M., Feng, L., Dreher, M., & Heber, D. (2008). Comparison of antioxidant potency of commonly consumed polyphenol-rich beverages in the United States. *J Agric Food Chem, 56*(4), 1415-1422. doi: 10.1021/jf073035s

Sellinger, M., Haag, K., Burckhardt, G., Gerok, W., & Knauf, H. (1990). Sulfated bile acids inhibit Na(+)-H+ antiport in human kidney brush-border membrane vesicles. *Am J Physiol, 258*(4 Pt 2), F986-991.

Sharma, K., Ix, J. H., Mathew, A. V., Cho, M., Pflueger, A., Dunn, S. R., . . . Kopp, J. B. (2011). Pirfenidone for diabetic nephropathy. *J Am Soc Nephrol, 22*(6), 1144-1151. doi: 10.1681/asn.2010101049

Sharma, K., Jin, Y., Guo, J., & Ziyadeh, F. N. (1996). Neutralization of TGF-beta by anti-TGF-beta antibody attenuates kidney hypertrophy and the enhanced extracellular matrix gene expression in STZ-induced diabetic mice. *Diabetes, 45*(4), 522-530.

Simsek, M., Naziroglu, M., & Erdinc, A. (2005). Moderate exercise with a dietary vitamin C and e combination protects against streptozotocin-induced oxidative damage to the kidney and lens in pregnant rats. *Exp Clin Endocrinol Diabetes, 113*(1), 53-59. doi: 10.1055/s-2004-830528

Spada, P. D., de Souza, G. G., Bortolini, G. V., Henriques, J. A., & Salvador, M. (2008). Antioxidant, mutagenic, and antimutagenic activity of frozen fruits. *J Med Food, 11*(1), 144-151. doi: 10.1089/jmf.2007.598

Sterling, K. A., Tehrani, T., & Rudnick, M. R. (2008). Clinical significance and preventive strategies for contrast-induced nephropathy. *Curr Opin Nephrol Hypertens, 17*(6), 616-623. doi: 10.1097/MNH.0b013e32830f45a3

Stocker, R., Glazer, A. N., & Ames, B. N. (1987). Antioxidant activity of albumin-bound bilirubin. *Proc Natl Acad Sci U S A, 84*(16), 5918-5922.

Stocker, R., Yamamoto, Y., McDonagh, A. F., Glazer, A. N., & Ames, B. N. (1987). Bilirubin is an antioxidant of possible physiological importance. *Science, 235*(4792), 1043-1046.

Sun, X., Seeberger, J., Alberico, T., Wang, C., Wheeler, C. T., Schauss, A. G., & Zou, S. (2010). Acai palm fruit (Euterpe oleracea Mart.) pulp improves survival of flies on a high fat diet. *Exp Gerontol, 45*(3), 243-251. doi: 10.1016/j.exger.2010.01.008

Suzuki, S., Hinokio, Y., Ohtomo, M., Hirai, M., Hirai, A., Chiba, M., . . . Toyota, T. (1998). The effects of coenzyme Q10 treatment on maternally inherited diabetes mellitus and deafness, and mitochondrial DNA 3243 (A to G) mutation. *Diabetologia, 41*(5), 584-588. doi: 10.1007/s001250050950

Swaminathan, S., Fonseca, V. A., Alam, M. G., & Shah, S. V. (2007). The role of iron in diabetes and its complications. *Diabetes Care, 30*(7), 1926-1933. doi: 10.2337/dc06-2625

Takahashi, M., Tsuboyama-Kasaoka, N., Nakatani, T., Ishii, M., Tsutsumi, S., Aburatani, H., & Ezaki, O. (2002). Fish oil feeding alters liver gene expressions to defend against PPARalpha activation and ROS production. *Am J Physiol Gastrointest Liver Physiol, 282*(2), G338-348. doi: 10.1152/ajpgi.00376.2001

Targher, G., Bosworth, C., Kendrick, J., Smits, G., Lippi, G., & Chonchol, M. (2009). Relationship of serum bilirubin concentrations to kidney function and albuminuria in the United States adult population. Findings from the National Health and Nutrition Examination Survey 2001-2006. *Clin Chem Lab Med,* Vol 47(9), 1055-1062.

Tepel, M., van der Giet, M., Schwarzfeld, C., Laufer, U., Liermann, D., & Zidek, W. (2000). Prevention of radiographic-contrast-agent-induced reductions in renal function by acetylcysteine. *N Engl J Med,* Vol 343(3), 180-184.

Tuttle, K. R., Bakris, G. L., Toto, R. D., McGill, J. B., Hu, K., & Anderson, P. W. (2005). The effect of ruboxistaurin on nephropathy in type 2 diabetes. *Diabetes Care,* Vol 28(11), 2686-2690.

Velasquez, M. T., Bhathena, S. J., Ranich, T., Schwartz, A. M., Kardon, D. E., Ali, A. A., . . . Hansen, C. T. (2003). Dietary flaxseed meal reduces proteinuria and ameliorates nephropathy in an animal model of type II diabetes mellitus. *Kidney Int,* Vol 64(6), 2100-2107. doi: 10.1046/j.1523-1755.2003.00329.x

von Schacky, C., Siess, W., Fischer, S., & Weber, P. C. (1985). A comparative study of eicosapentaenoic acid metabolism by human platelets in vivo and in vitro. *J Lipid Res, 26*(4), 457-464.

Wilcox, C. S., & Pearlman, A. (2008). Chemistry and antihypertensive effects of tempol and other nitroxides. *Pharmacol Rev,* Vol 60(4), 418-469.

Williams, M. E., Bolton, W. K., Khalifah, R. G., Degenhardt, T. P., Schotzinger, R. J., & McGill, J. B. (2007). Effects of pyridoxamine in combined phase 2 studies of patients with type 1 and type 2 diabetes and overt nephropathy. *Am J Nephrol,* Vol 27(6), 605-614.

Yokozawa, T., Nakagawa, T., Oya, T., Okubo, T., & Juneja, L. R. (2005). Green tea polyphenols and dietary fibre protect against kidney damage in rats with diabetic nephropathy. *J Pharm Pharmacol,* Vol 57(6), 773-780. doi: 10.1211/0022357056154

Zelle, D. M., Deetman, N., Alkhalaf, A., Navis, G., & Bakker, S. J. (2011). Support for a protective effect of bilirubin on diabetic nephropathy in humans. *Kidney Int,* Vol 79(6), 686; author reply 686-687.

Zhang, M., Hagiwara, S., Matsumoto, M., Gu, L., Tanimoto, M., Nakamura, S., . . . Tomino, Y. (2006). Effects of eicosapentaenoic acid on the early stage of type 2 diabetic nephropathy in KKA(y)/Ta mice: involvement of anti-inflammation and antioxidative stress. *Metabolism,* Vol 55(12), 1590-1598.

Ziyadeh, F. N., Hoffman, B. B., Han, D. C., Iglesias-De La Cruz, M. C., Hong, S. W., Isono, M., . . . Sharma, K. (2000). Long-term prevention of renal insufficiency, excess matrix gene expression, and glomerular mesangial matrix expansion by treatment with monoclonal antitransforming growth factor-beta antibody in db/db diabetic mice. *Proc Natl Acad Sci U S A,* Vol 97(14), 8015-8020.

13

Is Limb Loss Always Inevitable for Critical Neuro-Ischemic Foot Wounds in Diabetic Patients with End Stage Renal Disease and Unfit for Vascular Reconstructions?

Vlad Alexandrescu
Department of Thoracic and Vascular Surgery
Princess Paola Hospital
Marche-en-Famenne
Belgium

1. Introduction

End stage renal disease (ESRD) and diabetes mellitus are independently associated with advanced atherosclerosis with extended arterial wall calcifications and occlusions in inferior limb arteries (Norgreen et al., 2007). A severe arterial affectation was commonly documented in critical inferior limb ischemic (CLI) wounds, particularly located in the tibial trunks of these patients (Casserly, 2008; Norgreen et al., 2007). The association of CLI in subjects with impaired renal function and particularly ESRD leads to a notable higher rate of subsequent morbidity and mortality (Andreoli et al., 2008; Casserly, 2008; Mlekusch et al., 2004). Although revascularization indisputably represents the primary therapy for limb salvage (Casserly, 2008; Conrad et al., 2009; Norgreen et al., 2007), renal patients seem to require strikingly more challenging interventions, that focus hostile and diffusely diseased leg segments (Andreoli et al., 2008; Casserly, 2008; Conrad et al., 2009; Randon et al., 2010). Literature on arterial reconstruction (surgical and endovascular) reveals poor patency, tissue recovery and limb preservation data, coupled to high short and mid-term mortality rates for ESRD subjects (independently from other cardio-vascular risk factors) (Abou-Zamzam et al., 2007; Bradbury et al., 2010; Casserly, 2008; Leers et al., 1998). Similar observations were independently documented in diabetic ischemic limbs that have the metabolic and neuropathic background, local sepsis and important amount of tissue loss (Apelqvist et al., 1993; Dormandy et al., 1999; Edmonds, 2008; Norgreen et al., 2007). However, despite progresses in both surgical and endovascular approaches, in 14%-20% of these patients exhibiting advanced crural and pedal occlusive disease, neither of the available procedures can provide appropriate distal arterial supply, turning to amputation (Abou-Zamzam et al., 2007; Dormandy et al., 1999; Faglia et al., 2007). In these desperate cases, since all "conventional" arterial revascularization techniques were unsuccessful, the concept of *"venous arterialization"*, as extreme alternative for delivering the oxygenated blood to distal ischemic tissues was considered. These limb salvage alternatives for extreme CLI presentations (currently intended to amputation) were mostly described as using the available superficial veins of the affected limb (Jacop et al., 1999; Lengua et al., 2001).

While some reports claim encouraging limb salvage results (Jacop et al., 1999; Lengua et al., 2001; Lu et al., 2006), others remain reserved (Matzke et al., 1999).
Parallel efforts in CLI limb preservation were reported in the plastic reconstructive surgery field, by promoting the angiosomes model (AM) for reperfusion and tissue reconstruction upon specific arterial and venous bundles of blood supply (Attinger et al., 2001, 2006; Taylor & Pan, 1998).
A schematic description of these tissue irrigation areas in the foot is illustrated in **Fig. 1**.

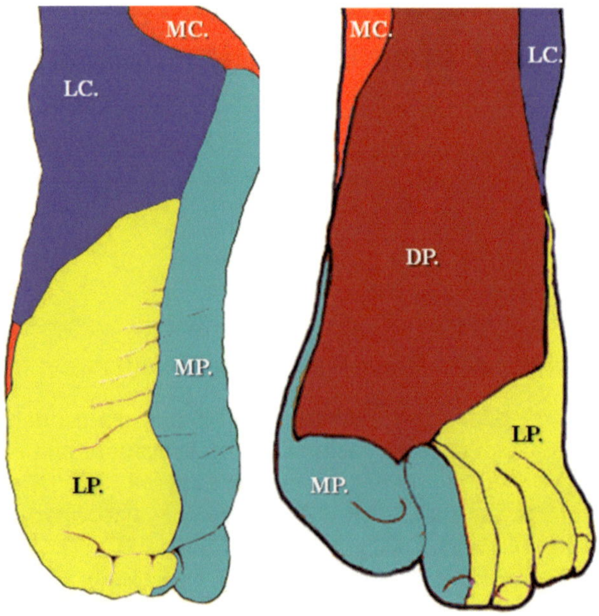

Fig. 1. A simplified illustration of the main angiosomes (and correspondent venosomes) related territories of the foot and ankle:
MC: The *Medial Calcaneal Artery*,
MP: The *Medial Plantar Artery* and **LP:** The *Lateral Plantar Artery* angiosomes, dependent from the *Posterior Tibial Artery* territory,
DP: The *Dorsalis Ppedis Artery* angiosome, from the *Anterior Tibial* arterial and venous bundle, and **LC:** The *Lateral Calcaneal Artery* angiosome from the *Peroneal arterio-venous* tract.

We propose to examine in this chapter the clinical efficacy of a new hybrid limb salvage technique (surgical and endovascular) for deep venous selective arterializations in extreme diabetic CLI presentations, unfit for any of the common arterial reconstructive methods (Alexandrescu et al., 2011). The method also proposes an appended AM strategy for revascularization, in the hope to enhance appropriate wound healing in these challenging situations (Alexandrescu et al., 2011; Attinger et al., 2006 Taylor & Pan, 1998).

2. Material and methods

Patients. From January 2003 until October 2010, a series of 28 limbs with threatening ischemic foot wounds in 26 diabetic and ESRD patients were retrospectively studied. All subjects were at high risk for major limb amputation with no feasible conventional arterial

revascularizations. They were treated by hybrid (surgical and endovascular) deep calf veins arterialization following the AM concept. This method allows **S**elective **A**rterio-**V**enous **E**ndoluminal **S**witch (the SAVES- technique, previously described by our group in the deep calf veins (Alexandrescu et al., 2011), following an AM strategy of perfusion (Attinger et al., 2001, 2006; Taylor & Pan, 1998). Two patients received a staged bilateral intervention at eight and twelve months interval, respectively. The method's aim is to provide a pulsatile flow to the foot by selective bypass arterialization of one of the paired either anterior, posterior or peroneal deep calf veins (according the AM distribution), with synchronous devalvulation and endoluminal coil-exclusion of the collaterals. The group gathered specific presentations with unfeasible or previously failed arterial reconstrucions, including lack of superficial vein material or inappropriate tissues conditions for distal bypasses (including eventual arterializations in the superficial venous network). Severe ischemic wounds (Rutherford categories 5-6.) (Dayal & Kent, 2005; Rutherford et al., 1997) confined to the foot (Wagner grades 3-4) (Driver et al., 2007) were noted in 22 limbs (79%), whereas 6 (21%) others presented complex below the knee trophic lesions. Advanced gangrene with irrecoverable tissue loss (Wagner grade 5 lesions) (Driver et al., 2007), preexisting severe cardiac insufficiency (LVEF < 30%) and eventual disagreement of patients for this type of intervention, represented the major exclusion criteria.
There were 20 men and the mean age was 73.7 years (in the range 56-89). Nine (32%) cases were insulin dependent.
Patient characteristics and risk factors are summarized in **Table I**:

PATIENTS CARACTERISTICS / RISK FACTORS	Nr. Limbs (n = 28).	(n%)
Age > 70 years	n = 12	43%
Smoking	n = 14	50%
Coronary Disease	n = 27	96%
Ejection Fraction = /< 35%	n = 18	64%
Cerebrovascular disease	n = 10	36%
COPD	n = 11	29%
LOCAL FEATURES IN TREATED	**/ LIMBS**	
3 Crural Arteries Occluded	n = 27	96%
Incomplete or occluded pedal arch	n = 22	78%
Failed previous femoral / distal bypass	n = 15	54%
Spread of Calcifications > 5cm	n = 24	86%
Associated Venuous Insufficiency OK	n = 10	35%
Inferior Limb Neuropathy	n = 26	93%
Osteomyelitis	n = 13	46%
Wagner score > 2	n = 23	82%

Table I.

The technical features of the 28 combined surgical and endovascular angiosome-oriented interventions are described in **Table II**:

The technical features of the 28 combined surgical /endovascular procedures.

Type of prosthetic bypass.		Localisation of the targeted venosome		Sites of collateral vein embolization	
FEMORO - POPLITEAL (P3)	(n = 17).	Anterior Tibial & forefoot	(n = 6)	TPt + collat. ATa.	(n = 3).
				TPa + collat. ATa.	(n = 3).
		Posterior Tibial & plantar/ heel	(n = 10).	ATa + collat. PTa.	(n = 10).
		Peroneal & lateral ankle	(n = 1).	ATa+PTa+collat. Peroneal	(n = 1).
POPLITEO (P1) - POPLITEAL (P3)	(n = 3).	Anterior Tibial & forefoot	(n = 3)	PTa + Peroneal	(n = 3).
FEMORO - TIBIAL	(n = 6).	Anterior Tibial & forefoot	(n = 2).	TPt + collat. ATa	(n = 1).
				PTa + collat. ATa	(n = 1).
		Posterior Tibial & heel	(n = 3).	Peroneal+collat. PTa	(n = 1).
				Collat. PTa	(n = 2).
		Peroneal & lateral ankle	(n = 1).	PTa + collat. Peroneal	(n = 1).
POPLITEO - TIBIAL	(n = 2).	Anterior Tibial & forefoot	(n = 1)	PTa+Peroneal+collat. ATa	(n = 1).
		Posterior Tibial & plantar	(n = 1).	ATa+Peroneal+collat. PTa	(n = 1).

ATa = Anterior Tibial artery

TPt = Tibio-Peroneal trunk

PTa = Posterior Tibial artery

Table II.

All patients were simultaneously followed in the nephrology-dialysis department. They underwent a preoperative complete inferior limbs arterial and venous Duplex scan, adding either DS-Arteriography (in our early experience) or preliminary Angio-CT assessment coupled to a per-operative angiography (in the recent years).
Complementary Duplex notification concerning the valvular competence and the anatomical distribution (the level of vein duplication) concerning the deep venous system were collected.
Following arterialization, adjuvant wound therapy was pursued in a multidisciplinary "diabetic-foot" clinic, according to each specific tissue defect presentation / **Table III**:

ADJUVANT WOUND TREATMENT	Nr. Limbs (n = 28).	(n%)
Vacuum-assisted wound closure	n = 8	28%
Biosynthetic skin substitutes	n = 2	7%
Maggot therapy	n = 5	18%
Hyperbaric oxygen therapy	n = 1	3%
Rotational skin flaps	n = 1	3%
PACE Technology	n = 2	7%
Epithelialization-stimulating dressings	n = 7	25%
Without local adjuvants: refuse or inability for treatment	n = 2	9%

Table III.

Definitions. Clinical grading of the inferior limb ischemia was evaluated according to the revised criteria of SVS/ISCVS (Rutherford et al., 1997) and the TASC (II) recommendations (Norgreen et al., 2007). Other specific clinical findings were guided by the Wagner revised classification (Driver et al., 2007) and the UK peripheral neuropathy screening score (Young et al., 1993).

The technical success was considered if a direct arterialized axis starting from the iliac level through the selected deep calf veins till the peri-malleolar or foot level network was present after devalvulation and selective embolizations of venous side branches. This implied lack of deep vein narrowing or major steal phenomena, induced by venous tibial collaterals or perforators.

Limb salvage implied no requirement of major amputation and if the functional autonomy of the patient was recovered (walking or standing) despite eventually minor amputations (at the metatarsal or toe level).

Endpoints and statistical analysis. All results were reported in an intention to treat analysis. Patency, clinical success, limb salvage and patients survival rates were studied using the Kaplan-Meier life-table method at sequential intervals.

The surgical and endovascular "SAVES" method for deep calf vein arterializations. The "hybrid" technique for vascular reconstruction (**S**elective **A**rterio-**V**enous **E**ndoluminal **S**witch - the "SAVES" method) followed a similar protocol, as previously described by our team (Alexandrescu et al., 2011). The pre-operative medication included a constant anti-platelet therapy (160 mg aspirin daily or clopidogrel 75 mg/day). In this cohort, the treatment was already started in all patients before the procedure for previous miscellaneous cardio-vascular problems. General anaesthesia was applied in 21 cases (75%), local anaesthesia and slight sedation in 6 (21%), while sole local anaesthesic products were preferred in 1 (4%) of interventions. In the *first stage* of the procedures (surgical), a classical protocol for femoro-infragenicular *PTFE bypass* was undertaken (**Fig. 2** and **3b**).

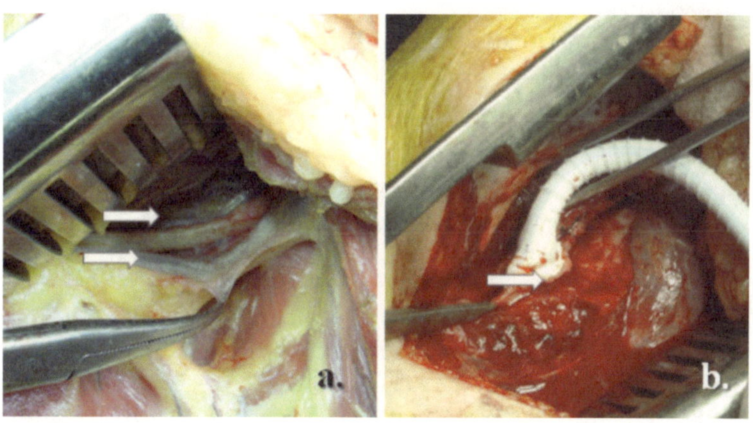

Fig. 2. Distal "PTFE- graft" anastomosis at the popliteal level:

a. The presence of a "twin popliteal veins" anatomical pattern white arrows),

b. Termino-lateral anastomosis as to arterialize one of the two popliteal veins in a femoro (arterial) - popliteal (venous) PTFE graft during *the first stage* of the procedure. The synthetic graft allows the passage of a long 6F introducer from the groin, further enhancing *the second stage* of the intervention: selective devalvulation and collateral embolization of specific tibial deep veins, following the AM distribution.

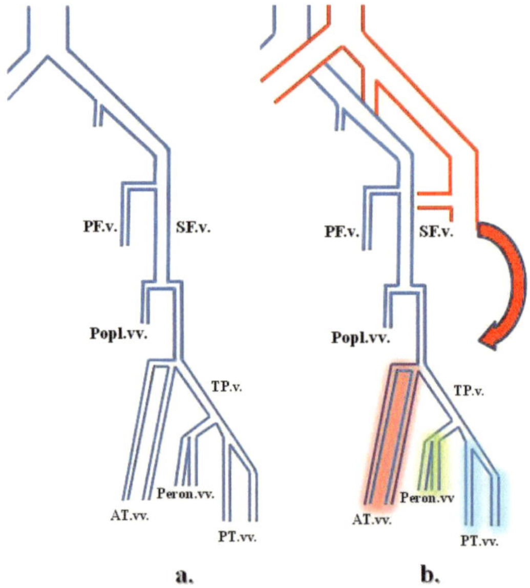

Fig. 3. a) A brief illustration of the main deep venous trunks in the leg:
PFv: *Profound Femoral* vein,
SFv: *Superficial Femoral* vein,
Popl. vv: *Popliteal* veins,
AT. vv: *Anterior Tibial* veins
Peron. vv: *Peroneal* veins
PT. vv: *Posterior Tibial* veins
b) The red curved arrow: schematic *arterial in-flow* from the groin. Below the knee twin veins and their correspondent venosomes:
In red: appended *Anterior Tibial Venosome*,
In yellow: correspondent *Peroneal Venosome*,
In blue: adjacent *Posterior Tibial Venosome*.

The common femoral artery was usually the chosen in-flow vessel (n= 16) albeit the SFA (n= 7) and the popliteal artery (n= 5) was seldom employed. The location of the distal anastomosis, to induce direct arterial flow toward the deep calf veins (**Fig. 2**), was planned upon the Duplex findings on the level of duplication (**Table II**) and topographical specificities of the wounds (the angiosomes distribution) (Attinger et al., 2001, 2006; Taylor et al., 1990, 1998). This distal anastomosis was realised on one of the doubled deep veins in a termino-lateral (n = 23) (**Fig. 2**) or termino-terminal way (n = 5). In all the cases, 8mm PTFE armed prosthesis (n = 21/ Distaflow BARD co. USA, and n = 7/ GORE Medical Products co.USA) were placed. Before clamping the femoral artery, a 2500 IU heparin amount was given in order to promote anticoagulation yet, minimizing possible interferences with the *second procedural stage* (endovascular), the *collateral embolizations*. The cephalad segment of the twin vein was ligated, while side anastomosis was chosen. Although the distal popliteal vein was found more often paired than single (**Fig. 2** and **3**) according to other similar observations (Wind et al., 1991), in ten cases (35%) the distal anastomosis was performed directly in selected venous tibial trunks **(Table II.)** and oriented toward the main corresponding foot angiosome (venosome) (**Fig. 1** and **3**). After releasing the flow in the

PTFE arterio-venous bypass, an 80cm / 6-F introducer sheath (Cook, inc. UK) was antegradely mounted via the common femoral artery traversing the prosthetic graft. A road-mapping of the infra-popliteal venous deep network was obtained, beyond the distal anastomosis. The competence of the deep valvular system was documented (often already affected by neuropathic "*idiosyncratic deep venous distension*" in this subset of patients) (Pureval et al., 1995). Although rarely needed, devalvulation was initially started by crossing each valve with a 0.035-inch hydrophilic guidewire (Terumo, Japan) and accomplished by the passage of the 6-F 80 cm long introducer sheath (occasionally necessitating few "back and forth" co-axially over the wire movements) (**Fig. 4a** and **5a**).

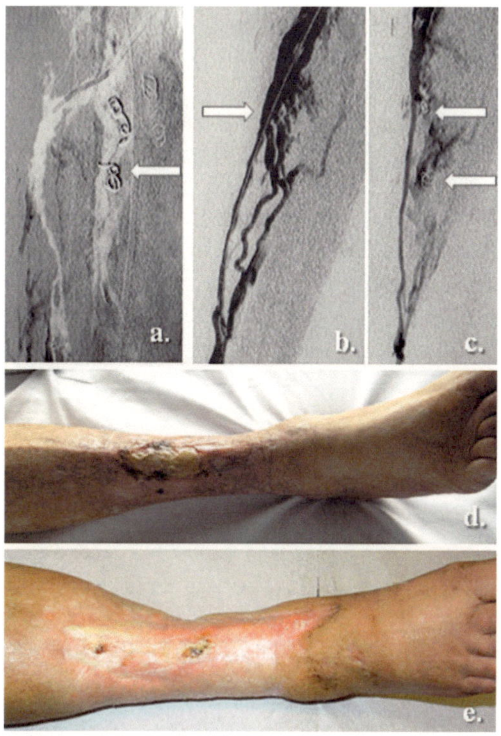

Fig. 4. Specific **Anterior Tibial** deep **veins** arterialization:

a. Initial selective embolization of the **Posteriof Tibial** and twin veins with peculiar canulation of the *Anterior Tibial* vein, enabling to direct the arterialization toward the *Anterior Tibial angiosome* and correspondent *venosome.*

b. Specific catheterization and devalvulation of the *Anterior Tibial* vein tovard the ankle,

c. The newly induced arterial flow in the *Anterior Tibial venosome*, after specific collateral embolization.

d. The initial clinical presentation featuring an extended ischemic and infected ulcer on the anterior tibial aspect of the calf.

e. The clinical outcome following specific anterior tibial veins arterialization, at seven months after multidisciplinary follow-up.

The long sheath was advanced until the ankle region in the angiosome-selected venous pathway. Contrast mapping demonstrated the principal collaterals or perforators of the chosen deep vein axis. Using a floppy tip 5-F vertebral or "Cobra 2-3" catheters (Cook inc.,

UK) or, in some other instances with a better adapted 4-F curved hydrophilic micro-catheter ("Slip-cath" selective catheter, Cook inc. UK), the main venous collaterals were selectively catheterized and occluded using coils embolization material (5-F "Tornado", "Nester" or stainless steel 5-8mm coils /Cook inc., Medical UK) (**Fig. 4 a, b, c,** and **5 a, b**). These coils were delivered mainly using the "*coaxial*" technique (and seldom only by the "*anchor*" method) (White & Pollak, 2006) in the principal deep venous ramifications. There was an average of 7.1 (n= 5-19) coils released per procedure. The side branches embolization stage was performed as distally as possible (**Fig. 4c** and **5c**), toward the clinical venosome-location of the wounds (White & Pollak, 2006). The progressing results were assessed by small contrast injections (**Fig. 4c** and **5c**). Not all the collaterals were approachable during this stage of the procedure, particularly the medium-sized to small diameter veins, usually located in the peri-malleolar deep network (**Fig. 5c**). To avoid prolonged time and contrast consuming interventions, the selective branch embolizations were restricted below the ankle level, as the distal blood pressure measured through the 6-F introducer sheath edge exceeded 50 mm Hg. This observation allowed exclusion of residual CLI hemodynamic features (Norgreen et al., 2007; Rutherford et al., 1997). Hemostasis was directly performed at the arterial puncture level after the withdrawal of sheaths. All patients were prescribed aspirin (160 mg/day) after the procedure, unless intolerant or previous treatment with clopidogrel, ticlopidin or oral anticoagulation, in which case these last ones were prolonged.

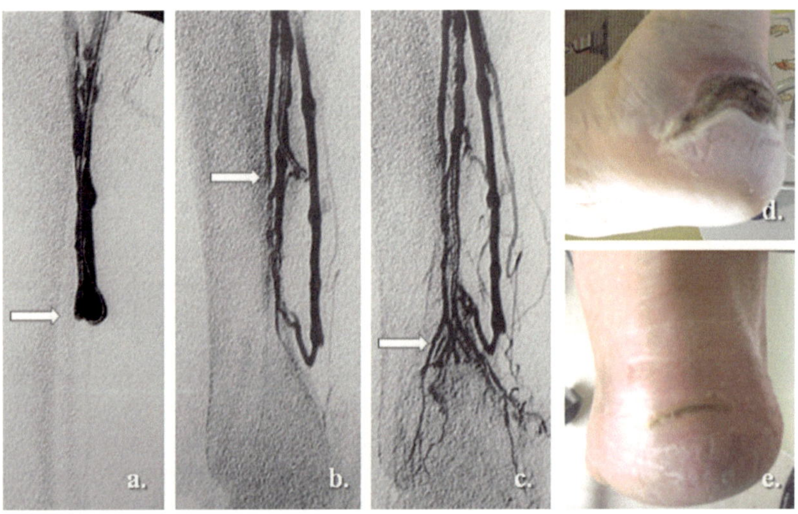

Fig. 5. Deep **Posterior Tibial veins** selective arterialization:

a. Devalvulation in the main vein trunk using the 0.035-inch guidewire and the passage of the 6F long introducer sheath.
b. Selective "coaxial" embolization of the main deep vein collaterals owing a 5F curved microcatheter.
c. Regain of the arterial flow in the vein collaterals around the heel targeting the *medial calcaneal angiosome* (and its appended *venosome*).
d. The initial heel neuro-ischemic wound.
e. Clinical result at five months providing the same multidisciplinary "diabetic foot" team surveillance.

Follow-up. In the post-operative period, patients were assessed by periodical clinical and hemodynamic (duplex scan) evaluations, focusing on tissue healing, bypass patency and the presence of arterial waves in the ankle or foot deep veins. Information was collected one month after discharge and every 6 months thereafter. In cases showing clinical tissue deterioration as primary end-point, corroborated by corresponding duplex findings, further Angio-CT or MRI evaluation was undertaken. Mean follow-up was 23.3 months (in the range 1-68 months).

3. Results

The initial technical success was achieved in 21/28 limbs (75%) with 96% corresponding thirty-day peri-operative mortality rate (one patient died from myocardial infarction). In seven instances, the procedure could not follow the scheduled protocol. In 2 cases, the distal venous anastomosis of the PTFE graft was unachievable either in a context of extensive fibrosis (multiple previous interventions) or by substantial inflammation. In 2 others, unexpected wall laceration of the selected venous conduit during the devalvulation stage required hemostasis by direct embolization of these veins. Since alternative deep veins arterializations without AM guidance were used, these cases were categorized as technical failures. There were 3 other situations when the distal embolization of collaterals could not be achieved: in two limbs, a rich network of fine branches with sharp angle and retrograde emergence rendered difficult all endovascular manoeuvres, while in other case the embolization stage was discontinued following an intolerance to contrast agents. For the whole 7 technical failures, 4 compulsory arterializations (non angiosomes-oriented) of miscellaneous deep or superficial veins, one minor and 2 major amputations were requested. During the first year of follow-up, there were 2 graft occlusions. In both instances, irregularities in the postoperative medication (modest compliance of patients) were noted. After eight months of surveillance one of these 2 limbs showed however, a correct tissue recovery despite the PTFE thrombosis, while major amputation was inevitable for the other.

The cumulative primary and secondary patency were (+/-SEM): 71% (+/- 9%), 59% (+/- 10%) and 59% (+/- 10%), at 12, 24 and 36 months, respectively. Limb salvage showed: 86% (+/- 7%) at one year and steady 77% (+/- 10%) afterwards, while the clinical success was: 82% (+/- 7%), 71% (+/- 10%) and 71% (+/- 10%) at identical time intervals (**Fig. 6**).

Deep venous system reflux was assessed in 19/28 (68%) limbs, whereas in only 10/28 (35%) previous evidence for clinical venous insufficiency was available. In all 28 treated limbs deep vein duplications were documented (preoperative Duplex) as follows: 20 in the distal popliteal (71%) (**Fig. 2**), 5 in the proximal popliteal (18%) and 3 concerning the superficial femoral (12%) deep veins. The overall 30-day peri-operative complication rate was 21% (6/28cases). Major complications were noted in three cases (11%): there were two temporary cardiac deficiencies after the initiation of the arterio-venous flow compensated by inotropic agents and diligent medical treatment and one secondary compartmental syndrome coupled to venous gangrene, ending in inevitable amputation. There were 3 other minor complication represented by 2 venous branch perforations of the collaterals with self limiting local effects and one causing secondary limb swelling, that needed prolonged postoperative physiotherapy before ambulation. Following the evoked AM strategy and appended venosome-model for arterialization (**Fig. 1**), we have noted: 10 limbs treated by preferential anterior tibial veins arterialization (trophic lesions located on the anterior leg and ankle, the forefoot, dorsum of the toes and foot) (**Fig. 4**), 16 others having revascularizations in the posterior tibial veins territory (ulcers of the medial calcaneal, plantar, hallux, medial malleolar and Achillean teguments) (**Fig. 5**), while the remnant 2 targeted a dominant peroneal in-flow (wounds located in the lateral calcaneal and lateral malleolar territories) (**Table II.**).

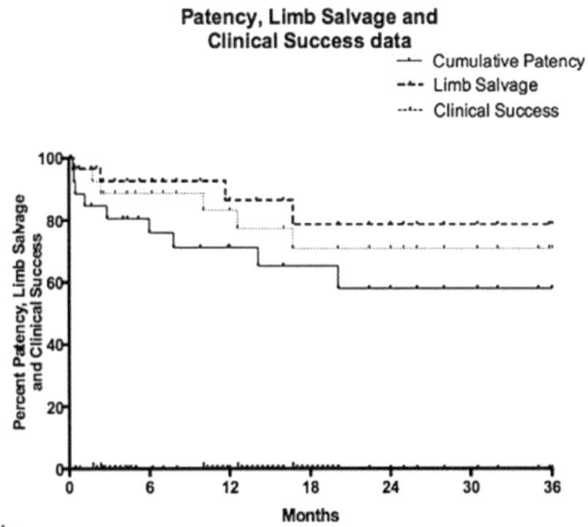

Subjects at risk:

	0	6	12	18	24	30	36
Cumulative Patency:	28	17	13	9	7	4	1
Limb Salvage:	28	19	14	10	8	4	1
Clinical Success:	28	19	15	11	9	5	1

Fig. 6. Patency, Limb Salvage and Clinical Success statistical data.

Although complete healing with or without minor amputations was documented in 15 treated limbs (54%) (**Fig. 4e** and **5e**), notable trends for tissue recovery without complete cicatrization were observed in 7 others (25%). Major amputations were however, inevitable in the remnant 6 presentations (21%). Cyclic relapses of the wounds, albeit without ischemic Duplex features were documented in 11 (39%) cases, mostly between the 10th -15th months of follow-up. These limbs were invariably associated a severe neuropathic background.

In the whole group of patients, six (21%) major amputations for miscellaneous clinical reasons were documented (2 technical failures, 2 major complications, 1bypass thrombosis and 1 progressively irreversible forefoot sepsis).

The thirty-day peri-operative mortality rate was 0%. The cumulative survival rates were 93%, 66% and 38% at 12, 24 and 36 months, respectively.

4. Discussion

The renal patient presents with unanimously recognized severe CLI features and consequent difficult revascularization patterns (Casserly, 2008; Conrad et al., 2009; Leers et al., 1998; Norgreen et al., 2007). A vast amount of contemporary literature shows the poor outcome commonly noted after surgical or endovascular arterial reconstruction in these patients (Arvela et al., 2010; Black et al., 2005; Casserly, 2008; Conrad et al., 2009; Leers et al., 1998). As the revascularization seems however feasible, particularly aggressive atherosclerosis coupled to long segment chronic occlusions, calcifications and depleted run-off, make further arterial patency and limb preservation quite questionable in ESRD subjects (Arvela et al., 2010; Black et al., 2005; Casserly, 2008; Leers et al., 1998). These poor clinical results are often associated with a high co-morbidity and mortality, independently from diabetes and other cardio-vascular risk factors (Leers et al., 1998; Mlekusch et al., 2004; Norgreen et al., 2007). Similar observations were described in the diabetic CLI context that adds the metabolic and neuropathic background, local sepsis, poor immune response and variable amounts of foot tissue loss (Abou-Zamzam et al., 2007; Apelqvist et al., 1993; Norgreen et al., 2007).

Moreover, the diabetic CLI "macro-angiopathic" atherosclerosis is characterised by enhance more aggressive and more distal occlusive lesions, with preferential tropism in the tibial trunks (Apelqvist et al., 1993; Dormandy et al., 1999; Faglia et al., 2007 Norgreen et al., 2007). A synchronous functional microcirculatory affectation induced by both neuropathic and septic entanglement, was also witnessed in this multifaceted pathology of the diabetic foot (Apelqvist et al., 1993; Boulton et al., 2006; Edmonds, 2008). Despite soaring progresses in technology and aggressive follow-up, long-term limb preservation seems however inferior in diabetic - ESRD subjects compared to other CLI patients, mainly due to extended infragenicular arterial thrombosis, calcifications and poor distal foot runoff (Abularrage et al., 2010; Dormandy et al., 1999).

While non-diabetic subjects seem to express intima-layer, eccentric and patchy wall arterial calcifications, prevailing in the coronary also the peripheral vessels (the « *type I* » calcifications) (Irvin & Guzman, 2009), the diabetic also ESRD patients have media-layer, concentric and rather continuous wall calcifications (the "Mönckeberg sclerosis" or « *type II* » calcifications) (Irvin & Guzman, 2009). These particularly dense « *type II* » calcific deposits featuring the below-knee arterial trunks were independently associated with more severe CLI presentations (Irvin & Guzman, 2009 ; Leskinen et al., 2002), requiring additional technical challenges (Abou-Zamzam et al., 2007; Alexandrescu et al., 2011; Casserly, 2008; Leers et al., 1998) and consequent higher technical failures. They were also connected with low patency and discouraging limb loss rates (Casserly, 2008; Combe et al., 2009; Leers et al., 1998; Ohtake et al., 2011).

The reported 1-year survival rate after major amputations ranges between 50%-60% and seems to be worse for patients undergoing above- the-knee versus below-the-knee interventions (Dormandy et al., 1999; Toursarkissian et al., 2002). Despite undeniable progresses in both surgical and endovascular approaches, in about 14%-20% of patients featuring severe crural and pedal occlusive disease, neither of the available techniques can afford appropriate distal arterial supply, resulting amputation (Abou-Zamzam et al., 2007; Apelqvist et al., 1993; Combe et al., 2009 Norgreen et al., 2007; Toursarkissian et al., 2002). This assertion seems particularly valid regarding the ESRD subjects suffering from CLI (Abou-Zamzam et al., 2007; Apelqvist et al., 1993; Arvela et al., 2010; Black et al., 2005; Casserly, 2008; Conrad et al., 2009).

Complementary efforts for limb preservation were achieved in the plastic reconstructive surgery field, by applying the AM policy for perfusion in tissue rebuilding. The concept delineates the human body in specific 3D blocks of tissue, fed by peculiar arterial and venous bundles of blood supply (Attinger et al., 2001, 2006; Taylor et al., 1990, 1998). Originally pioneered for the pediculated flaps techniques, the AM strategy (Attinger et al., 2006; Taylor et al., 1998) was also applied to improve healing in lower limb ischemic ulcers (Alexandrescu et al., 2008; Neville et al., 2009; Varela et al., 2010; Setacci et al., 2010). Based on the anatomical studies of Taylor (Taylor et al., 1990, 1998) and Attinger (Attinger et al., 2001, 2006), new preferential strategies for vascular access, revascularization or amputation were described. Schematically, in the foot and lower ankle were initially allocated 5 angiosomes (Attinger et al., 2006; Taylor et al., 1998) depending on the three main tibial trunks : the anterior, the posterior tibial and the peroneal arteries. A succinct exemplification of the corresponding skin sectors is showed in **Fig. 1**. Each angiosome encompasses an arterial (arteriosome) and correspondent venous (venosome) participation (Taylor et al., 1990, 1998). Particularly for this chapter, a specific *venosome*-orientation (concerning the venous facet of each angiosome) (Alexandrescu et al., 2011; Taylor et al., 1990) in deep calf veins arterialization was designed (**Fig. 3b**).

Deep veins arterialization in ESRD and diabetic CLI patients may offer the advantage to direct flow in the deep calf venous conduits *spared from typical type II calcifications* (Irvin & Guzman, 2009) and extended chronic occlusions (Lu et al., 2006; Toursarkissian et al., 2002). This may enable to *deliberately choose* specific distal territories (**Fig. 4** and **5**) to be reperfused (Alexandrescu et al., 2011). It may also fit selected extreme situations for limb salvage, despite irrecoverable occlusions of the arterial network (Alexandrescu et al., 2011; Lu et al., 2006). The concept of venous arterialization to treat advanced CLI presentations has emerged as an extreme therapeutic alternative in cases with impracticable conventional arterial reconstructions (Jacop et al., 1999; Lu et al., 2006). In **Table I,** are schematized the main features of the patients addressed for this technique. The majority of arterializations for "hopeless" CLI presentations intended for amputation were described in the literature using the available superficial venous system (Jacop et al., 1999; Lengua et al., 2001; Lu et al., 2006). A growing number of contemporary reports seem to provide rather encouraging (Lengua et al., 2001; Lu et al., 2006) than pessimistic results (Matzke et al., 1999) concerning this evolving technique. In most of the published studies, the arterialized venous conduit and the distal anastomosis are located at different levels in the superficial saphenous system, usually adding destruction of the appended valves (Lengua et al., 2001; Lu et al., 2006; Ozbek et al., 2005). In this setting, the arterialization of the superficial venous network carries however, some possible limitations: a) its availability (particularly in ESRD, diabetic CLI patients with huge dialysis-access and cardio-vascular surgical past) and b) the presence of surrounding inflammation, sepsis and edema. This latest factor affects the "quality" of the surounding venous bed and hampers further graft preparation or its accessibility to the distal foot anastomosis (Alexandrescu et al., 2011; Lu et al., 2006). Furthermore, in these situations the eventual affiliation of the AM concept may be problematic, as the saphenous network offers only limited choices in targeting specific areas for foot arterializations (Alexandrescu et al., 2011). Only odd reports are focusing until yet, on alternative deep veins arterialization for CLI limb salvage. This strategy was however previously proposed, either in experimental (Ozek et al. 1997) or as staged interventions (Chen et al., 1998; Lu et al., 2006), without systematic valvular avulsion.

Although rational, the genuine concept for distal valves destruction in newly arterializated venous conduits, has give rise to different techniques assembling either metallic olives, retrograde balloon PTA or 0.035-inc guidewire-enhanced valvular disruption, sustained or not by Fogarty catheters (Lu et al., 2006). Other authors have promoted the sole hydraulic effect of the new arterial pulsatile flow, as to be adequate enough for counteracting the venous valves barrier, especially in the deep venous circulation (Chen et al., 1998; Krisnan & Rayman, 2008; Lu et al., 2006). In spite of recent supportive observations [44], this latest hypothesis remains controversial (Lu et al., 2006).

In the author's group experience, we stressed the concept of restoring limb perfusion in the deep venous pathway, for untreatable ESRD ischemic lesions deemed for "classical" arterial reconstructions. Most of these cases featured characteristic infrapopliteal extensive occlusions (Casserly, 2008; Conrad et al., 2009; Norgreen et al., 2007; Toursarkissian et al., 2002) and calcifications (Alexandrescu, 2009; Irvin & Guzman, 2009; Krisnan & Rayman, 2008; Leskinen et al., 2002), when all types of conventional reconstructions have previously failed or were impracticable (**Table I.).**

In this setting, bypassing the deep venous network towards the distal foot circulation seemed unconditioned neither by tegumental integrity, swelling or tissue infection, nor by the availability of saphenous versus other autologous bypass conduits. The current calf venous duplication (Wind et al., 1991), may offer the possibility to enhance precise arterializations (**Fig. 3-5**) in one of the twin tibial veins (Alexandrescu et al., 2011), by following a specific AM strategy (Alexandrescu et al., 2011; Taylor et al., 1990). To achieve this aim, acquiring effective valvular incompetence also proved to be indispensable in our experience. This was either primary induced by the first crossing of the 0.035-inch hydrophillic guidewire (**Fig. 5**), or complementary obtained with the passage of a 6-F, 80 cm long introducer sheath through the distal deep vein (**Fig. 4b** and **5b**). Nevertheless, the lack of residual valvular tensile stress was documented in all the cases by injecting a small amount of contrast before proceeding to the embolization stage. A preexistent valvular incompetence by vein walls enlargement was witnessed in more than 25% of cases, oftentimes without previous evidence for chronic venous insufficiency. This finding may correlate the presence of up to 93% neuropathic limbs in this cohort (**Table I.),** that exhibit the previously described *"idiosyncratic deep venous distension"* context (Alexandrescu et al., 2011; Boulton et al., 2006; Edmonds, 2008; Pureval et al., 1995). The existence of neuropathy-associated capillary shunting in diabetic ESRD subjects (Krisnan & Rayman, 2008; Pureval et al., 1995), seems to allow local redistribution of the dermal, sub-dermal and muscular blood flow and by additional ascendant venous collectors (Calota et al., 2007). This makes possible the blood mass transfer from deep calf to the surface, especially as moderate venous hypertension appears (Calota et al., 2007; Edmonds, 2008; Krisnan & Rayman, 2008). Duplication in tibial veins may allow the arterialized flow to be deliberately oriented towards specific ulcerated zones of the distal leg (Alexandrescu et al., 2011; Taylor et al., 1990) according to the AM policy (**Fig. 1** and **2**). First described by Taylor et al. (Taylor et al., 1990, 1998), the "angiosomes model" for perfusion was further developed by Attinger et al. (Attinger et al., 2001, 2006) also in the plastic reconstructive surgery field. Although with limited contemporary evidence for CLI applications at the present time, this concept seems to gain more acceptance in the limb salvage domain (Neville et al., 2009; Varela et al., 2010; Setacci et al., 2010) and represents one of the current concerns of our multidisciplinary diabetic "foot-team" (Alexandrescu et al., 2008, 2009, 2011). According to their initial description, each angiosome encompasses twin *arteriosomes* and *venosomes* for blood supply, all being interconnected in a vast compensatory system (the"*choke vessels*") (Attinger et al., 2006; Taylor et al., 1998). The *arterial side* of this "rescue network" relying on adjacent angiosomes seems particularly damaged in ESRD/diabetic patients exhibiting peculiar medium-sized collaterals depletion by aggressive atherosclerosis joined to small arterial septic thrombosis (the already reported "*end artery occlusive disease*" pattern) (O'Neal, 2008). Unlike the arteries, deep calf veins and collaterals seem less affected by this occlusive process (Alexandrescu et al., 2011; Krisnan & Rayman, 2008). This important aspect may enable deep vein arterialization to access specific leg territories (angiosomes), throughout their appended venous communicants (venosomes), in areas although deprived from direct arterial connections (Alexandrescu et al., 2011).

We used the venosomes orientation (Taylor et al., 1990) joined to the SAVES technique (Alexandrescu et al., 2011) in all these marginal candidates for common revascularizations and observed correct healing with or without minor amputations in 15 treated limbs (54%). Notable trends for tissue recovery however without complete cicatrization were documented in 7 others (25%). Major amputation were inevitable in the remnant 6 presentations (21%).

It has been stipulated that the "venosomes" allocation may be prone to anatomical variations (Taylor et al., 1990) according to the individual distribution of the deep venous system (Calota et al., 2007; Taylor et al., 1990; Wind et al., 1991) (**Fig. 3**). We believe that systematic preoperative Duplex assessment joining « on table » road-mapping, may provide important information in detecting these venous pecularities (26% limbs in our cohort). We also observed that staged embolizations of the major vein collaterals were technically more demanding in the posterior tibial territory (**Fig. 5**), by steady large perforators or communicants, sometimes appointing sharp retrograde emergences with more arduous cannulation.

All treated patients expressed discrete to moderate lower limb edemas after arterializations. This phenomenon showed generally a spontaneous resolution during the postoperative first month. Similar observations in dedicated literature suggest that the more distal the location of the outflow anastomosis in long arterio-venous fistulas (femoro-infrapopliteal in our technique), the higher likelihood to enhance a better cardiac tolerance (Lengua et al., 2001; Ozek et al. 1997).

As noticed, in one case (4%) persistent limb swelling joining calf compartmental syndrome and venous gangrene were documented, unfortunately ending with major amputation. In two other cases (8%), cardiac insufficiency symptoms were perceived: one precocious and reversible manifestation (in the 30-day complications subset) and one insidious and retarded presentation (two months after the procedure), in a severe and inoperable coronary context.

The study presented in this chapter may express some clear limitations: beyond its retrospective nature and the small number of cases included, the results in terms of limb salvage are not easy to be compared with other series of conventional arterial reconstructions or venous arterializations, since the technique itself and the selection criteria are different.

In addition, the "SAVES" method represent only an evolving therapeutic option, since specific difficulties and related complications (notably the collateral embolization stage), may be subject for further technical improvements. A larger clinical experience and skills, joining more sophisticated devices for endovascular navigation and collateral occlusion (like modular micro-catheters, specific pro-thrombotic substances or embolic microspheres) may probably contribute to further technical refinements. Finally, to accurately evaluate and compare limb preservation in this subset of diabetic and renal patients oftentimes implies (beyond reestablishing limb perfusion) the undeniable implication of multi-disciplinary team surveillance (Abularrage et al., 2010; Alexandrescu et al., 2008; Apelqvist et al., 1993; Boulton et al., 2006; Driver et al., 2007; Edmonds, 2008; Norgreen et al.).

5. Conclusion

Deep calf venous arterialization (the SAVES-method) may represent an extreme alternative for limb salvage in selected, inoperable presentations for conventional arterial revascularization. The association of an angiosome strategy seems, at this stage of the available clinical experience, a possible useful method to enhance distal ulcer healing. Larger studies, providing comparative and randomized data are thus needed, as to ascertain these preliminary observations.

6. Acknowledgments

We would like to acknowledge in the first place all the members of the « Dialysis and Nephrology » department, also all those exercing a constant multidisciplinary activity in our institutional "*Diabetic-Foot Group*".
Equal acknowledgements the *Princess Paola Hospital's* radiology, cardiology and endocrinology departments for their assiduous assessment and punctual support in managing these challenging cases.

7. References

Abou-Zamzam AM Jr, Gomez NR, Molkara A, Banta JE, Teruya TH, Killeen JD, et al. A prospective analysis of critical limb ischemia: factors leading to major primary amputation versus revascularization. *Ann Vasc Surg.* 2007; 21(4): 458-463.

Abularrage CJ, Conrad MF, Hackney LA, Paruchuri V, Crawford RS, Kwolek CJ, et al. Long-term outcomes of diabetic patients undergoing endovascular infrainguinal interventions. *J Vasc Surg.* 2010 ;52 : 314-322.

Alexandrescu V, Hubermont G, Philips Y, Guillaumie B, Ngongang C, Vandenbossche P, et al. Selective angioplasty following an angiosome model of reperfusion in the treatment of Wagner 1-4 diabetic foot lesions: practice in a multidisciplinary diabetic limb service. *J Endovasc Ther.* 2008; 15: 580-593.

AlexandrescuVA.Commentary:Below-the-ankle subintimal angioplasty: how far can we push this application for lower limb preservation in diabetic patients? *J Endovasc Ther.* 2009;16: 617–8.

Alexandrescu V, Hubermont G, Vincent G. Diabetic neuro-ischemic foot wounds: does primary angioplasty following an angiosome model of perfusion can improve the fate of minor amputations and influence the global limb preservation rates? In: *Advances in Medicine and Biology* (Vol. 15) N.Y. Nova Science Publish. 2011: 17-37.

Alexandrescu V, Ngongang C, Vincent G, Ledent G, Hubermont G. Deep calf veins arterialization for inferior limb preservation in diabetic patients with extended ischaemic wounds, unfit for direct arterial reconstruction: preliminary results according to an angiosome model of perfusion. *Cardiovasc Revasc Medicine.* 2011;12: 10-19.

Andreoli M, Galli G, Arienzo A, Nora A, Tedoli M, Guidetti G, et al. Prevention and therapy of critical ischemia in hemodialyzed patients. *G Ital Nefrol.* 2008;26, Suppl 45: S28-S31.

Apelqvist J, Larsson J, Agardh CD. Long-term prognosis for diabetic patients with foot ulcers. *J Intern Med.* 1993;233(6):485-91.

Arvela E, Soderstrom M, Korhonen M, Halmesmaki K, Alback A, Lepantalo M, et al. Finnvasc score and modified Prevent III score predict long-term outcome after infrainguinal surgical and endovascular revascularization for critical limb ischemia. *J Vasc Surg.* 2010; 52: 1218-1225.

Attinger CE, Evans KK, Bulan E, et al. Angio- somes of the foot and ankle and clinical implications for limb salvage: reconstruction, incisions and revascularization. *Plast Reconstr Surg.* 2006;117(7 Suppl):261S–293S.

Attinger CE, Cooper P, Blume P, et al. The safest surgical incision and amputations applying the angiosomes principle and using the Doppler to assess the arterial-arterial connec- tions of the foot and ankle. *Foot Ankle Clin North Am.* 2001; 6:745–801.

Black JH, LaMuraglia GM, Kwolek CJ, Brewster DC, Watkins MT, Cambria RP. Contemporary results of angioplasty-based infrainguinal percutaneous interventions. *J Vasc Surg.* 2005; 42: 932-939.

Boulton AJM, Armstrong DG. The diabetic foot. In : *Clinical diabetes, translating research into practice.* Philadelphia, Saunders Elsevier, 2006 : 179-195.

Bradbury AW, Adam DJ, Bell J, Forbes JF, Fowkes FG, Gillespie I, et al. Bypass versus angioplasty in severe ischaemia of the leg (BASIL) trial: An intention to treat analysis of amputation-free and overall survival in patients randomized to a bypass surgery-first or balloon angioplasty-first revascularization strategy. *J Vasc Surg.* 2010; 51(5 Suppl): 5S-17S.

Calota F, Mogoanta S, Intorcaciu M, Pasalega M, Popescu CF, Vasile I, et al. The venous system of the lower limbs. *Rom J Morphol Embriol.* 2007; 48(4): 355-360.

Casserly IP. Interventional management of critical limb ischemia in renal patients. *Adv Chronic Kidney Dis.* 2008;15(4): 384-395.

Chen XS, Lin T, Chen DL, Guan YB. Venous arterialization of posterior tibial vein channel for extensive arterial occlusion of lower extremities. *J Surg Concepts Pract.* 1998; 3:219-221.

Combe C, Albert JM, Bragg-Gresham JL, Angreucci VE, Disney A, Fukuhara S, et al. The burden of amputation among hemodialysis patients in the Dialysis Outcomes and Practice Patterns Study (DOPPS). *Am j Kidney Dis.* 2009; 54: 680-692.

Conrad MF, Kang J, Cambria RP, Brewster DC, Watkins MT, Kwolek CJ, et al. Infrapopliteal balloon angioplasty for the treatment of chronic occlusive disease. *J Vasc Surg.* 2009, 50(4): 799-805.

Dayal R, Kent C. Standardized reporting practices. In Rutherford Vascular Surgery 6th edition. Philadelphia. Elsevier Saunders Inc. 2005: 41-52.

Driver V, Landowski MA, Madsen JL. Neuropathic Wounds: The diabetic wound. In: Acute and Chronic Wounds-Current Management Concepts. Philadelphia, by Mosby Elsevier Inc. 2007: 307-336.

Dormandy J, Heek L, Vig S. Major amputations: clinical patterns and predictors. *Semin Vasc Surg.* 1999;12:154-161.

Edmonds M. A natural history and framework for managing diabetic foot ulcers. *Br J Nurs,* 2008, 17(11): S20, S22, S24-S29.

Faglia E, Clerici G, Caminiti M, Quarantiello A, Curci V, Morabito A. Predictive values of transcutaneous oxygen tension for above-the- ankle amputation in diabetic patients with critical limb ischemia. *Eur J Vasc Endovasc Surg.* 2007(33):731–736.

Irvin CL, Guzman RJ. Matrix metalloproteinases in medial arterial calcification: potential mechanisms and actions. *Vascular.* 2009. 17, Suppl 1; S40-S44.

Jacop S, Nassef A, Belli AM, Dormandi JA, Taylor RS. Vascular surgery society of Great Britain and Ireland: distal venous arterializations for nonreconstructable arterial disease. *Br J Surg.* 1999;86(5):694-698.

Krisnan SM, Rayman G. Microcirculation and the diabetic foot. In: "The foot in diabetes" 4th edition. London. Wiley & Sons Ltd, 2008: 41-51.

Leers SA, Reifsnyder T, Delmonte R, Caron M. Realistic expectations for pedal bypass grafts in patients with end-stage renal disease. *J Vasc Surg.* 1998;28(6):976-980.

Lengua F, La Madrid A, Acosta C, Barriga H, Maliqui C, Arauco R et al. Arterialization of the distal veins of the foot for limb salvage in arteritis. Technique and results. *Ann Chir.* 2001;126:629-638.

Leskinen Y, Salenius JP, Lehtimaki T, Huhtala H, Saha H. The prevalence of peripheral arterial disease and medial arterial calcification in patients with chronic renal failure: requirements for diagnostics. *Am J Kidney Dis.* 2002;40: 472-479.

Lu XW, Idu MM, Ubbink DT, Legemate DA. Meta-analysis of the clinical effectiveness of venous arterializations for salvage of critically ischaemic limbs. *Eur J Vasc Surg.* 2006;31:493-499.

Matzke S, Pitkanen J, Lepantalo M. Does saphenous vein arterializations prevent major amputation in critical leg ischemia? A comparative study. *J Cardiovasc Surg. (Torino)* 1999;40:845-847.

Mlekusch W, Exner M, Sabeti S, Amighi J, Schlager O, Wagner O, et al. Serum creatinine predicts mortality in patients with peripheral artery disease: infuence of diabetes and hypertension. *Atherosclerosis.* 2004; 175 (2): 361-367.

NevilleRF, Attinger CE, Bulan EJ, Ducic I, Thomassen M, Sidawy AN. Revascularization of a specific angiosome for limb salvage: does the target artery matter? *Ann Vasc Surg.* 2009; 23(3): 367-373.

Norgreen L, Hiatt WR, Dormandy JA, Nehler MR, Harris KA, Fowkes FGR on behalf of the TASC II Working Group. Inter-Society Consensus for the management of peripheral arterial disease (TASC II.). *Eur J Vasc Endovasc Surg.* 2007; 33, Suppl.1:S32-55.

Ohtake T, Oka M, Ikee R, Mochida Y, Ishioka K, Moryia H, et al. Impact of lower limbs' arterial calcification on the prevalence and severity of PAD in patients on hemodialysis. *J Vasc Surg.* 2011; 53: 676-683.

O'Neal LW. Surgical pathology of the foot and clinicopathologic correlations. In: *Levin and O'Neal's The Diabetic Foot.* Philadelphia, Mosby Elsevier. 2008: 367-401.

Ozbek C, Kestelli M, Emrecan B, Ozsoyler I, Bayatli K, Yasa H, et al. A novel approach: ascending venous arterialization for atherosclerosis obliterans. *Eur J Vasc Endovasc Surg* 2005; 29:47–51

Ozek C, Zhang F, Lineaweaver WC, Chin BT, Newlin L, Eiman T, et al. Arterialization of the venous system in a rat lower limb model. *Br. J Plast Surg.* 1997; 50(6): 402-406.

Pureval TS, Goss DE, Watkins PJ, Edmonds ME. Lower limb venous pressure in diabetic neuropathy. *Diabetes Care.* 1995; 18(3): 377-338.

Randon C, Jacobs B, De Ryck F, Vermassen F. Angioplasty or primary stenting for infrapopliteal lesions: results of a prospective randomized trial. *Cardiovasc Intervent Radiol.* 2010; 33(2): 260-269.

Rutherford RB, Baker JD, Ernst C, Johnston KW, Porter JM, Ahn S, et al. Recommended standards for reports dealing with lower extremity ischemia : revised version. *J Vasc Surg.* 1997; 26(3): 517-38. Erratum in: *J Vasc Surg.* 2001; 33(4): 805.

Setacci C, De Donato G, Setacci F, et al. Ischemic foot: definition, etiology and angio- some concept. *J Cardiovasc Surg (Torino).* 2010; 51: 223–231.

Taylor GI, Caddy CM, Watterson PA, Crock JG. The venous territories (venosomes) of the human body: experimental study and clinical implications. *Plast Reconstr Surg.* 1990;86(2):185-213.

Taylor GI, Pan WR. Angiosomes of the leg: anatomic study and clinical implications. *Plast Reconstr Surg.* 1998; 102(3): 599-616.

Toursarkissian B, Shireman PK, Harrison A, D'Ayala M, Schoolfield J, Sykes MT. Major lower- amputation: contemporary experience in a single veterans affairs institution. *Am Surg.* 2002;68:606-610.

Varela C, Acín F, de Haro J, Bleda S, Esparza L, March JR. The role of foot collateral vessels on ulcer healing and limb salvage after successful endovascular and surgical distal procedures according to an angiosome model. *Vasc Endovascular Surg.* 2010; 44(8): 654-660.

White RI, Pollak JS. Controlled delivery of pushable fibered coils for large vessel embolotherapy. In: Vascular Embolotherapy a comprehensive approach, Volume 1, general principles, chest, abdomen and great vessels. Springer, 2006: 35-43.

Wind GG, Valentine RJ. Popliteal artery. In: Anatomic exposures in vascular surgery. Baltimore: William&Wilkins, 1991: 373-410.

Young MJ, Boulton AJ, Macleod AF, Williams DR, Sonksen PH. A multicenter study of the prevalence of the diabetic peripheral neuropathy in the United Kingdom hospital clinic population. *Diabetologia.* 1993; 150-154.

14

Diabetes and Renal Disease

Rodica Mihăescu, Corina Şerban, Simona Drăgan,
Romulus Timar, Ioana Mozoş, Marius Craina and Adalbert Schiller
University of Medicine and Pharmacy „Victor Babeş" Timişoara
Romania

1. Introdution

Diabetes and its devastating complications reduce life expectancy and adversely affect quality of life amongst those affected, thus, posing immense challenges to many societal sectors. The upsurge in the prevalence of diabetes from 171 million in 2000 to 366 million by 2030 as projected by the World Health Organization threatens to overwhelm the economic and healthcare system globally.

In type 1 diabetes the prevalence gradually increases from onset of disease (6% after 1-3 years), reaching over 50% after 20 years [Warram, 1996]. In type 2 diabetes the prevalence is 20-25% in both newly diagnosed and established diabetes [Mogensen, 1994]. Approximately 40% of patients with type 1 diabetes and 20 to 40% of those with type 2 diabetes will eventually develop diabetic nephropathy, although the reason why not all patients with diabetes develop this complication is unknown.

In both types of diabetes, chronic hyperglycemia is the primary cause of the disease. In type 1 diabetes hyperglycemia starts in the first decades of life and is usually the only recognized cause of nephropathy. On the contrary, in type 2 diabetes hyperglycemia starts after the forties, usually when the kidneys have already suffered the long-term consequences of ageing and of other recognized promoters of chronic renal injury such as arterial hypertension, obesity, dyslipidemia, and smoking [Ruggenenti, 2000]. Similar histological and clinical courses in all diabetic individuals indicated that the pathogenesis of nephropathy is similar in patients with type 1 and type 2 diabetes mellitus.

The kidney is an extremely complex organ with broad ranging functions in the body, including, but not restricted to, waste excretion, ion and water balance, maintenance of blood pressure, glucose homeostasis and generation of erythropoietin or activation of vitamin D. With diabetes, many of these integral processes are interrupted via a combination of hemodynamic and metabolic changes; hyperglycemia also activates a series of changes leading to glomerular and tubular dysfunction and accelerates glomerular cell apoptosis [Forbes, 2010]. Different pathogenetic, hemodynamic and metabolic processes can lead to diabetic kidney disease. In recent years, great progress has been made in understanding the risk factors and pathogenetic processes in diabetic nephropathy. In addition, new insight into the pathophysiology of this chronic disease has lead to better preventive therapies, treatment possibilities and reduced progression to end stage renal disease.

Diabetic kidney disease refers to a characteristic set of *structural and functional kidney abnormalities* in patients with diabetes. Classic glomerulosclerosis is characterized by increased glomerular basement membrane width, diffuse mesangial sclerosis, hyalinosis, microaneurysm, and hyaline arteriosclerosis [Mauer, 1981]. The structural abnormalities include hypertrophy of the kidney, increase in glomerular basement membrane thickness, nodular and diffuse glomerulosclerosis, tubular atrophy, and interstitial fibrosis. The functional alterations include an early increase in glomerular filtration rate with intraglomerular hypertension, subsequent proteinuria, systemic hypertension, and eventual loss of renal function [Ayodele - 2004].

The management of patients with type 2 diabetes and progressive kidney disease requires a comprehensive approach that includes aggressive blood pressure control with agents that also lower urinary protein excretion and optimization of glucose and lipid control, considering the therapeutic limitations imparted by renal dysfunction. Clinicians must also address the comorbidities associated with renal failure such as anemia and secondary hyperparathyroidism. Diabetic nephropathy typically follows a slowly progressive course from albuminuria to azotemia. Consequently, optimal care includes planning for the management of impending renal failure long before the patient requires dialysis or transplantation.

The aim of this chapter is to provide a comprehensive review about the risk factors, the histological changes and the pathogenic mechanisms that lead to diabetic nephropathy/diabetes kidney disease, diagnosis, new biomarkers and recent developments in the prevention and treatment of diabetes kidney disease, targeting the main risk factors and resulting in renal protection and reduced disease progression.

2. Diabetic nephropathy or diabetic kidney disease?

The phenomenon of albuminuria has been recognized for more than 200 yr, and its association with kidney disease dates to the epochal insights of Richard Bright in 1827 [Cameron, 1988]. The presence of microalbuminuria is associated with increased cardiovascular morbidity and mortality, and regular screening is recommended in guidelines for diabetes care. Albuminuria reflects functional and potentially reversible abnormalities initiated by glomerular hyperfiltration, proteinuria, a size-selective dysfunction of the glomerular barrier normally associated with glomerular filtration rate (GFR) decline that may result in end-stage renal disease [Ruggenenti, 2006].

The Diabetes and Chronic Kidney Disease work group of the National Kidney Foundation Kidney Disease Outcomes Quality Initiative suggested that chronic kidney disease considered to be caused by diabetes should be named "*diabetic kidney disease*" and the term "*diabetic nephropathy*" should be reserved for kidney disease attributed to diabetes with histopathological changes, demonstrated by renal biopsy [Cavanaugh - 2007]. Progression from normoalbuminuria to microalbuminuria defines *the initiation* of diabetic nephropathy, and the transition from microalbuminuria to overt diabetic nephropathy resulting in deterioration of renal function and end-stage renal disease constitutes its *progression*.

Diabetic kidney disease is characterized by persistent albuminuria (>300 mg/dl or >200 µg/min) that is confirmed on at least 2 occasions 3 to 6 months apart, with a progressive decline in the glomerular filtration rate (GFR), elevated arterial blood pressure, and an increased risk for cardiovascular morbidity and mortality.

3. The initiation of diabetic kidney disease

Generalized endothelial dysfunction and inflammation are important antecedents of microalbuminuria in both types of diabetes. Markers of endothelial dysfunction, including elevated serum von Willebrand factor (vWF) and increased transcapillary albumin escape rate, are present before the onset of microalbuminuria in type 1 diabetes and worsen in association with it. Type 2 diabetes is often complicated by the presence of other risk factors for vascular disease, and discerning the contribution of hyperglycemia and its sequel to endothelial dysfunction in this condition is more difficult [Satchell, 2008]. While in some type 2 diabetic patients microalbuminuria may occur in the absence of evidence of endothelial dysfunction, in others, vWF levels predict its development [Stehouwer, 2002]. Markers of chronic low-grade inflammation, including C-reactive protein (CRP), are also correlated with microalbuminuria in type 1 and type 2 diabetes [Schalkwijk, 1999].

4. The natural progression of diabetic kidney disease

In an initial phase, diabetic kidney disease is characterized by glomerular hyperfiltration due to a reduction in the resistance of the afferent and efferent glomerular arterioles, and consequent increased renal perfusion. The natural progression of diabetic nephropathy has been well studied in type 1 diabetes by Mogenson et al. There are 5 stages of diabetic kidney disease:

Stage 1: Stage of hyperfiltration is characterized by renal hypertrophy and renal hyperfiltration. Increased glomerular filtration leads to increased urinary albumin excretion rate (increases by 20- 40 percent) along with increase in renal blood flow by 9 -14 percent.

Stage 2: Renal hyperfiltration with increased glomerular filtration pressure persists, but there is normalization of urinary albumin excretion rate and normal blood pressure.

Stage 3: Incipient nephropathy or stage of microalbuminuria is characterised by urinary albumin excretion rate of 30 -300 mg per day, with a rise of blood pressure. More characteristic is the impaired nocturnal dip in blood pressure. Microscopically, the renal biopsy (or histology) shows increased basement membrane thickness and increased mesangium.

Stage 4: Overt nephropathy is characterized by progressive drop in glomerular filtration rate by 10 ml per minute per year, while proteinuria increases at the rate of 15 - 40 percent per year and hypertension ensues.

Stage 5: End stage renal disease occurs at about 7 -14 years from stage 4 requiring renal replacement therapy.

However, it is often difficult to document these various stages in a diabetic patient in clinical practice because of confounding factors, such as blood pressure medications, which modify the natural course of diabetic nephropathy.

A greater proportion of patients with type-2 diabetes compared with type-I diabetes have microalbuminuria and overt nephropathy at or shortly after diagnosis of diabetes. This is because the disease may have been present for several years before the diagnosis. In addition, concomitant presence of hypertension at the time of diagnosis also contributes to the high prevalence of microalbuminuria in type-2 diabetes. Progression from microalbuminuria to overt nephropathy occurs in 20-40% of Caucasians within a 10-year period, with approximately 20% of those with overt nephropathy progressing to ESRD over a period of 20 years [Ayodele, 2004].

5. Epidemiology

Diabetic kidney disease is one of the most serious complications of diabetes mellitus and is the leading cause of end stage renal disease both in the USA and in Europe, requiring renal replacement therapy. As the population of patients with diabetes of long duration grows, reports of a dramatically increasing burden of diabetic nephropathy are appearing. Globally the burden of diabetes is expected to double between 2000 and 2030, with the greatest increases in prevalence expected to occur in the Middle East, sub-Saharan Africa, and India (KDOQI Clinical Practice Guidelines). This increased risk and more rapid progression of diabetic nephropathy also has been reported in immigrants from developing to developed countries (KDOQI Clinical Practice Guidelines) [Burney, 2009].

Diabetic kidney disease affects males and females equally and rarely develops before 10 years' duration of type 1 DM. The peak incidence (3%/year) is usually found in persons who have had diabetes for 10-20 years. The mean age of patients who reach end-stage kidney disease is about 60 years. Although in general, the incidence of diabetic nephropathy is higher among elderly persons who have had type 2 diabetes for a longer period, the role of age in the development of diabetic kidney disease is unclear. In Pima Indians with type 2 diabetes, the onset of diabetes at a younger age was associated with a higher risk of progression to end-stage kidney disease.

6. Risk factors

Although diabetes is often accompanied by hyperglycemia, hypertension, and altered lipid profile, surprisingly, most individuals with type 1 or type 2 diabetes do not develop diabetic nephropathy. This suggests that other factors are involved [Hall, 2006]. Persuasive evidences have implicated also nontraditional risk factors including lipid disorders, chronic inflammation and anemia in the development of diabetic kidney disease.

6.1 Race

The incidence and severity of diabetic kidney disease are increased in blacks, Mexican Americans, Pima Indians, and Hispanics compared with Caucasians. Even after adjusting for confounding factors such as lower socioeconomic status and increased incidence of hypertension in blacks, there is still a 4.8 times greater risk of ESRD in blacks compared to Caucasians [Ayodele, 2004].

6.2 Aging

Ageing is *per se* a cause of progressive glomerulosclerosis and combined with the risk factors may contribute to the specific arteriolosclerotic changes, that often coexist with, and occasionally overwhelm, the typical features of diabetic glomerulopathy, in particular in type 2 diabetes [Ruggeneti, 1998]. Renal blood flow and GFR diminish over time in elderly persons, minimized by a rise in the filtration fraction. In older diabetic patients, the decrease in kidney mass, particularly the renal cortex, and the histological changes of diabetic nephropathy are compounded by advanced vascular changes. Pathologically, the aging kidney may be associated with basement membrane thickening and mesangial expansion that are also key histological features of diabetic glomerulopathy. Global glomerulosclerosis affecting the kidneys of elderly persons may relate to hyperperfusion, also observed in diabetes. However, studies about the diagnosis and prevalence of diabetic kidney disease in the elderly are lacking [Williams, 2009].

6.3 Smoking

Smoking is a risk factor for diabetic nephropathy and might contribute to its progression [64]. Although some studies did not confirm these observations, it is strongly recommended to quit smoking in any phase of DN, also aiming to reduce the associated cardiovascular and cancer risk [Luk, 2008].

6.4 Genetic risk factors

Genetic susceptibility is one of the determinants of progression and severity in diabetic kidney disease. Several genes predisposing to type 2 diabetes have recently been identified. In addition to the recognized and powerful effects of environmental factors, there is abundant evidence in support of genetic susceptibility to the microvascular complication of nephropathy in individuals with both type 1 and type 2 diabetes. Familial aggregation of phenotypes such as end-stage renal disease, albuminuria, and chronic kidney disease have routinely been reported in populations throughout the world, and heritability estimates for albuminuria and glomerular filtration rate demonstrate strong contributions of inherited factors. Recent genome-wide linkage scans have identified several chromosomal regions that likely contain diabetic nephropathy susceptibility genes, and association analyses have evaluated positional candidate genes under these linkage peaks. These complimentary approaches have demonstrated that polymorphisms in the carnosinase 1 gene on chromosome 18q, the adiponectin gene on 3q, and the engulfment and cell motility gene on 7p are likely associated with susceptibility to diabetic nephropathy [Freedman - 2007].

6.5 Arterial hypertension

Increase of arterial blood pressure is an early and frequent phenomenon in diabetic nephropathy as well as in the development of macrovascular lesions. There has been some recent evidence that genetic predisposition to hypertension may predispose to the development of diabetic kidney disease. In diabetic kidney disease hypertension is not merely the result of relentless kidney damage. There is considerable clinical evidence that the elevated arterial pressure is also important in the genesis of the glomerular lesion. Indeed the development of proteinuria is paralleled in most cases by a gradual increase in systemic blood pressure, and there is a significant correlation between the blood pressure levels and the rate of decline in glomerular filtration rate [Mogensen, 1985]. In type 2 diabetes, lowering blood pressure, regardless of the used agent, retards the onset and progression of diabetic nephropathy [Schrier, 2002]. In type 1 diabetes, Lurbe et al. have noted that an insufficient decline in nighttime blood pressure (nondipping) preceded the onset of microalbuminuria [Lurbe, 2002]. Although the type 2 diabetic patient is usually hypertensive before the onset of nephropathy, nephropathy aggravates the severity of hypertension.

6.6 Hyperglycemia

The hyperglycemic state itself is a strong risk factor for diabetic kidney disease and causes the proliferation of mesangial cells and their matrix, as well as the thickening of the basement membrane. In recent years, many discoveries elucidated the mechanisms by which hyperglycemia affect the renal glomerular and tubulointerstitial cells and suggested that podocyte injury have a pivotal role in the pathogenesis of diabetic glomerulopathy. Molecular pathogenesis of diabetic podocyte injury is likely multifactorial involving a number of interrelated signaling pathways that have yet to be well understood. Sustained hyperglycemia affects the glomerular cells by various mechanisms. The changes lead to altered structure and function in the glomerulus.

6.7 Lipid disorders

Patients with diabetes have a variety of disorders of plasma lipids. These lipid abnormalities are known to contribute to cardiovascular risk. The role of lipids in diabetic nephropathy is not clear [Hall, 2006]. In type 2 DM, elevated serum cholesterol is a risk factor for the development of DN. In type 1 DM patients increased serum triglycerides, total and LDL-cholesterol were associated with micro- and macroalbuminuria. High serum cholesterol also seems to be a risk factor for GFR loss in macroalbuminuric type 1 diabetic subjects [Zelmanovitz - 2009].

For many decades, obesity has been known to cause structural changes to the renal parenchyma, and biopsies from obese subjects consistently showed glomerulomegaly with or without focal segmental glomerulosclerosis. Several mechanisms have been proposed to explain obesity-related renal changes. One explanation is the greater work load imposed on the kidneys as a direct result of larger body mass, as increased tissue turnover and toxic output place additional strains on the nephrons. Another hypothesis is lipotoxicity: the exposure of renal tissues to excess free fatty acid leads to generation of oxidative stress and cytotoxic lipid products. Recent attention has focused on adipose tissue as a rich source of pro-inflammatory cytokines and growth factors such as tumor necrosis factor a, interleukin-6 and leptin. The plethora of circulating cytokines is believed to have direct effects on renal hemodynamics and glomerular cellularity [Luk, 2008].

Ravid et al. found that the level of cholesterol both at onset and after a five-year follow-up period was positively related with the subsequent increase in urinary albumin excretion in microalbuminuric patients with type-2 diabetes [Ravid, 1995]. Gall et al. found that total serum cholesterol was significantly associated with development of abnormally increased urinary albumin excretion [Gall, 1997]. Klein et al. in a study of type-I individuals, found that higher total serum cholesterol and lower HDL cholesterol were associated with incidence of renal insufficiency [Klein, 1999].

6.8 Increased protein intake

Protein intake: 0.8 - 1.0 gram per kilogram body weight per day in patients with normal renal functions and decrease to 0.6-0.8 gram per kilogram body weight per day once proteinuria sets in. High intakes of animal protein have been shown to increase renal blood flow and glomerular filtration rate (GFR) whereas soy protein does not appear to have this effect. Substituting soy protein for animal protein has been found to decrease hyperfiltration in subjects with diabetes and may reduce urine albumin excretion [Song, 2004].

6.9 Chronic inflammation

With the recognition of the central role played by inflammatory processes in cardiovascular disease and both type 1 and type 2 diabetes, the association between potentially modifiable inflammatory biomarkers and clinical outcomes such as nephropathy and cardiovascular disease in diabetes is of interest. Moreover, although diabetic nephropathy has traditionally not been considered an inflammatory nephritis, more recent evidence that macrophage accumulation is characteristic for diabetic glomerulosclerosis has challenged this perception [Foruta, 1993].

Recent studies suggested that inflammatory processes and immune cells might be involved in the development and progression of diabetic nephropathy. Infiltrated macrophages are found within renal diabetic tissues, and recent studies demonstrated that macrophage-derived products can induce further inflammation in the diabetic kidney. Furthermore, activated T lymphocytes have been associated with diabetic nephropathy. One of the most striking features of leukocytes from patients with diabetes is the activated status of blood neutrophils. There is no doubt that immune cells participate in the vascular injury in the conditions of diabetic nephropathy, and their migration into the kidney is a crucial step in the progression of this disease [Galkina - 2006]. A few cross-sectional studies of individuals with type 1 diabetes have reported associations between increased albumin excretion rate and elevated levels of inflammatory markers including high-sensitivity (hs) C-reactive protein (CRP), soluble (s) tumor necrosis factor-α receptor-1 (TNFR-1), intercellular adhesion molecule-1 (ICAM-1), and vascular cell adhesion molecule-1 (VCAM-1), but whether the elevation of these inflammatory markers precedes nephropathy progression is not well described.

Inflammatory cytokines and growth factors, mainly VEGF, TGF-ß, IL-1, IL-6, and IL-18, as well as TNF-α, are also involved in the development and progression of DKD [Navarro-Gonzales, 2008]. If inflammation contributes to the development of nephropathy, it would represent a potential therapeutic target for slowing the microvascular and macrovascular complications of diabetes [Lin, 2008].

6.10 Anemia

Anemia is a common finding in patients with diabetes, particularly in those with overt nephropathy or renal impairment. Anemia in patients with diabetes is not restricted to those with renal impairment, as about half have normal renal function. Failure to up-regulate erythropoietin production in response to a declining hemoglobin level has been suggested to be the primary mechanism leading to chronic anemia. Accordingly, the presence of anemia may be a distinctive marker for renal tubulointerstitial dysfunction even before overt nephropathy manifests [Luk, 2008]. The precise mechanisms by which diabetes impairs the renal erythropoietin response to reduced Hb remain to be established. While functional erythropoietin deficiency is clearly linked to renal dysfunction in diabetes, the reduction in synthesis of erythropoietin in response to anemia appears to be beyond that seen in other renal (and particularly glomerular) diseases. A number of mechanisms potentially contribute to the preferential development of anemia in patients with diabetes. For example, the predominance of damage to specific cells and to the vascular architecture of the renal tubulo-interstitium, and the resulting systemic inflammation, autonomic neuropathy, and induction of inhibitors of erythropoietin release, have all been suggested as contributors to impaired renal erythropoietin production and release [Thomas, 2006]. Although anemia can be considered a marker of kidney damage, reduced hemoglobin levels independently identify diabetic patients with an increased risk of microvascular complications, cardiovascular disease and mortality. Nevertheless, a direct role in the development or progression of diabetic complications remains to be clearly established and the clinical utility of correcting anemia in diabetic patients has yet to be demonstrated in randomized controlled trials. Correction of anemia certainly improves performance and quality of life in diabetic patients [Thomas, 2007].

6.11 Hyperuricemia

Uric acid has been associated with renal disease, even though hyperuricemia may be a marker of or by itself be responsible for microvascular disease in diabetes. In animal models, elevated level of uric acid can lead to arteriolopathy of preglomerular vessels, impaired autoregulation, glomerular hypertension, as well as endothelial dysfunction. Kidney damage in hyperuricemic rats is not dependent on blood pressure, and instead involves the renin-angiotensin system. In patients with diabetes, serum uric acid early in the course of diabetes is significantly, and independent of confounders, associated with later development of persistent macroalbuminuria. Therefore, uric acid may be a novel and important player in the pathogenesis of microvascular complications in diabetes. A dose-response relationship between serum uric acid and early decline in renal function has recently been demonstrated in patients with type-1 diabetes [Hovind, 2011].

6.12 Aldosterone

Another deleterious factor that has been underappreciated until recently is aldosterone. In addition to the classic effects of promoting sodium retention and volume expansion, aldosterone promotes inflammation, production of cytokines, growth factors and endothelial dysfunction, which acts on the renal vasculature, glomeruli and tubules and favors the emergence of proteinuria. In the setting of diabetes and longstanding hyperglycemia, free amino groups of proteins are non-enzymatically modified by glucose and its metabolites to form Schiff bases that eventually lead to the formation of advanced glycation end products (AGEs).

6.13 The use of oral contraceptives

Oral contraceptive (OC) use is associated with increased intrarenal renin–angiotensin-aldosterone system (RAA System) activity and risk of nephropathy, though the contribution of progestins contained in the OC in the regulation of angiotensin-dependent control of the renal circulation has not been elucidated [Sarna, 2009].

7. Pathogenic mechanisms

Multiple mechanisms contribute to the development and outcomes of diabetic nephropathy, such as an interaction between hyperglycemia induced metabolic and hemodynamic changes and genetic predisposition, which sets the stage for kidney injury [Dronavalli - 2008]. Extracellular matrix accumulation is one of the hallmarks in the development of the disease that leads to the formation of glomerular and interstitial lesions [Deckert, 1981]. Multiple biochemical pathways have been postulated that explain how hyperglycemia causes tissue damage: nonenzymatic glycosylation that generates advanced glycosylation end products, activation of protein kinase C, and acceleration of the polyol pathway.

8. Increased advanced glycation end products (AGEs)

Advanced glycation end products (AGEs) are diverse group of molecules and are well known heterogeneous compounds formed nonenzymatically through an interaction of reducing sugar with free amino group of proteins, lipids and nucleic acids [Krishan, 2010]. AGEs form at a constant rate in the normal body; however, in diabetes, this process is drastically increased. Accumulation of AGEs in the kidney may contribute to the progressive alteration in renal architecture and loss of renal function in patients and rodents via various mechanisms, including their cross-linking properties of matrix proteins and activation of the downstream signaling. AGEs may produce functional changes in the kidney by cross-linking with the glomerular basement membrane and other vascular membranes. AGE binding proteins may also be involved. The best defined is the receptor for AGEs (RAGE). Three main consequences have been found in association with AGEs inside cells: (1) functional alterations of intracellular proteins, (2) altered interaction with AGE receptors, and (3) altered interactions with matrix and other cells. Binding of AGEs to RAGEs activates cell signaling mechanisms coupled to increased transforming growth factor-ß (TGF-ß) and vascular endothelial growth factor (VEGF) expression, which are increased in diabetic nephropathy and are thought to contribute to diabetes complications.

8.1 Increased transforming growth factor ß1

Studies in rodent models have suggested that reduction in renal transforming growth factor (TGF)-β1 may underlie the renoprotective effects of the renin-angiotensin system (RAS) blockade [Langham, 2006]. Over the past several years, experimental evidence consistently has suggested a key role for TGF-β in the pathogenesis of the extracellular matrix accumulation that characterizes diabetic nephropathy and closely correlates with declining renal function [Mauer, 1984]. Angiotensin II potently induces synthesis of transforming growth factor (TGF)-β, a profibrotic growth factor consistently implicated in the pathogenesis of diabetic nephropathy [Border, 1996]. The mechanisms for this fibrogenic or prosclerotic action of TGF-β are multiple and include both stimulation of extracellular matrix synthesis and inhibition of its degradation [Bruijn, 1996].

8.2 Activation of protein kinase Cß (PKCß)

Other proposed mechanisms by which hyperglycemia promotes the development of diabetic nephropathy include activation of PKC that involves de novo formation of diacylglycerol and oxidative stress. Hyperglycemia also increases the generation of advanced products of nonenzymatic glycosilation of proteins through activation of aldol reductase pathway and protein kinase C (PKC). The final products of non-enzymatic glycosilation are bound to collagen and proteins that constitute the glomerular basement membrane and make the glomerular barrier more permeable to the passage of proteins, resulting in increased urinary albumin excretion [Zelmanovitz, 2009]. Two clinical observations explain the possible mechanisms involved. The first is that the hyperglycemic state seems to sensitize the endothelium to injury from elevated blood pressure. The second observation is that successful pancreas transplant that results in normal insulin regulation and normoglycemia is associated with a reversal of the lesions of diabetic nephropathy [Lurbe, 2002]. Specifically, activation of this enzyme leads to increased secretion of vasodilatory prostanoids, which contributes to glomerular hyperfiltration. By activation of TGF-β1, PKC might also increase production of extracellular matrix by mesangial cells. PKC activation induces the activity of mitogen-activated protein kinases (MAPK) in response to extracellular stimuli through dual phosphorylation at conserved threonine and tyrosine residues. The coactivation of PKC and MAPK in the presence of high glucose concentrations indicates that these two families of enzymes are linked [Dronavalli, 2008].

8.3 Aldose reductase pathway/polyol pathway

Aldose reductase (AR) is a monomeric reduced nicotinamide adenine dinucleotide (NAD) phosphate (NADPH)-dependent enzyme and a member of aldo-keto reductase superfamily. Aldose reductase (AR) is widely expressed aldehyde-metabolizing enzyme. The polyol pathway is implicated in the pathogenesis of diabetic nephropathy. A number of studies have shown a decrease in urinary albumin excretion in animals administered aldose reductase inhibitors, but in humans these agents have not been studied widely and the results are inconclusive [Tilton, 1989]. The reduction of glucose by the AR-catalyzed polyol pathway has been linked to the development of secondary diabetic complications [Srivastava - 2005].

8.4 The protein kinase C (PKC) pathway

The protein kinase C (PKC) superfamily comprises proteins that are activated in response to various pathogenic stimuli in the diabetic state. Hyperglycemia is the predominant stimulus that induces the activation of distinct PKC isoforms within a cell, each mediating specific functions, probably through differential subcellular localization. Craven and DeRubertis [Craven, 1989] and Lee et al. [Lee, 1989] were the first to provide data indicating that activation of the PKC system by hyperglycemia may represent an important pathway by which glucotoxicity is transduced in susceptible cells in diabetic nephropathy. The putative intracellular mechanism is the glucose induced de novo synthesis of diacylglycerol that is one of the intracellular activators of PKC [Menne, 2009]. PKC activation is involved in the regulation of vascular permeability and contractility, endothelial cell activation and vasoconstriction, extracellular matrix (ECM) synthesis and turnover, abnormal angiogenesis, excessive apoptosis, leukocyte adhesion, abnormal growth factor signaling and cytokine action, as well as abnormal cell growth and angiogenesis, all of which are involved in the pathophysiology of diabetic vascular complications [Meier, 2009].

8.5 Vascular endothelial growth factor (VEGF) pathway

Vascular endothelial growth factor (VEGF) is a key regulator of vascular permeability and angiogenesis and is implicated in the pathogenesis of diabetic retinal neovascularisation. In the glomerulus it is produced in large amounts by podocytes and is thought to be important in maintaining glomerular endothelial cell fenestrations [Satchell, 2006]. Hyperglycemia increases the expression of vascular endothelial growth factor (VEGF) in podocytes causing increased vascular permeability. VEGF has the potential to induce the new vessel growth seen in early diabetic nephropathy and to alter the permeability characteristics of the endothelium [Kanesaki, 2005]. In human type 1 diabetes, serum VEGF concentrations vary according to glycemic control, and higher levels are associated with microvascular complications, including microalbuminuria [Chiarelli, 2000]. In type 2 diabetes, VEGF is upregulated early in the course of disease and urinary VEGF levels are correlated with microalbuminuria [Kim, 2005]. Further studies have confirmed initial upregulation of VEGF signalling in type 2 diabetes followed by a down-regulation with podocyte loss and sclerosis development [Hohenstein, 2006].

8.6 Oxidative stress pathway

A large body of evidence indicates that oxidative stress is the common denominator link for the major pathways involved in the development and progression of diabetic micro- as well as macrovascular complications of diabetes nephropathy. Both hyperglycemia and activation of the renin-angiotensin system play a role in the generation of reactive oxygen species (ROS) [Anjaneyulu, 2004]. There are a number of macromolecules that have been implicated for increased generation of reactive oxygen species (ROS), such as, NAD(P)H oxidase, advanced glycation end products (AGE), defects in polyol pathway, uncoupled nitric oxide synthase (NOS) and mitochondrial respiratory chain via oxidative phosphorylation. Excess amounts of ROS modulate activation of protein kinase C, mitogen-activated protein kinases, and various cytokines and transcription factors which eventually cause increased expression of extracellular matrix (ECM) genes with progression to fibrosis and end stage renal disease. Activation of renin-angiotensin system (RAS) further worsens the renal injury induced by ROS in diabetic nephropathy. Buffering the generation of ROS may represent a promising therapeutic to ameliorate renal damage from diabetic kidney disease; however, various studies have demonstrated minimal reno-protection by these agents [Kashihara - 2010]. These derangements, along with hemodynamic changes, activate various cytokines and growth factors such as vascular endothelial growth factor, transforming growth factor-β, Interleukin 1 (IL 1), IL-6 and IL-18.

8.7 The activation of the transcription factor NF-kB

Patients with diabetic kidney disease have higher monocyte NFκB activity than diabetic patients without renal complications. The transcription factor NF-kB helps to control the expression of numerous genes activated during inflammation. NF-kB is induced by various cell stress–associated stimuli including growth factors, vasoactive agents, cytokines, and oxidative stress. NF-kB in turn controls the regulation of genes encoding proteins involved in immune and inflammatory responses (i.e., cytokines, chemokines, growth factors, immune receptors, cellular ligands, and adhesion molecules) [Schmid - 2006]. Inhibition of NFκB reduces interstitial monocyte infiltration in rats with proteinuria, and NFκB is believed to play a key role in proteinuria-induced tubulointerstitial damage in diabetes [Remuzzi, 1998].

9. The histological changes

Three major histological changes occur in the glomeruli of persons with diabetic kidney disease. First, mesangial expansion is directly induced by hyperglycemia, perhaps via increased matrix production or glycosylation of matrix proteins. Second, thickening of the glomerular basement membrane occurs. Third, glomerular sclerosis is caused by intraglomerular hypertension (induced by dilatation of the afferent renal artery or from ischemic injury induced by hyaline narrowing of the vessels supplying the glomeruli). These different histological patterns appear to have similar prognostic significance. All of these are part and parcel of microvascular complications of diabetes. A large body of evidence indicates that oxidative stress is the common denominator link for the major pathways involved in the development and progression of diabetic micro- as well as macro-vascular complications of diabetes.

Light microscopy findings show an increase in the solid spaces of the tuft, most frequently observed as coarse branching of solid (positive periodic-acid Schiff reaction) material (diffuse diabetic glomerulopathy). Large cellular accumulations also may be observed within these areas. These are circular on section and are known as the Kimmelstiel-Wilson lesions/nodules.

Electron microscopy provides a more detailed definition of the structures involved. In advanced disease, the mesangial regions occupy a large proportion of the tuft, with prominent matrix content. Further, the basement membrane in the capillary walls (ie, the peripheral basement membrane) is thicker than normal. Immunofluorescence microscopy may reveal deposition of albumin, immunoglobulins, fibrin, and other plasma proteins along the GBM in a linear pattern most likely as a result of exudation from the blood vessels, but this is not immunopathogenetic or diagnostic and does not imply an immunologic pathophysiology. The renal vasculature typically displays evidence of atherosclerosis, usually due to concomitant hyperlipidemia and hypertensive arteriosclerosis.

The severity of diabetic glomerulopathy is estimated by the thickness of the peripheral basement membrane and mesangium and matrix expressed as a fraction of appropriate spaces (eg, volume fraction of mesangium/glomerulus, matrix/mesangium, or matrix/glomerulus). The glomeruli and kidneys are typically normal or increased in size initially, thus distinguishing diabetic nephropathy from most other forms of chronic renal insufficiency, wherein renal size is reduced (except renal amyloidosis and polycystic kidney disease).

10. Clinical diagnosis of diabetic kidney disease

The clinical diagnosis of diabetic kidney disease is, mainly, based on detection of albuminuria from spot urine is recommended because the albumin-creatinine ratio by spot urine sample has demonstrated excellent correlation with the 24-hour urine albumin measurements. Estimated glomerular filtration rate (eGFR), has been added to the albuminuria also as a renal biomarker. Both are indeed associated with renal and cardiovascular disease in individuals with diabetes and may be used to identify individuals at risk of long-term complications.

Microalbuminuria, which is an indicator of endothelial dysfunction, and an independent marker for cardiovascular morbidity and mortality in individuals with and without diabetes is defined as an albumin-creatinine ratio of 30-300 mg/g from a spot urine collection, urinary albumin excretion 30-300 mg/24 hours in a 24-hour urine collection, or 20-200 µg/min in a timed urine collection.

Macroalbuminuria is defined as an albumin/creatinine ratio (ACR) > 300 mg/g from a spot urine collection, urinary albumin excretion > 300 mg/24 hours in a 24-hour urine collection, or >200 µg/min in a timed urine collection. For initial screening of diabetic kidney disease, the measurement of albuminuria from spot urine is recommended because the ACR by spot urine sample has demonstrated excellent correlation with the 24-hour urine albumin measurements.

If the determination of albuminuria cannot be performed at diagnosis, we can measure proteinuria. *Microproteinuria* is defined by a value between 300-500 mg/24 hours and *macroproteinuria* is defined by a value higher than 500 mg/24 hours. Serum markers of glomerular filtration rate and microalbuminuria identify renal impairment in different segments of the diabetic population, indicating that serum markers as well as microalbuminuria tests should be used in screening for nephropathy in diabetic patients.

There is accumulating evidence suggesting that the risk for developing diabetic nephropathy and cardiovascular disease starts when UAE values are still within the normoalbuminuric range [Gerstein, 2001]. After the diagnosis of micro- or macroalbuminuria is confirmed, patients should undergo a complete evaluation, including a work-up for other etiologies and an assessment of renal function and the presence of other comorbid associations [Gross - 2005].

10.1 Glomerular filtration rate

Although the best measure for glomerular filtration rate (GFR) is obtained by techniques that involve infusion of exogenous substances, GFR is usually estimated in clinical practice by various formulae based on serum creatinine concentration, since this is much less invasive and time-consuming. The most popular equation used today is the Modification of Diet in Renal Disease (MDRD) equation [Levey, 1999].

Recent efforts to identify novel biomarkers in the diabetic population have been evolving either to detect early kidney injury or repair that ultimately lead to progression of diabetic kidney disease.

10.2 Cystatin-C

Cystatin-C, a cysteine protease inhibitor that is produced by virtually all nucleated cells and released into the bloodstream is entirely filtered by the kidney glomerulus and metabolized by the proximal tubule. Recently interest has developed in cystatin-C and was proposed as a potential endogenous filtration marker of GFR because it is a more sensitive indicator of mild renal impairment and may better estimate the GFR than serum creatinine.

10.3 Retinol-binding protein 4 (RBP-4)

Retinol-binding protein 4 (RBP-4) is a small visceral protein, mainly synthesized in the liver and catabolized in the kidneys after glomerular filtration. Initially reported as an adipokine that impairs insulin sensitivity, the concentrations of this adipokine are increased in diabetic patients as compared to normal subjects.

Mechanistic studies have suggested that RBP-4 impaired insulin sensitivity by inhibition of insulin receptor substrate-1 phosphorylation and phosphatidylinositol 3-kinase activation in muscle and by induction of glucose production in liver via cytosolic phosphoenolpyruvate carboxykinase (PEPCK) stimulation [Yang, 2005]. Interestingly, urinary RBP-4 excretion is increased in early diabetic nephropathy and might even be a marker of early renal damage preceding microalbuminuria [Hong, 2000].

10.4 Connective tissue growth factor (CTGF)

Connective tissue growth factor (CTGF) is a polypeptide with functions in extracellular matrix production and other profibrotic activity mediated by transforming growth factor-β1. Other biological functions of CTGF include angiogenesis, chondrogenesis, osteogenesis, and cell adhesion, migration, proliferation, and differentiation. The upregulation of CTGF has been observed in human and experimental diabetic nephropathy.

10.5 Pigment epithelium-derived factor (PEDF)

Pigment epithelium-derived factor (PEDF) is a glycoprotein that belongs to the superfamily of serine protease inhibitors with complex neurotrophic, neuroprotective, anti-angiogenic, anti-oxidative and anti-inflammatory properties, any of which could potentially be exploited as a therapeutic option for the treatment of vascular complications in diabetes. Recent studies suggest that PEDF could reduce proteinuria by suppressing podocyte damage and decreased nephrin as well as increased VEGF expression in the glomeruli of ADN rats. It has been reported that PEDF counteracts the effects of VEGF [Liu, 2004] and advanced glycation end products [Inagaki, 2003]. It is noteworthy in the future to determine whether PEDF may be used as a specific marker for screening incipient DN.

10.6 Pentoxifylline (PTF)

Pentoxifylline (PTF) is a methylxanthine derivative with favorable effects on microcirculatory blood flow as a result of its rheological properties. Recent studies have shown that PTF reduces urinary protein excretion in individuals with diabetes, both with normal renal function and with renal insufficiency. In a previous study in patients with diabetes and nephropathy, was found that TNF-α concentrations were significantly elevated and related to the urinary protein excretion and, moreover, that the levels of this cytokine decreased after PTF administration, with a significant correlation between the decrease of TNF-α and the reduction of proteinuria. It was demonstrated in rats that Pentoxifylline reduces the accumulation and proliferation of glomerular macrophages in mesangial proliferative glomerulonephritis, and the recruitment of macrophages, lymphocytes, and major histocompatibility complex (MHC) class II antigen-positive cells into remnant kidney interstitium [Lin, 2002].

Emerging roles of urinary biomarkers have proven beneficial due to the ability to standardize the various markers to creatinine or peptides already present in the urine. The role of neutrophil gelatinase-associated lipoprotein, kidney injury molecule-1 and podocin derivatives have gained enormous significance in the process of early identification of kidney injury in the diabetic population [Buddineni - 2011].

11. Differential diagnosis

Differential diagnosis is usually based on the history, physical examination, laboratory evaluation, and imaging of the kidneys. Renal biopsy is only recommended in special situations. The diagnosis of diabetic nephropathy is easily established in long-term type 1 diabetic patients (>10 years diabetes duration), especially if retinopathy is also present. Typical diabetic nephropathy is also likely to be present in proteinuric type 2 diabetic patients with retinopathy. However, diagnostic uncertainty exists in some patients with type 2 diabetes since the onset of diabetes is unknown and retinopathy is absent in a significant proportion (28%) of these patients [Christensen, 2001].

Imaging of the kidneys, usually by ultrasonography, should be performed in patients with symptoms of urinary tract obstruction, infection, or kidney stones or with a family history of polycystic kidney disease [Levey, 2003].

12. Prevention and treatment of diabetic nephropathy

Monitoring of type 2 diabetic patients for microalbuminuria at least once per year is recommended. Microalbuminuria in type 2 diabetic patients is not as potent a real risk predictor as in type 1 diabetic patients, but it is certainly the best available tool to identify patients in need of intensified treatment [Rugenetti, 1998].

13. Glycemic and blood pressure control

The interventions which proved to prevent the onset or attenuate the progression of diabetic nephropathy includes a combination of tight control of blood glucose (goal is < 7%), tight control of blood pressure (goal < 130/80 mmHg), lowering of urine albumin, and stopping of smoking (a well-established endothelial cell toxin that also affects progression of kidney disease), the specific blockage of the renin-angiotensin-aldosteron system (RAAS), with either angiotensin-converting enzyme inhibitors (ACEI) or angiotensin II receptor blockers (ARB) and lipid-lowering therapy, especially statins and fibrates.

There is evidence that early therapeutic intervention in patients with chronic kidney disease or diabetes can delay onset of complications and improve outcomes [Atkins, 2010]. For example, the UKPDS [Holman, 2008 Bilous, 2008], STENO-2 [Gaede, 2008], and ADVANCE studies [Patel, 2007, Patel, 2008, Zoungas, 2009] demonstrated that tight control of blood glucose level, blood pressure (and lipids in STENO-2) significantly reduced incidence and progression of diabetic kidney disease. In people with type 2 diabetes, inhibition of the renin-angiotensin-aldosterone system using an ACE inhibitor or an ARB decreased the progression from normoalbuminuria to microalbuminuria [Ruggenenti, 2004], reduced the progression from micro albuminuria to macroalbuminuria, [Parving, 2001] and slowed the development of ESRD [Lewis, 2001]. Thus the use of an ACE inhibitor or ARB is now standard therapy for patients with diabetic nephropathy as well as glucose, lipid and blood pressure control. Effective management using evidence-based therapies is the fourth step in tackling diabetic kidney disease.

Like other microvascular complications of diabetes, there are strong associations between glucose control (as measured by hemoglobin A1c [A1C]) and the risk of developing diabetic nephropathy. Patients should be treated to the lowest safe glucose level that can be obtained to prevent or control diabetic nephropathy [Fowler - 2008]. Glycemic control in both type 1 and type 2 diabetes has been associated with reduced appearance of diabetic nephropathy (microalbuminuria) [Hall, 2006]. Control of glycemia in type 2 diabetic patients with nephropathy represents some peculiar aspects. Today there is no longer any doubt that tight glycemic control prevents the onset or progression of diabetic nephropathy in type 2 diabetic patients as it does in type 1 diabetic patients. In the past, it had been thought that once clinically manifest nephropathy had developed, a point of no return was reached beyond which tight glycemic control failed to prevent the further decline in renal function. Nevertheless recent studies from the Steno Hospital showed that glycemic control had some, although less pronounced compared with tight BP control, effect on the rate of progression [Wolf, 2003].

The Diabetes Control and Complications Trial, the United Kingdom Prospective Diabetes Study and the Japanese Diabetes Intervention Study have confirmed that tight glycemic control can prevent the development of all microvascular complications including nephropathy [Looke, 2008].

Once albuminuria occurs, controlling blood pressure assumes critical importance. The use of renin–angiotensin blockade has been a major advance in the management of diabetic nephropathy. Major landmark studies including the Irbesartan Diabetic Nephropathy Trial [Louis, 2001] and RENAAL study [Brenner, 2001] have provided compelling evidence to support the renoprotective effect of angiotensin-II receptor antagonists, independent of blood pressure lowering [Looke, 2008].

The renin–angiotensin system (RAAS) is an important target for hemodynamic disturbances in diabetic kidney disease. Blocking the renin–angiotensin system in diabetes has pluripotent effects on modifying the systemic and glomerular hemodynamic as well as attenuating the pro-inflammatory and pro-fibrotic changes in renal parenchyma [Look, 2008]. The pharmacological agents which block the RAAS slow the progression of renal dysfunction more effectively than other classes of antihypertensive agents. In addition to normalization of systemic and glomerular hypertension, it is now clear that inhibition of the RAAS at various levels have several renoprotective effects, including anti-inflammatory and antifibrotic mechanisms.

Currently available therapies for this blockade are angiotensin converting enzyme inhibitor (ACE-I), angiotensin II type 1 receptor blocker (ARB) and direct renin inhibitor. If the treatment with ACEI and/or ARB does not reach the blood pressure target levels, then they can be combined with other drug classes, even before maximizing the dose of each agent. The combination of agents may include calcium channel blockers (especially nondihydropyridine), β-blockers, diuretics or central α_2-agonist.

Another concept of a dual blockade of the RAAS has been developed by Mogensen in 2000. Since ACEI and ARB interrupt the RAAS at different levels, the combination of these classes of drugs may have an additive effect on renoprotection. The renoprotective effects of dual blockade of the RAAS with ARB and direct renin inhibitor (aliskiren) may also be effective.

Addition of diuretics has been strongly recommended by KDOQI guidelines to achieve target blood pressures of < 130 mmHg in cases of recalcitrant hypertension in diabetes kidney disease patients. The role for aldosterone antagonist (spironolactone) and statins in prevention of metabolic derangements consequent to RAAS overactivity in DKD is emerging.

The BP-lowering arm of the Action in Diabetes and Vascular disease: preterAx and diamicroN-MR Controlled Evaluation (ADVANCE) study recently reported that the routine administration of a fixed combination of the angiotensin converting enzyme inhibitor perindopril and the diuretic indapamide to a broad cross-section of patients with type 2 diabetes reduced the risk for cardiovascular and kidney outcomes, regardless of initial BP level. More recently, the glucose-lowering arm of ADVANCE reported that intensive glucose lowering based on gliclazide (modified release) reduced the risk for new or worsening nephropathy.

While good glycemic control ameliorates the development of microalbuminuria in type 1 and type 2 diabetes there is increasing evidence that angiotensin-converting enzyme inhibition and angiotensin receptor blockade are ineffective as primary prevention strategies. Blood pressure control remains the mainstay of treating established diabetic renal disease and a multi-factorial intervention approach in those with type 2 diabetes and microalbuminuria appears to be effective in reducing mortality based on data from one study [Walker, 2010].

14. Aldosterone receptor antagonists

Experimental studies supporting aldosterone antagonists have shown anti-inflammatory effect, anti-fibrotic properties and suppression of markers of tubular injury, interstitial fibrosis and glomerulosclerosis [Kramer, 2007]. Aldosterone antagonists have generally been considered to have an antiproteinuric effect, and addition of spironolactone to an ACE inhibitor or ARB is associated with a marked and sustained antiproteinuric effect, with the rate of hyperkalemia being similar to placebo. These results are based on studies with small numbers of patients, mostly of very short follow-up. There are no long term data regarding benefit with the combination of ACE inhibitor or ARB and aldosterone antagonists in terms of slowing the progression of diabetic kidney disease. In clinical practice, the use of this combination of agents in patients with low GFR should be undertaken with careful instructions for dietary potassium restriction and avoidance of nonsteroidal anti-inflammatory drugs and cyclooxy-genase-2 inhibitors [Satirapoj, 2010].

15. Peroxisome proliferator-activated receptors (PPAR)-gamma agonists

Peroxisome proliferator activated receptor-γ (PPARγ) is a ligand activated transcription factor that regulates cell growth, inflammation, lipid metabolism and insulin sensitivity, appear to have a role in regulating adipogenesis and blood pressure [Satirapoj, 2010]. PPARγ agonists may indirectly suppress the systemic production of a proinflammatory milieu mainly via inhibiting TNF-α, PAI-1, and IL-6 expression in adipose tissue. Additionally, PPARγ seems to have anti-inflammatory effects on monocytes. PPARγ activation can reduce the production of cytokines (TNF-α, IL-1, IL-6), probably through inhibiting the activity of proinflammatory transcription factors such as NF-κB. PPARs have also been implicated in many renal pathophysiological conditions, including diabetic nephropathy and glomerulosclerosis [Ruan, 2008]. Recently it was demonstrated that peroxisome proliferator activated receptor-γ (PPARγ) agonists block the deleterious effects of AGEs and exert beneficial actions on diabetic nephropathy. It has been successfully shown that PPAR-γ agonists limit high glucose-induced inflammation in proximal tubular cells. PPAR-γ agonists also exert anti-fibrotic effects in human proximal tubular cells under high glucose conditions by attenuating the increase in AP-1, TGF-β1 and downstream production of the extracellular matrix protein, fibronectin. PPAR-γ agonists can improve insulin sensitivity, reduce triglyceride levels and decrease the risk of atherosclerosis. PPARγ agonists have been shown to lower blood pressure in animals and humans, perhaps by suppressing the renin-angiotensin (Ang)-aldosterone system (RAAS), including the inhibition of Ang II type 1 receptor expression, Ang-II-mediated signaling pathways, and Ang-II-induced adrenal aldosterone synthesis/secretion [Sugawara, 2011].

16. Protein restriction

Animal studies have shown that restriction of dietary protein intake also reduces hyperfiltration and intraglomerular and retards the progression of several models of renal disease, including diabetic glomerulopathy. Reduction of dietary protein has long been proposed as a treatment for CRF and this intervention has shown a modest benefit in slowing loss of filtration function, but adherence to this form of therapy is difficult in diabetes.

17. Lipid control

Clinical studies in patients with diabetic nephropathy showed that lipid control can be associated with an additional effect of reduction in proteinuria. Lipid-lowering agents (statins) showed renoprotection in a variety of proteinuric glomerular diseases [Agarwal, 2007]. Although lipid-lowering treatment has been shown to be effective in reducing cardiovascular morbidity and mortality in diabetic patients with hyperlipidemia, their effects on diabetic nephropathy are still unclear due to lack of prospective randomized intervention studies [Chen, 2005]. Early studies have demonstrated that treatment with the HMG CoA reductase inhibitor pravastatin decreases albuminuria in patients with type 2 diabetes [Sasaki, 1990]. Experimental studies demonstrated that lipid-lowering agents exerted a certain degree of renoprotection, through both indirect effects from lipid lowering and a direct effect on cell protection. Therefore, lipid control appears to be important in the prevention and treatment of diabetic nephropathy [Chen, 2005].

18. Antioxidants

There have been multiple trials using vitamin E, vitamin C, probucol, taurine, n-acetylcysteine, lipoic acid, and other antioxidant drugs in animals. Animal studies using these compounds have been shown to be effective in reducing the development of diabetic kidney disease. It's hard to translate these animal results to humans as many trials in mice and rats are very effective in the particular animal but often ineffective in humans. This may be due to short duration of animal studies, dose differences between animals and humans, and different pathophysiologic processes between animals and humans. Human studies with antioxidants for diabetic nephropathy are limited and have had variable results [Stanton, 2011].

Despite receiving optimal care to control blood pressure and metabolic risk factors as well as inhibition of the renin–angiotensin system in a clinical trial setting, there is a considerable residual risk for cardio-renal complications in patients with diabetic kidney disease. Understanding the molecular milieu of diabetic podocyte injury, an early event in diabetic nephropathy, remains a primary target in identifying novel avenues for early intervention and prevention of severe late complications of this increasingly prevalent disease. Decreasing hyperglycemia's toxic effects, stimulating the endogenous protective factors, controlling obesity and low grade inflammation as well as correction of anemia may represent also areas where novel strategies can be developed and tested to curb this rising global burden of cardio-renal complications in diabetic patients. Correction of anemia improves renal tissue oxygenation, reduces hypoxic damage and associated oxidative stress. There have been several reports suggesting that early erythropoietin treatment may retard the progression of renal diseases and delay the commencement of renal replacement therapy.

Annual screening for microalbuminuria will allow the identification of patients with nephropathy at a point very early in its course. Improving glycemic control, aggressive antihypertensive treatment, and the use of ACE inhibitors or ARBs will slow the rate of progression of nephropathy. In addition, protein restriction and other treatment modalities such as phosphate lowering may have benefits in selected patients.

In conclusion, there are very compelling reasons to better understand the mechanisms underlying diabetic kidney disease, to develop new treatments that can both prevent the development of kidney disease and slow or stop the progression.

19. References

[1] ADVANCE Collaborative Group, Patel A, MacMahon S, Chalmers J, Neal B, Woodward M, Billot L, Harrap S, Poulter N, Marre M, Cooper M, Glasziou P, Grobbee DE, Hamet P, Heller S, Liu LS, Mancia G, Mogensen CE, Pan CY, Rodgers A, Williams B: Effects of a fixed combination of perindopril and indapamide on macrovascular and microvascular outcomes in patients with type 2 diabetes mellitus (the ADVANCE trial): A randomised controlled trial. Lancet 370: 829–840, 2007

[2] ADVANCE Collaborative Group, Patel A, MacMahon S, Chalmers J, Neal B, Billot L, Woodward M, Marre M, Cooper M, Glasziou P, Grobbee D, Hamet P, Harrap S, Heller S, Liu L, Mancia G, Mogensen CE, Pan C, Poulter N, Rodgers A, Williams B, Bompoint S, de Galan BE, Joshi R, Travert F: Intensive blood glucose control and vascular outcomes in patients with type 2 diabetes. N Engl J Med 358: 2560– 2572, 2008

[3] Agarwal R. Effects of statins on renal function. Mayo Clin Proc 2007; 82: 1381-90.

[4] Anjaneyulu M, Chopra K: Effect of irbesartan on the antioxidant defense system and nitric oxide release in diabetic rat kidney. Am J Nephrol 24: 488–496, 2004
[5] Atkins RC, Zimmet P. Diabetic Kidney disease: act now or pay later. Kidney Int. 2010 Mar;77(5):378- 80.
[6] Ayodele OE, Alebiosu CO, Salako BL: Diabetic nephropathy--a review of the natural history, burden, risk factors and treatment. J Natl Med Assoc 96:1445 - 1454, 2004.
[7] B.M. Brenner, M.E. Cooper, D. de Zeeuw, W.F. Keane, W.E. Mitch, H.H. Parving, et al., Effects of losartan on renal and cardiovascular outcomes in patients with type 2 diabetes and nephropathy, N. Engl. J. Med. 345 (2001) 861–869.
[8] Bilous R. Microvascular disease: what does the UKPDS tell us about diabetic nephropathy? Diabet Med, 2008; 25:25-9.
[9] Border WA, Yamamoto T, Noble NA: Transforming growth factor-β in diabetic nephropathy. Diabetes Metab Rev 12: 309–339, 1996
[10] Bruijn JA, Roos A, de Geus B, de Heer E: Transforming growth factor-beta and the glomerular extracellular matrix in renal pathology. J Lab Clin Med 123: 34–47, 1994
[11] Burney B, Kalaitzidis R, Bakris G. Novel therapies of diabetic nephropathy. Curr Opin Nephrol Hypertens, 2009; 18:107-11.
[12] Cameron JS: The nephrotic syndrome: A historical review. In: The Nephrotic Syndrome, edited by Cameron JS, Glassock RJ, New York, Marcel Dekker, 1988, pp 3–56
[13] Chiarelli F, Spagnoli A, Basciani F et al (2000) Vascular endothelial growth factor (VEGF) in children, adolescents and young adults with type 1 diabetes mellitus: relation to glycaemic control and microvascular complications. Diabet Med 17:650–656
[14] Christensen PK, Larsen S, Horn T, Olsen S, Parving HH: Renal function and structure in albuminuric type 2 diabetic patients without retinopathy. Nephrol Dial Transplant 16:2337–2347, 2001.
[15] Craven P, DeRubertis F (1989) Protein kinase C is activated in glomeruli from streptozotocin diabetic rats. J Clin Invest 83:1667–1675
[16] Deckert T, Poulsen JE: Diabetic nephropathy: Fault or destiny? Diabetologia 21: 178–183, 1981
[17] Dronavalli S, Duka I, Bakris GL. The pathogenesis of diabetic nephropathy. Nat Clin Pract Endocrinol Metab 2008; 4: 444–452
[18] E.J. Lewis, L.G. Hunsicker, W.R. Clarke, T. Berl, M.A. Pohl, J.B. Lewis, et al., Renoprotective effect of the angiotensinreceptor antagonist irbesartan in patients with nephropathy due to type 2 diabetes, N. Engl. J. Med. 345 (2001) 851–860.
[19] Forbes JM, Cooper ME. Glycation in diabetic nephropathy. Amino Acids 2010 [Epub ahead of print].
[20] Fowler MJ. Microvascular and macrovascular complications of diabetes. Clin Diabetes. 2008;26(2):77–82.
[21] Freedman BI, Bostrom M, Daeihagh P, et al. Genetic factors in diabetic nephropathy. Clin J Am Soc Nephrol 2007;2:1306–1316.
[22] Furuta T, Saito T, Ootaka T, Soma J, Obara K, Abe K, Yoshinaga K: The role of macrophages in diabetic glomerulosclerosis. Am J Kidney Dis 21:480 - 485, 1993.
[23] Gaede P, Lund-Andersen H, Parving HH et al. Effect of a multifactorial intervention on mortality in type 2 diabetes. N Engl J Med, 2008; 358:580-91.

[24] Gall M-A, Hougaard P, Borch-Johnsen K, et al. Risk factors for development of incipient and overt diabetic nephropathy in patients with noninsulin-dependent diabetes mellitus: prospective observational study. BMJ.1997;314:783-788.
[25] Gerstein H, Mann J, Yi Q, Zinman B, Dinneen S, Hoogwerf B, Halle J, Young J, Rashkow A, Joyce C, Nawaz S, Yusuf S: Albuminuria and risk of cardiovascular events, death, and heart failure in diabetic and nondiabetic individuals. JAMA 286:421-426, 2001
[26] Hall PM. Prevention of pregression in diabetic nephropathy. Diab. Spectr. 2006;19:18–24
[27] Hohenstein B, Hausknecht B, Boehmer K, Riess R, Brekken RA, Hugo CP (2006) Local VEGF activity but not VEGF expression is tightly regulated during diabetic nephropathy in man. Kidney Int 69:1654–1661
[28] Holman RR, Paul SK, Bethel MA et al. 10-year follow-up of intensive glucose control in type 2 diabetes. N Engl J Med, 2008; 359:1577-89.
[29] Hong CY, Chia KS, Ling SL: Urinary protein excretion in type 2 diabetes with complications. J Diabetes Complications 14:259 –265, 2000.
[30] Hovind P, Rossing P, Johnson RJ, Parving HH, Serum Uric Acid as a New Player in the Development of Diabetic Nephropathy, Journal of Renal Nutrition, 21 (1): 124-127, 2011.
[31] Inagaki Y, Yamagishi S, Okamoto T, Takeuchi M, Amano S: Pigment epithelium-derived factor prevents advanced glycation end products-induced monocyte chemoattractant protein-1 production in microvascular endothelial cells by suppressing intracellular reactive oxygen species generation. Diabetologia 2003; 46: 284–287.
[32] Janssen B et al. (2005) Carnosine as a protective factor in diabetic nephropathy: association with a leucine repeat of the carnosinase gene CNDP1. Diabetes 54: 2320–2327
[33] Jones CA, Krolewski AS, Rogus J, Xue JL, Collins A, Warram JH. Epidemic of end-stage renal disease in people with diabetes in the United States population: do we know the cause? Kidney Int 2005;67:1684-1691.
[34] Kanesaki Y, Suzuki D, Uehara G et al (2005) Vascular endothelial growth factor gene expression is correlated with glomerular neovascularization in human diabetic nephropathy. Am J Kidney Dis 45:288–294
[35] Kashihara N, Haruna Y, Kondeti VK, Kanwar YS. Oxidative stress in diabetic nephropathy. Curr Med Chem. 2010;17:4256-4269.
[36] Kim NH, Oh JH, Seo JA et al (2005) Vascular endothelial growth factor (VEGF) and soluble VEGF receptor FLT-1 in diabetic nephropathy. Kidney Int 67:167–177
[37] Klein R, Klein BEK, Moss SE, et al. The 10-year incidence of renal insufficiency in people with type-I diabetes. Diabetes Care. 1999;22:743-751.
[38] Kramer AB, van der Meulen EF, Hamming I, van Goor H, Navis G. Effect of combining ACE inhibition with aldosterone blockade on proteinuria and renal damage in experimental nephrosis. Kidney S240 J Med Assoc Thai Vol. 93 Suppl. 6 2010 Int 2007; 71: 417-24.
[39] Krishan P, Chakkarwar VA, Diabetic nephropathy: Aggressive involvement of oxidative stress, J Pharm Educ Res Vol. 2, Issue No. 1, June 2011

[40] Langham RG, Kelly DJ, Gow RM, Zhang Y, Cordonnier DJ, Pinel N, Zaoui P, Gilbert RE: Transforming growth factor-beta in human diabetic nephropathy: Effects of ACE inhibition. Diabetes Care 29: 2670–2675, 2006.

[41] Lee TS, MacGregor LC, Fluharty SJ, King GL (1989) Activation of protein kinase C by elevation of glucose concentration: proposal for a mechanism in the development of diabetic vascular complications. PNAS 86:5141–5145

[42] Levey AS, Bosch JP, Lewis JB, Greene T, Rogers N, Roth D; Modification of Diet in Renal Disease Study Group. A more accurate method to estimate glomerular filtration rate from serum creatinine: a new prediction equation. Ann Intern Med 1999; 130:461–470.

[43] Levey AS, Coresh J, Balk E, Kausz AT, Levin A, Steffes MW, Hogg RJ, Perrone RD, Lau J, Eknoyan G: National Kidney Foundation practice guidelines for chronic kidney disease: evaluation, classification, and stratification. Ann Intern Med 139:137–147, 2003.

[44] Lewis EJ, Hunsicker LG, Clarke WR et al. Renoprotective effect of the angiotensin-receptor antagonist irbesartan in patients with nephropathy due to type 2 diabetes. N Eng J Med, 2001; 345:851-60.

[45] Lin J, Glynn RJ, Rifai N, et al. Inflammation and progressive nephropathy in type 1 diabetes in the diabetes control and complications trial. Diabetes Care 2008;31:2338–43. [PubMed: 18796620]

[46] Liu H, Ren JG, Cooper WL, Hawkins CE, Cowan MR, Tong PY: Identification of the antivasopermeability effect of pigment epithelium- derived factor and its active site. Proc Natl Acad Sci USA 2004; 101: 6605- 6610.

[47] Luk A, Chan JC. Diabetic nephropathy—what are the unmet needs? Diabetes Res Clin Pract. 2008; 82(suppl 1):S15-S20.

[48] Lurbe E, Redon J, Kesani A, Pascual JM, Tacons J, Alvarez V, Batlle D: Increase in nocturnal blood pressure and progression to microalbuminuria in type 1 diabetes. N Engl J Med 347:797–805, 2002.

[49] Lurbe L, Redon J, Kesani A, Pascual JM, Tacons J, Alvarez V, Battle D: Increase in nocturnal blood pressure and progression to microalbuminuria in type 1 diabetes. N Engl J Med 347: 797–805, 2002

[50] Mauer SM, Steffes MW, Brown DM: The kidney in diabetes. Am J Med 70:603–612, 1981.

[51] Mauer SM, Steffes MW, Ellis EN, Sutherland DE, Brown DM, Goetz FC: Structural-functional relationships in diabetic nephropathy. J Clin Invest 74: 1143–1155, 1984

[52] Meier M, Menne J, Haller H. Targeting the protein kinase C family in the diabetic kidney: lessons from analysis of mutant mice. Diabetologia 52: 765–775, 2009.

[53] Menne J, Meier M, Park JK, Haller H. Inhibition of protein kinase C in diabetic nephropathy—where do we stand? Nephrol Dial Transplant 2009; 24: 2021-3.

[54] Mogensen CE, Christiansen CK. Blood pressure changes and renal function changes in incipient and overt diabetic nephropathy. Hypertension 1985;7:II64–II73.

[55] Mogensen CE, Poulsen PL (1994) Epidemiology of microalbuminuria in diabetes and in the background population. Curr Opin Nephrol Hypertens 3:248–256

[56] Mogensen CE. Defintion of diabetic renal disease in insulin dependent diabetes mellitus based on renal function tests. In The Kidney and Hypertension in diabetes mellitus . 3rd ed. Mogensen CE ,ed. London, Kluwer,1996 pp.11
[57] Navarro-Gonzalez JF, Mora-Fernandez C. The role of inflammatory cytokines in diabetic nephropathy. J Am Soc Nephrol 2008; 19: 433-42.
[58] Parving HH, Lehnert H, Jens Bröchner-Mortensen et al. The effect of irbesartan on the development of diabetic nephropathy in patients with type 2 diabetes. N Engl J Med, 2001; 345:870-8.
[59] Patel A, MacMahon S, Chalmers J et al. and ADVANCE Collaborative Group. Effects of a fixed combination of perindopril and indapamide on macrovascular and microvascular outcomes in patients with type 2 diabetes mellitus (the ADVANCE trial): a randomised controlled trial. Lancet, 2007; 370:829-40.
[60] Patel A, MacMahon S, Chalmers J et al. and ADVANCE Collaborative Group. Intensive blood glucose control and vascular outcomes in patients with type 2 diabetes. N Engl J Med, 2008; 358:2560-72.
[61] Ravid M, Neumann L, Lishner M. Plasma lipids and the progression of nephropathy in diabetes mellitus type-2: effect of ACE inhibitors. Kidney Int. 1995;47:907-910.
[62] Remuzzi G, Bertani T. Pathophysiology of progressive nephropathies. N Engl J Med 1998;12:1448–1456.
[63] Ruan, X., Zheng, F. and Guan, Y. (2008) PPARs and the kidney in metabolic syndrome. Am. J. Physiol. Renal Physiol. 294, F1032–F1047
[64] Ruggenenti P, Fassi A, Ilieva AP et al. Preventing microalbuminuria in type 2 diabetes. N Engl J Med., 2004; 351(19):1941-51.
[65] Ruggenenti P, Gambara V, Perna A, Bertani T, Remuzzi G: The nephropathy of non-insulin-dependent diabetes: Predictors of outcome relative to diverse patterns of renal injury. J Am Soc Nephrol 9: 2336–2343, 1998
[66] Ruggenenti P, Remuzzi G. Nephropathy of type 2 diabetes mellitus. J Am Soc Nephrol1998; 9: 2157–2169
[67] Ruggenenti P, Remuzzi G. Time to abandon microalbuminuria? Kidney Int. 2006;70:1214-22.
[68] Ruggenenti P, Remuzzi G: Nephropathy of type 1 and type 2 diabetes: diverse pathophysiology, same treatment? Nephrol Dial Transplant 15:1900–1902, 2000
[69] Sasaki T, Kurata H, Nomura K, et al: Amelioration of proteinuria with pravastatin in hypercholesterolemic patients with diabetes mellitus. Jpn J Med 29:156–163, 1990
[70] Satchell SC, Tasman CH, Singh A et al (2006) Conditionally immortalized human glomerular endothelial cells expressing fenestrations in response to VEGF. Kidney Int 69:1633–1640
[71] Satchell SC, Tooke JE. What is the mechanism of microalbuminuria in diabetes: a role for the glomerular endothelium? Diabetologia 51: 714–725, 2008
[72] Satirapoj B. Review on pathophysiology and treatment of diabetic kidney disease. J Med Assoc Thai. 2010;93 (suppl 6):S228 -S241.
[73] Schalkwijk CG, Poland DC, van Dijk W et al (1999) Plasma concentration of C-reactive protein is increased in type I diabetic patients without clinical macroangiopathy and correlates with markers of endothelial dysfunction: evidence for chronic inflammation. Diabetologia 42:351–357

[74] Schmid H, Boucherot A, Yasuda Y, Henger A, Brunner B, Eichinger F, Nitsche A, Kiss E, Bleich M, Grone HJ, Nelson PJ, Schlondorff D, Cohen CD, Kretzler M: Modular activation of nuclear factor-kappaB transcriptional programs in human diabetic nephropathy. Diabetes 55: 2993–3003, 2006

[75] Schrier RW, Estacio RO, Esler A, Mehler P: Effects of aggressive blood pressure control in normotensive type 2 diabetic patients on albuminuria, retinopathy and strokes. Kidney Int 61:1086–1097, 2002.

[76] Song Y, Manson JE, Buring JE, Liu S. A prospective study of red meat consumption and type 2 diabetes in middle-aged and elderly women: the Women's Health Study. Diabetes Care. 2004;27:2108–2115.

[77] Srivastava SK, Ramana KV, Bhatnagar A. Role of aldose reductase and oxidative damage in diabetes and the consequent potential for therapeutic options. Endocr Rev. 2005;26:380 -392.

[78] Stanton RC Oxidative stress and diabetic kidney disease. Curr Diab Rep 2011 Aug;11(4):330-6.

[79] Stehouwer CD, Gall MA, Twisk JW, Knudsen E, Emeis JJ, Parving HH (2002) Increased urinary albumin excretion, endothelial dysfunction, and chronic low-grade inflammation in type 2 diabetes: progressive, interrelated, and independently associated with risk of death. Diabetes 51:1157–1165

[80] Sugawara A, Uruno A, Kudo M, Matsuda K, Yang CW, Ito S. Sugawara A, Uruno A, Kudo M, Matsuda K, Yang CW, Ito S., Korean J Intern Med 26:19 (2011)

[81] The Diabetes Control and Complications Trial Research Group, The effect of intensive treatment of diabetes on the development and progression of longterm complications in insulin-dependent diabetes mellitus, N. Engl. J. Med. 329 (1993) 977–986.

[82] The United States Renal Data System. http://www.usrds.org/ Annual Data Report 2010

[83] Thomas M.C. Anemia in diabetes: marker or mediator of microvascular disease? Nat. Clin. Pract. Nephrol. 2007;3:20–30.

[84] Thomas MC, Cooper ME, Rossing K, Parving HH: Anaemia in diabetes: is there a rationale to TREAT? Diabetologia 49: 1151–1157, 2006.

[85] Tilton RG et al. Prevention of hemodynamic and vascular filtration changes in diabetic rats by aldose reductase inhibitors. Diabetes 1989; 38: 1258-1270.

[86] United Kingdom Prospective Diabetes Study (UKPDS) Group, Intensive blood-glucose control with sulphonylureas or insulin compared with conventional treatment and risk of complications in patients with type 2 diabetes, Lancet 352 (1998) 837–853.

[87] Walker JD, An update on diabetic renal disease, Br J Diabetes Vasc Dis 2010;10:219-223.

[88] Warram JH, Gearin G, Laffel L, Krolewski AS (1996) Effect of duration of type I diabetes on the prevalence of stages of diabetic nephropathy defined by urinary albumin/creatinine ratio. J Am Soc Nephrol 7:930–937

[89] Y. Ohkubo, H. Kishikawa, E. Araki, T. Miyata, S. Isami, S. Motoyoshi, et al., Intensive insulin therapy prevents the progression of diabetic microvascular complications in Japanese patients with non-insulin dependent diabetes mellitus: a randomized prospective 6-year study, Diabetes Res. Clin. Prac. 28 (1995) 103–117.

[90] Zoungas S, de Galan BE, Ninomiya T et al. The combined effects of routine blood pressure lowering and intensive glucose control on macrovascular and microvascular outcomes in patients with type 2 diabetes; new results from ADVANCE. Diabetes Care, 2009; 32:2068-74

15

Diabetic Nephropathy: A Cardiovascular Risk Factor

Caroline Jane Magri[1,3] and Stephen Fava[2,3]
[1]*Department of Cardiac Services, Mater Dei Hospital, Tal- Qroqq, Msida*
[2]*Diabetes & Endocrine Centre, Department of Medicine*
Mater Dei Hospital, Tal- Qroqq, Msida
[3]*University of Malta Medical School*
University of Malta, Tal- Qroqq, Msida
Malta

1. Introduction

Diabetic nephropathy (DN) is an important and often life-threatening microvascular complication of diabetes mellitus (DM). It is usually first manifested as an increase in urinary albumin excretion (microalbuminuria), which progresses to overt albuminuria and then to renal failure (Mogensen et al., 1983). However, the EDIC/DCCT study showed that a significant number of patients develop renal insufficiency without the presence of microalbuminuria (Molitch et al., 2006).

The incidence of end-stage renal disease (ESRD) and type 2 DM as a co-morbid condition has increased continuously during the past decades (Ritz & Stefanski., 1996; Ritz & Orth., 1999a) and has been named a medical catastrophe of worldwide dimensions (Ritz et al., 1999b). Thus, the proportion of diabetic patients among patients with treated ESRD ranges between 12 and 95%, depending on nations and ethnicities investigated, with the majority (43-95%) usually being type 2 diabetic subjects (Ismail & Cornell, 1999).

A similar increase in the incidence of ESRD secondary to DM has been demonstrated following analyses of the United States Renal Data System data (USRDS 2004 Annual Data Report). Between 1999 and 2003, diabetes was responsible for >44.8% of all new cases of ESRD in the United States. This increase could not be fully explained by changes in assignment of causes of ESRD, rising prevalence of DM, increased access to renal replacement therapy (RRT), increased acceptance of individuals with DM to ESRD programs, or increased survival of patients with DM (Jones et al., 2005). It has been suggested that external factors might be responsible for this growth in DN incidence.

Although diabetes has long been identified as a cardiovascular disease (CVD) risk equivalent, only recently has chronic kidney disease (CKD) been more widely recognized as an independent risk factor for CVD and all-cause mortality (Kidney Disease Outcomes Quality Initiative, 2004; Levey et al., 2003; Weiner et al., 2004; Go et al., 2004). In a study of more than 1 million ambulatory adult patients, the risk of a cardiovascular event and death due to any cause increased at every level of CKD below a GFR of 60 mL/min per 1.73 m^2, with a nearly 3.5-fold increased risk of a cardiovascular event and a 6-fold increased risk of death for those with a GFR of less than 15 mL/min/1.73 m2 (i.e. CKD stage 5) (Go et al., 2004). This has also been confirmed in diabetic subjects (Nag et al., 2007). In addition, microalbuminuria has been associated with an increased risk of CVD, both in patients with and without DM (Klausen et al., 2004; Gerstein et al., 2001; Dinneen & Gerstein, 1997). Therefore, in patients with DN, the increased cardiovascular risk associated with diabetes and with CKD are additive and increase as DN progresses (Adler et al., 2003; Miettinen et al., 1996). Thus, in a retrospective claims-based study of more than 1 million Medicare enrollees aged 65 years and older, the risk of cardiovascular events was significantly increased in those with either CKD or diabetes alone, but cardiovascular risk was greatest when both conditions were present (Foley et al., 2005). Interestingly, many patients with CKD, particularly elderly patients, may be several times more likely to die of CVD before progression to ESRD (Collins et al., 2003). In view of all this, one realizes that early preventive measures and effective therapy are crucial. For this to achieved, the mechanisms underlying cardiovascular organ damage in patients with DN have to be better understood. A better understanding may further help to identify biomarkers for early detection of patients at high risk.

2. Methods

A comprehensive systematic review focusing on diabetic nephropathy as a cardiovascular risk factor was performed. Pubmed and Embase were used as electronic search engines. The search included all published papers and was not limited to human studies or to papers published in English. Cross-sectional, case-control and cohort studies, systematic reviews and meta-analyses were analysed to assess types of cardiovascular events observed in patients with DN, potential pathogenetic mechanisms, cardiac consequences of disturbed renal function, links between DN and CVD, possible biomarkers, as well as therapeutic strategies to deal with DN and CVD, as discussed below.

3. Cardiovascular disease in subjects with diabetic nephropathy

The evaluation of DN, from research and clinical viewpoints, depends on the assessment of two continuous variables, albumin excretion rate (AER) and glomerular filtration rate (GFR). Both have been associated with the increased CVD noted in DN, as discussed below.

3.1 Cardiovascular disease in diabetic patients with macroalbuminuria

The role of macroalbuminuria in CVD has been outlined in the post-hoc analyses of the Irbesartan Diabetic Nephropathy Trial (IDNT) and the Reduction of End points in NIDDM with the Angiotensin II Antagonist Losartan (RENAAL) studies. The IDNT enrolled subjects with type 2 DM, hypertension, and macroalbuminuria (Lewis et al., 2001). Irbesartan proved to be superior to amlodipine or placebo with respect to renoprotection but no difference was detected between treatment groups on the secondary outcome of cardiovascular (CV) events. A post hoc analysis was performed by Anavekar et al. (2004) to assess the relationship between baseline AER and the CV composite (CV death, nonfatal myocardial infarction (MI), hospitalization for heart failure, stroke, amputation, and coronary and peripheral revascularization). Univariate analysis revealed that CV events progressively increased with increasing quartiles of baseline AER while multivariate analysis confirmed albuminuria as an independent risk factor for cardiovascular events with a 1.3-fold increased relative risk for each natural log increase of 1 U in urine albumin-creatinine ratio (ACR).

Similar results were noted in the Reduction of End points in NIDDM with the Angiotensin II Antagonist Losartan (RENAAL) whereby losartan was superior to placebo with regards to renoprotection in type 2 diabetic, hypertensive patients with macroalbuminuria. However it conferred no statistically significant benefit on the secondary CV outcomes (Brenner et al., 2001), although de novo heart failure was less frequently noted in the losartan group. Nevertheless, in a post-hoc analysis of RENAAL, baseline albuminuria was again shown to be a predictor of both the prespecified composite CV end point (composite of MI, stroke, first hospitalization for heart failure or unstable angina, coronary or peripheral revascularization, or CV death) as well as of heart failure alone. With subjects stratified into 3 groups on the basis of baseline ACR, comparison of the highest tertile with the lowest revealed an adjusted hazard ratio of 1.92 for the composite CV end point and 2.70 for heart failure. In multivariate analysis, baseline albuminuria was the strongest independent predictor of both outcomes. In addition, the change in AER from baseline to 6 months was the only dynamic correlate of adverse CV outcomes. A 50% reduction in baseline albuminuria translated into an 18% reduction in the composite CV end point and a 27% reduction in the risk of heart failure. It has thus been suggested that albuminuria serve as an indicator of therapeutic response.

3.2 Cardiovascular disease in diabetic patients with microalbuminuria

Microalbuminuria also correlates with adverse CV events. In a type 2 diabetic population, Mattock et al. (1998) reported that microalbuminuria was the strongest predictor of adverse CV outcomes with an odds ratio of 10.02. In addition, in the HOPE study, a baseline ACR >2.0 mg/mmol (present in 32.6% of the diabetic cohort and 14.8% of the non-diabetic cohort) increased the adjusted relative risk of CV events (1.83), all-cause death (2.09), and hospitalization for congestive heart failure (3.23). In addition, the impact of microalbuminuria on the primary composite outcome of CV death, MI, or stroke was significant in both diabetic (relative risk 1.97) and non-diabetic (relative risk 1.61) subjects (Mann et al., 2004).

3.3 Cardiovascular disease in diabetic patients with renal impairment

Declining renal function plays an important role in CVD in diabetic patients, as demonstrated in the Valsartan in Acute Myocardial Infarction (VALIANT) trial. This was a multicentre, double-blind randomized controlled trial that enrolled patients with acute myocardial infarction (MI) complicated by either clinical or radiologic signs of heart failure and/or left ventricular dysfunction. Patients were randomly assigned to receive captopril, valsartan, or both. GFR was estimated using the 4-component MDRD equation. It was shown that the likelihood of experiencing the primary end-point of all-cause mortality was higher in patients with than without DM for each level of renal function. In addition, a decrease in eGFR of 10 units was associated with hazards of 1.09 (95% confidence interval 1.06 to 1.12, $p < 0.001$) in patients with DM and 1.08 (95% confidence interval 1.06 to 1.10, $p < 0.001$) in patients without DM for risk of fatal and nonfatal CV outcomes independent of treatment assignment (Anavekar et al., 2008).

The importance of renal impairment in predicting outcome following myocardial infarction in diabetic patients was also investigated by Ahmed et al. (2008). It was shown that the combination of renal impairment and DM was associated with a particularly high risk of MI and death/MI following a non-ST elevation MI, suggesting that attention to preserving renal function may be of particular benefit for reducing cardiovascular risk in diabetic patients.

3.4 Diabetic nephropathy & peripheral arterial occlusive disease

Peripheral arterial occlusive disease (PAOD) is a major cause of morbidity, especially affecting the elderly population (1-3). In addition, the main cause of mortality in patients with PAOD is ischaemic heart disease (IHD) as has been shown in several studies, while subgroup analyses suggest that PAOD carries a particularly poor prognosis in diabetes (Davis et al., 2006; Li J et al., 2007).

DN has been reported to be associated with PAOD in both type 1 and type 2 diabetic subjects (Zander et al., 2002). Both albuminuria and declining GFR are probably associated with increased risk. Various studies have shown that PAOD is more prevalent in type 2 diabetic patients with increased albumin excretion rate (Mostaza et al., 2006; Bianchi et al., 2007). It is likely that microalbuminuria reflects widespread vascular damage. In addition, a reduction in GFR has been shown to be associated with PAOD in both non-diabetic (O'Hare et al., 2004) and diabetic patients (Mostaza et al., 2006; Bianchi et al., 2007). Albuminuria and declining renal function are also independent predictors of the occurrence of PAOD in non-Caucasian populations in both genders (Hsieh et al., 2009).

Interestingly, in a type 2 diabetic population with advanced microvascular disease, as evidenced by proliferative diabetic retinopathy requiring laser treatment, we have shown that increasing age, total cholesterol levels, and vibration perception thresholds, together with declining renal function and lower BMI are independent predictors of PAOD, whilst microalbuminuria was not (Magri et al., In press). This implies that the association between impaired renal function and PAOD is not solely mediated by microvascular disease. The lack of association of microalbuminuria with PAOD in our study is probably best explained by the fact that all our patients had advanced microvascular disease, as evidenced by proliferative diabetic retinopathy, and had been suffering from diabetes for a long duration (18.6 ± 9.1 years). Therefore normoalbuminuric patients in our study probably represented a cohort which was genetically protected from diabetic renal disease. This suggests that the association of PAOD and microalbuminuria observed in other studies is mediated through shared environmental predisposing factors (example poor blood pressure and glycaemic control) in individuals who are genetically susceptible to develop renal disease.

Yoshimura et al. (2008) have shown that in type 2 diabetic patients with normal ankle-brachial indices (ABIs), eGFR correlated positively with flow volume ($p=0.002$) and negatively with brachial-ankle pulse wave velocity ($p=0.0258$) and with resistive index ($p=0.0029$) in patients with albuminuria but not in those with normoalbuminuria. This implies an association between nephropathy and impaired lower limb circulation secondary to higher arterial stiffness and increased vascular resistance in type 2 DM. Similar results were shown in Japanese type 2 diabetic patients with normal ABIs where the major risk factors for reduced flow volume were age, hypertension, and DN ($r^2 = 0.303$, $p < 0.001$) (Suzuki et al., 2003). These results indicate that DN plays an important role in the early stages of PAOD in diabetes by altering vascular resistance and arterial stiffness.

A high ABI (>1.40) has been found to be associated with an increased risk of CKD (defined as eGFR <60ml/min/1.73m^2) in diabetic individuals at high cardiovascular risk (OR 2.4; 1.0-6.4) but not in non-diabetic patients (Liu et al., 2010). A high ABI is a marker of generalised stiffening of the lower limb arteries and is probably mediated through medial arterial calcification (MAC) in the majority of cases. MAC has been associated with increased left ventricular mass and aortic pulse-wave velocity in ESRD, leading to cardiac fibrosis and increased arrhythmia risk. Similar associations might be present in DM patients with high ABI but without severe renal disease, thus leading to increased cardiovascular morbidity and mortality. Nonetheless, Liu et al. conclude that further studies are needed to clarify the link between high ABI, CKD and CVD in diabetes.

3.5 Diabetic nephropathy & cerebral infarction

CKD is a known risk factor for cerebrovascular disease. In addition, stroke is more common in type 2 diabetic subjects with nephropathy compared to type 2 diabetic subjects without nephropathy (Alwakeel et al., 2009; Alebiosu et al., 2004). The independent effects of albuminuria and eGFR on stroke and silent cerebral infarction in type 2 DM have been investigated by Bouchi et al. (2009 & 2010, respectively). While a lower eGFR was associated with an increased risk of stroke in univariate analysis, it lost its significance in multivariate analysis. Clinical albuminuria remained a significant risk factor for stroke, with an adjusted HR of 2.40 (1.46-3.95, P=0.001) compared with normoalbuminuria (Bouchi et al., 2009). Miettinen et al. (1996) have previously shown an association between proteinuria and incident stroke in type 2 diabetic patients. Similarly, in Japanese type 2 diabetic patients, both a high urinary albumin creatinine ratio and a low eGFR were significantly associated with silent cerebral infarction (SCI) (lacunar infracts) in univariate analysis; however only albuminuria remained a significant risk factor for SCI in multivariate analysis (Bouchi et al., 2010). SCI predicts incident clinically evident stroke, cardiovascular disease and dementia. Bouchi et al. (2010) conclude that the association between albuminuria and cerebrovascular disease could be explained either by common aetiological factors, including oxidative stress, inflammation, endothelial dysfunction, obesity, thrombotic state, hypertension and dyslipidaemia, or by similarities between the haemodynamic and anatomical aspects of renal and cerebral small vessel disease.

In type 1 DM subjects, it has been shown that parents of patients with diabetic nephropathy have reduced survival which seems to be largely explained by an increase in vascular deaths, in particular, a four-fold increase in the number of strokes (Lindsay et al., 1999). Likewise, Thorn et al. (2007) have shown that type 1 diabetic patients with diabetic nephropathy had a higher prevalence of maternal (41 vs. 35%, p =0.046) and paternal (62 vs. 55%, p =0.044) hypertension, maternal stroke (7.6 vs. 5.1%, P = 0.044), and paternal (4.3 vs. 2.9%, p =0.030) type 1 diabetes, compared to type 1 diabetic subjects without nephropathy. Similarly, parental hypertension has been associated with nephropathy in type 2 diabetic Pima Indians (Nelson et al., 1996).These data suggest that there is a shared hereditary risk factor predisposing diabetic patients to nephropathy and their parents to an increased risk of vascular disease, in particular stroke. This is likely to be largely mediated through a genetic predisposition to higher blood pressure, but other factors may also be involved.

4. Cardiovascular consequences of diabetic nephropathy

Disturbed renal function in DN leads to a multitude of adverse cardiovascular effects, as outlined in Figure 1. Increased blood pressure together with accelerated large vessel disease and increased arterial stiffening and calcification lead to increased afterload whilst hypervolaemia and anaemia lead to increased preload with consequent adverse effects on the heart. These cardiac abnormalities are further augmented by the local activation of the renin-angiotensin system (RAS) and endothelin (ET) system, amongst others. The RAS plays a role in the activation of the sympathetic nervous system, the dysregulation of endothelial function and progression of atherosclerosis, and inhibition of the fibrinolytic system, while direct profibrotic actions of angiotensin II and aldosterone in the kidney and heart promote end-organ injury. On the other hand, serum ET-1 levels were found to be associated with left ventricular hypertrophy.

Increased blood pressure is an early feature of renal disease and undoubtedly contributes to the excess cardiovascular risk (reviewed by Ritz et al., 2010). High blood pressure also predisposes to renal disease and predates the onset of diabetic nephropathy (Nelson et al., 1993). Therefore patients with high blood pressure are at risk of developing both renal and cardiovascular disease. However high blood pressure is also a consequence of renal disease, thereby initiating a vicious cycle resulting in progression of CKD as well as in CKD being causally related to increased cardiovascular risk. An extensive discussion of the mechanisms of these inter-relationships between blood pressure and kidney disease is beyond the scope of this review.

Left ventricular hypertrophy (LVH) is an important risk factor for adverse cardiovascular outcomes in patients with CKD. LVH has been demonstrated to be an important predictor of cardiovascular mortality in type 2 diabetic subjects with and without DN (Astrup et al., 2007). In addition, there is increasing LVH with progression of nephropathy (Alebiosu et al., 2008; Suzuki K et al., 2001). A potential pathogenic role of parathyroid hormone on LVH has been suggested, together with its effect on interstitial fibrosis and thickening of intramyocardial arterioles (Amann et al., 1994). This is consistent with several clinical findings showing a positive correlation between parathyroid hormone concentration and cardiovascular morbidity and mortality in dialysis patients (Block et al., 1998). Interestingly, cardiovascular autonomic neuropathy (CAN) as indicated by impaired parasympathetic nervous system function, has been shown to be associated with the presence of LVH in diabetic patients on haemodialysis. This suggests that the co-existence of CAN and LVH may be one of the key factors for the high incidence of cardiovascular events in diabetic haemodialysis patients (Nishimura et al., 2004). Likewise, Weinrauch et al. (2006) have demonstrated regression of LVH in DN patients occurring in parallel with improvement in cardiac autonomic function, as determined from heart rate variability. The authors conclude that there is a common mechanism linking LV mass and CAN, such that improvement in LV mass might be predicted through analysis of baseline heart rate variation.

In a study in patients with CKD stages 2-4, approximately half of whom were diabetic, McQuarrie et al. (2010) have shown that the degree of albuminuria is independently and significantly associated with left ventricular mass, as assessed using volume-independent cardiac magnetic resonance imaging; this relationship was shown to be independent of blood pressure. These findings suggest that the increased left ventricular mass provides a potential link between elevated protein excretion, left ventricular hypertrophy (LVH) and the increased mortality seen in patients with CKD.

Left ventricular diastolic dysfunction is another adverse cardiac effect (Figure 2). In a study of 67 patients with non-dialysis CKD, Miyazoto et al. (2005) found that DN is a significant predictor of LV diastolic dysfunction in CKD subjects, independent of other influencing factors such as age, blood pressure, renal function, anaemia and LV hypertrophy. LV diastolic dysfunction is characterized by elevated left ventricular end-diastolic pressure or left arterial pressure, ultimately leading to LV systolic dysfunction and overt heart failure symptoms.

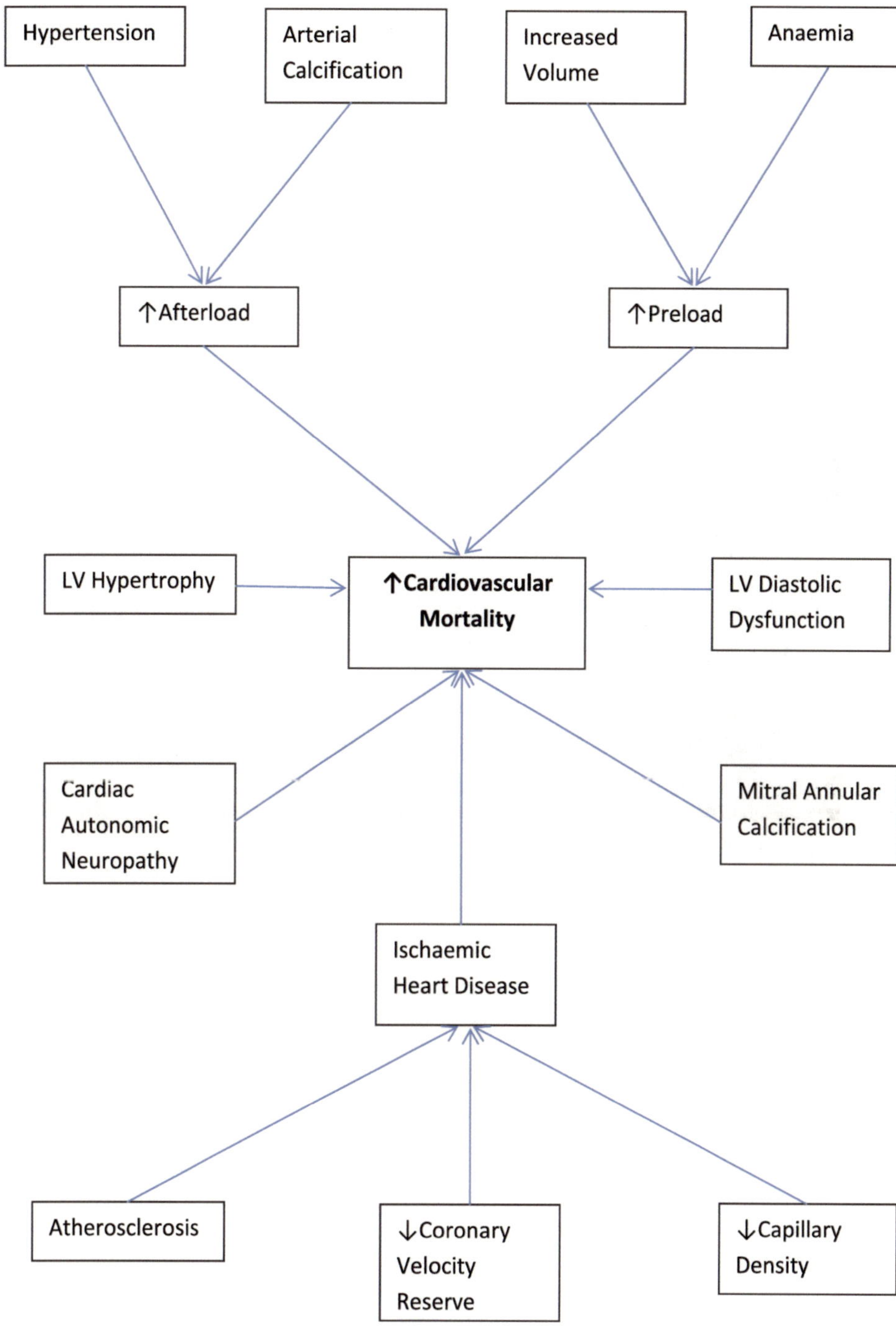

Fig. 1. Cardiovascular Consequences of Diabetic Nephropathy

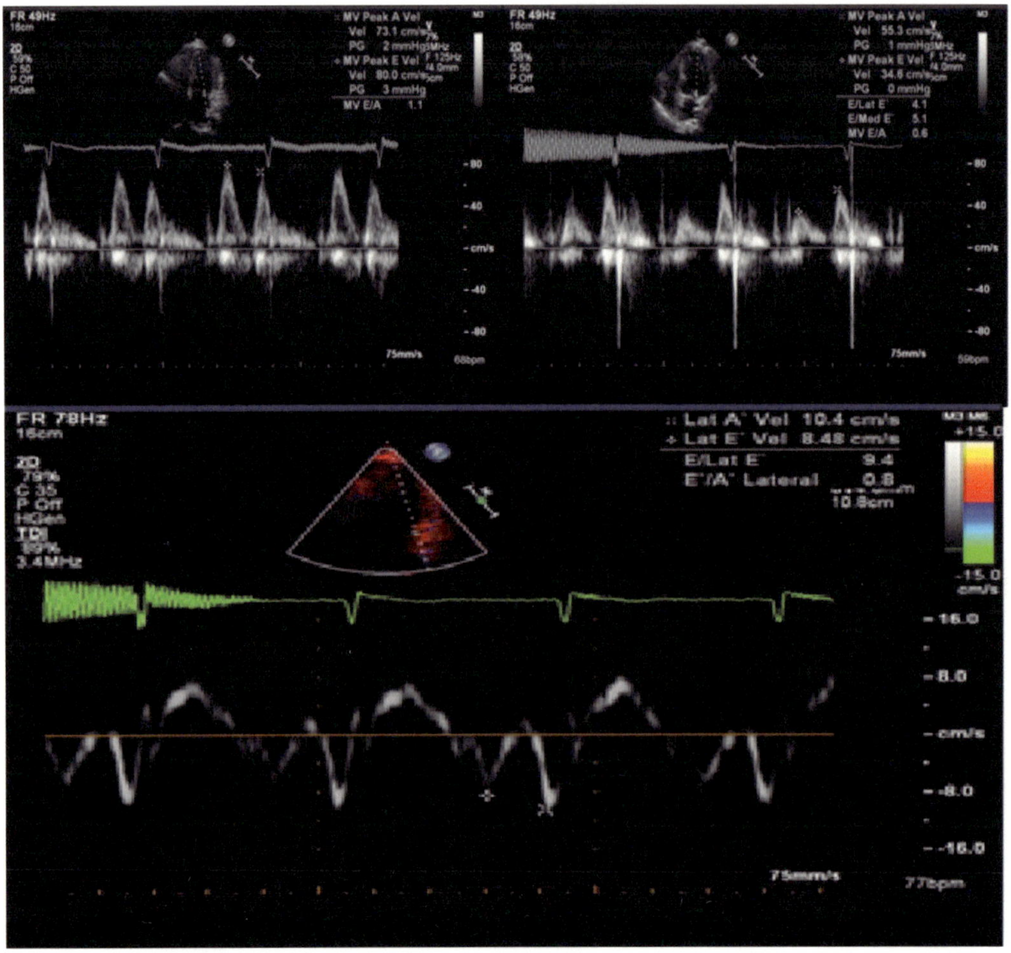

Fig. 2. Doppler evidence of left ventricular diastolic dysfunction. (A) Mitral inflow pattern during normal breathing (B) Mitral inflow pattern during Valsalva manoeuvre showing reversibility of inflow pattern (E<A), typical of restrictive pattern of diastolic dysfunction (C) Tissue Doppler evidence indicating diastolic dysfunction

Mitral annular calcification (MiAC) is another important cardiac abnormality found in patients with CKD. This is because MiAC has been shown to predict atrial fibrillation, stroke and cardiovascular disease morbidity and mortality. In the Framingham Heart Study (Fox et al., 2006), 3047 participants (some of whom had CKD secondary to diabetes) were assessed for the presence of mitral annular calcification (MiAC), aortic sclerosis and aortic annular calcification. It was demonstrated that the combination of both CKD and MiAC was associated with a three-fold increased risk of death compared with those with neither CKD nor MiAC (p= 0.0004), following adjustment for age and gender. Interestingly, the association between CKD and MiAC occurred before the onset of ESRD; however, no significant association was found between CKD and either aortic sclerosis or aortic annular calcification (odds ratio 1.1 and 1.1, respectively). It is still unclear whether MiAC is a causal mechanism that mediates this association or a risk marker; further research is needed to unveil underlying pathophysiologic mechanisms.

Ischaemic heart disease (IHD) is strongly associated with DN. Patients with both ESRD and diabetes mellitus carry an increased risk of coronary atherosclerosis. The possible mechanisms are discussed in section 5. In addition to coronary atherosclerosis, abnormalities in myocardial blood flow and in coronary flow reserve could be responsible for cardiovascular morbidity in DN. Ragosta et al. (2004) have demonstrated that subjects with DN and normal coronary arteries had abnormalities in **coronary velocity reserve** (CVR). Abnormal CVR was caused by an elevation of baseline arterial peak velocity in 66% of these cases. The elevated baseline velocity may be caused by an increase in LV mass from associated long-standing hypertension, or by circulating humoral factors with vasodilator properties present in renal failure, for example nitric oxide. In addition, the baseline heart rate and the presence of diabetes mellitus with renal failure were independent predictors of abnormal CVR by multivariable analysis. Therefore, in the presence of end-organ damage caused by diabetes mellitus, abnormalities in coronary physiology may be seen in the absence of overt epicardial coronary artery disease.

In addition to arterial changes, reduction in **capillary density** is another important factor in CKD which interferes with oxygen delivery. In uraemic subjects with LVH, there is a significant decrease in capillary density, leading to an increase in intercapillary distance, and potentially compromising the blood and oxygen supply of the myocardium under conditions of increased demand, thus rendering the myocardium more prone to ischaemic injury. LVH is common in diabetic subjects secondary to concomitant hypertension. These findings suggest that in uraemic patients with LVH, there is probably decreased expression of vascular endothelial growth factor or increased expression of inhibitors of capillary angiogenesis, such that capillary growth does not keep pace with cardiomyocyte growth (reviewed by Amann et al., 2006). It is possible that low capillary density or poor capillary recruitment puts subjects at risk of developing hypertension, kidney disease as well as cardiovascular disease. Further studies are needed to clarify the pathological mechanisms underlying the decrease in cardiac capillary supply.

5. Potential pathogenic mechanisms

Various mechanisms account for the cardiovascular dysfunction present in renal disease, as outlined below.

5.1 Endothelial cell dysfunction

The vascular endothelium is a versatile multifunctional tissue having many synthetic and metabolic properties (Figure 3). Endothelial cell dysfunction seems to be central in the genesis of many different aspects of cardiovascular dysfunction in subjects with DN, such as increased pulse wave velocity (Yokoyama et al., 2004) and decreased flow-mediated dilation (FMD) of the brachial artery (Yilmaz et al., 2008). Table 1 outlines the various factors leading to endothelial cell dysfunction.

Yilmaz et al. (2008) have demonstrated that endothelium-dependent vascular dysfunction, as assessed using FMD, correlates with proteinuria in type 2 diabetic subjects with early DN. Interestingly, no correlation was found between proteinuria and nitroglycerine-mediated dilation (NMD) of the brachial artery. This suggests that there decreased bioavailability of nitric oxide (NO), but that the vessels remain responsive to it in DN. In addition, a positive association was found between proteinuria and the intracellular protein nicotinamide-phosphoribosyltransferase (NAMPT)/visfatin, which is thought to be a marker of endothelial cell damage. On the other hand, there were negative associations between proteinuria and two vasoprotective molecules, namely adiponectin and fetuin-A. The authors suggest that proteinuria might lead to endothelial dysfunction via increasing serum levels of the NO-synthase inhibitor ADMA, probably secondary to increased protein turnover, together with loss of vasoprotective circulating proteins such as adiponectin and fetuin.

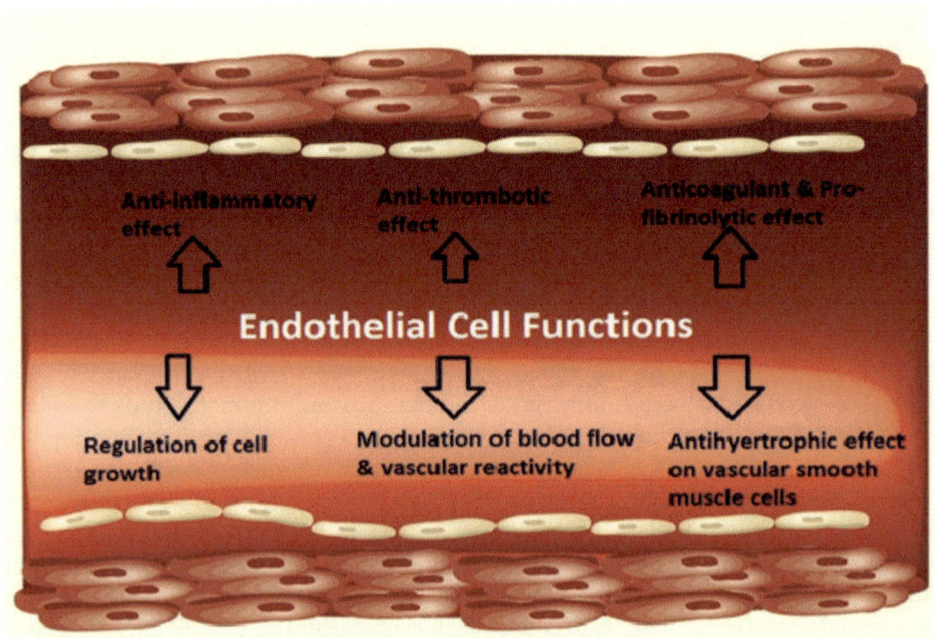

Fig. 3. Endothelial Cell Properties & Functions (Reproduced from Expert Review of Cardiovascular Therapy, October 2011, Vol. 9, No. 10, Page 1280 with permission of Expert Reviews Ltd)

• ↑ Asymmetrical dimethylarginine
• ↓Adiponectin levels
• ↓Fetuin levels
• Insulin resistance
• ↑soluble receptor for AGE
• Renin-angiotensin system activation
• ↑uric acid levels
• ↑homocysteine levels

Table 1. Factors leading to endothelial cell dysfunction

Asymmetrical dimethylarginine (ADMA) is an endogenous competitive nitric oxide (NO) synthase inhibitor. It can be metabolized by dimethylarginine dimethylaminohydrolase (DDAH) or excreted by the kidneys (Leiper et al., 2006). It is increased in patients with increased cardiovascular risk (Kielstein et al., 1999; Zoccali et al., 2002; Surdacki et al., 1999) and predicts future cardiovascular events (Schnabel et al., 1995). Accumulation of ADMA in CKD could promote atherosclerosis and is related to a history of myocardial infarction and/or stroke in patients with type 1 DM and macroalbuminuria (Tarnow et al., 2004). In type 2 diabetic patients with albuminuria, increased ADMA was also shown to be linked to macrovascular disease, and is associated with declining GFR and subclinical inflammation, as assessed using high senstivity C-reactive proten (hsCRP) (Krzyzanowska et al., 2007).

In addition to its direct inhibitory effect on endothelial NO synthase, ADMA may cause endothelial dysfunction via other mechanisms. These include increased superoxide production by activation of the NAD(P)H-oxidase, thereby interfering with NO bioavailability; activation the local RAS, thus contributing to the development of arteriolar dysfunction and increased tone; and a decrease in the number of circulating endothelial progenitor cells (EPCs), possibly interfering with vascular repair mechanisms (reviewed by Fliser, 2010).

Insulin resistance also plays an important role in endothelial dysfunction. Insulin resistance has been associated with renal disease in both types 1 (Yip J et al., 1993) and 2 (Groop et al., 1993) diabetes, thereby offering another possible explanation of the association between cardiovascular disease and DN. Furthermore, endothelial cell injury has recently been linked to increased shear stress (Boulanger et al., 2007). The latter is known to be associated with high blood pressure.

Plasma levels of the soluble receptor for advanced glycation end-products (RAGE) are strongly associated with CVD in patients with DN (Nin et al., 2010). RAGE has been shown to induce the production of adhesion molecules and inflammatory cytokines, thus promoting endothelial and renal dysfunction, low grade inflammation and vascular remodeling. Through these mechanisms, RAGE may contribute to both DN and cardiovascular disease.

Activation of the renin-angiotensin system in DN results in endothelial dysfunction. When angiotensin II acts through the AT1 receptor, it stimulates the generation of reactive oxygen species by NAD(P)H oxidase and other enzyme systems, leading to upregulation of inflammatory mediators, which include cytokines, chemokines, adhesion molecules, and plasminogen activator inhibitor 1, and superoxide scavenging of NO. These events promote endothelial dysfunction, vascular remodeling, and the progression of atherosclerosis (Schiffrin et al., 2004).

There is also evidence that hyperuricaemia induces endothelial dysfunction by inhibiting NO production (Khosla et al., 2005), modulates inflammatory response (Kang et al., 2005), and stimulates vascular smooth muscle cell proliferation. In a study by Correa Leite (2011), a decline in GFR was associated with an increase in CVD risk factors (increased fibrinogen and hematocrit levels) only among subjects with higher uric acid levels. These alterations may promote thrombotic disorders via a hypercoagulable state and increase in blood viscosity. Consequently, serum uric acid measurement in patients with mild renal impairment may serve as a potentially useful means of identifying subjects at risk of developing CVD.

Hyperhomocysteinaemia may also play a role in endothelial dysfunction. Elevated plasma homocysteine levels are associated with albuminuria in both type 1 (Soedamah-Muthu et al.,

2005) and type 2 diabetic patients (Aso et al., 2004). It has been suggested that elevated total homocysteine levels cause vascular complications secondary to oxidative stress, endothelial damage and decreased nitric oxide bioavailability. In addition, the increased susceptibility of diabetic subjects to hyperhomocysteinaemia may be secondary to an acceleration of glucose-induced oxidative stress on endothelial cells (Soedamah-Muthu et al., 2005). This hypothesis is supported by animal studies showing that homocysteine-induced endothelial dysfunction occurs much more readily in the presence of diabetes than in its absence (Schukla et al., 2002).

5.2 Endothelial progenitor cells

Bone marrow-derived EPCs in peripheral circulation contribute to re-endothelialization of injured vessels as well as to neovascularization of ischaemic lesions and therefore play a key role in maintaining the integrity of the vascular system. Various factors influence the number and function of EPCs. Mild-to-moderate renal dysfunction accompanying stable angina has been shown to be associated with EPC depletion, irrespective of angiographic CAD extent. This may exacerbate an imbalance between endothelial injury and EPC-mediated repair, thus contributing to high cardiovascular risk in CAD coexisting with renal insufficiency. In addition, the number of EPCs is decreased in both patients with type 1 and type 2 DM, and EPCs from patients with DM have impaired function of adhesion, proliferation, and tubulization. All these findings indicate that EPCs play an important role in the pathogenesis of DN.

Interestingly, erythropoietin (EPO) has been shown to be a potent stimulator of EPC proliferation and differentiation. In addition, EPO has important direct biological effects on mature endothelial cells, including protection against ischemia and apoptosis, modulation of endothelial cell-cell and cell-matrix contacts, enhancement of endothelial cell migration and formation of primitive vascular structures in vitro. Mature endothelial cells do not lose their EPO receptors, unlike erythrocytes; hence, antiapoptotic signaling persists much longer, making endothelial cells more resistant to ischemia-induced cell death. Fliser (2010) thus suggests that EPO might be a key regulator of vascular protection. The adverse effects noted with use of recombinant human EPO (rHuEPO) could be attributed to the abrupt increase in the hematocrit level in CKD patients with serious vascular problems. In addition, rHuEPO increases the number and activation of thrombocytes, while increasing platelet adherence to the injured endothelium. However, the increase in hematocrit related to rHuEPO treatment is not associated with an increased risk for thrombosis as long as endothelial NO production serves as the compensatory mechanism. Consequently, there is ongoing research for an optimal rHuEPO dose that is safe, or EPO analogues (example the carbamylated form of EPO) that maintain tissue protective effects but lack the adverse effect on erythropoiesis and thrombopoiesis (Fliser, 2010).

5.3 Inflammation

CKD results in a chronic, low-grade inflammatory process that becomes evident even in the early stages of the disease. Circulating levels of inflammatory markers, such as C-reactive protein (CRP) and interleukin-6 (IL-6), are elevated in CKD patients. Navarro et al. (2008) have recently shown a relationship between inflammatory activation of peripheral blood mononuclear cells (reflected by enhanced mRNA expression of TNF-alpha and IL-6) and renal involvement (reflected by increased urinary albumin excretion) in type 2 diabetic patients. Increased inflammation could thus play a role in accelerated atherosclerosis and increased cardiovascular risk associated with DN.

5.4 Advanced glycation end-products

Advanced glycation end-products (AGEs) are products of non-enzymatic glycation and oxidation of proteins and lipids. They are increased in situations with hyperglycemia and oxidative stress such as DM. The kidney plays an important role in clearance and metabolism of AGEs. In CKD, AGE concentrations increase, partly by an increase in oxidative and carbonyl stress, leading to structural renal changes with further CKD progression, thus creating a vicious circle.

AGEs and their receptors play an important role in the pathophysiology of DN (reviewed by Busch et al., 2010). Besides vascular damage, RAGE drives the development of glomerulosclerosis and promotes podocyte activation in DN. Accumulation of AGEs affects almost all renal structures, including basement membranes, mesangial and endothelial cells, podocytes and tubules. In addition, medial smooth muscle cell injury in intrarenal arteries is caused by interaction between glycoxidation and complement activation, leading to progression of DN. AGEs and RAGE also are thought to play a key role in predisposing to cardiovascular disease in CKD patients (Noordzij et al., 2008; Lindsey et al., 2009).

However, even though AGEs and their receptors are involved in the pathogenesis of vascular and kidney disease, the role of circulating AGEs as biomarkers for cardiovascular risk estimation is questionable. In a post-hoc analysis of type 2 DM patients having DN from the IDNT cohort (Lewis et al., 2001; Berl et al., 2003), serum concentration of carboxymethyl-lysine (an important AGE) was not found to be an independent cardiovascular or renal risk factor (Busch et al., 2006). This may be due to the fact that serum concentrations failed to correlate with AGEs deposited in target tissues. Nonetheless, further research is needed to elucidate the role of AGEs and their receptors in the pathophysiology of DN and associated co-morbidities. In addition, there is ongoing research on the possible therapeutic benefit of inhibitors of AGE formation and putative breakers of already formed AGEs in the prevention and treatment of patients with DN and diabetic cardiovascular disease.

5.5 Lipoprotein abnormalities

Lipoprotein abnormalities also play a role. DN is characterized by low high-density lipoprotein (HDL)-concentrations and elevated intermediate-density lipoprotein (IDL), both of which contribute to an increased cardiovascular risk. Shoji et al. (2001) have demonstrated that elevated serum creatinine has greater impact than albuminuria on abnormalities in IDL and HDL. In addition, in diabetic patients, serum lipoprotein (a) concentration is associated with albuminuria, further contributing to the elevated cardiovascular risk (Hernández et al., 2000).

5.6 Adhesion molecules

Elevated plasma concentrations of soluble adhesion molecule concentrations in patients with DN could play an important role in the development of atherosclerosis and increased cardiovascular risk. Thus, plasma concentration of soluble intercellular adhesion molecule (sICAM)-1 is elevated in type 1 diabetic patients with microalbuminuria and the concentrations of sICAM-1 as well as soluble vascular adhesion molecule (sVCAM)-1 are elevated in patients with macroalbuminuria and normal serum creatinine (Clausen et al., 2000).

5.7 Hyperfibrinogenaemia

Hyperfibrinogenaemia is a cardiovascular risk factor. Tessari et al. (2006) have shown an upregulation of hepatic secretory proteins, albumin and fibrinogen, in albuminuric type 2 DM subjects compared with type 2 DM normoalbuminuric patients. Such an upregulation seems to be responsible for the hyperfibrinogenaemia observed in the albuminuric diabetic patients, and could thus play a role in the adverse cardiovascular effects noted in this high risk population.

5.8 Cardiac autonomic neuropathy

Cardiac autonomic neuropathy (CAN) is another important mechanism. In type 2 DM patients, CAN and DN were found to be independently associated with asymptomatic CAD (Beck et al., 1999). In type 1 DM patients with nephropathy, CAN assessed as heart-rate variation during deep breathing was shown to be an independent risk factor for cardiovascular morbidity and mortality (Astrup et al., 2006). In addition, autonomic neuropathy may be associated with increased central arterial stiffness (Nemes et al., 2010). The mechanisms by which CAN increases cardiovascular morbidity and mortality are still under debate. Suggested mechanisms include impaired central control of respiration in patients with CAN (Sobotka et al., 1986); exercise intolerance with a reduced response in heart rate and blood pressure and decreased cardiac output during exercise; and possibly QT prolongation (Whitsel et al., 2000; Veglio et al., 2000).

6. Other possible links between cardiovascular disease & diabetic nephropathy

Several hypotheses have been proposed to explain the link between the kidney and cardiovascular disease. These have been reviewed by Amann et al. (2006) and are outlined below.

Local factors may play a role in the cross-talk between the kidney and the cardiovascular system. The original Steno hypothesis (Deckert et al., 1989) suggested that enzymes involved in the metabolism of anionic components of the extracellular matrix (e.g. heparan sulphate proteoglycan) vulnerable to hyperglycaemia are probably the primary cause of albuminuria and the associated complications. Genetic polymorphisms of these enzymes could explain the variation in susceptibility to diabetic nephropathy and cardiovascular disease. However, there is little evidence supporting this hypothesis. An alternative hypothesis is a common glycocalyx defect in the glomerulus and in the systemic circulation. This is because the endothelial glycocalyx plays a significant role in the genesis of vascular pathology and controls vascular permeability (Gouverneur et al., 2006; Henry & Duling, 1999). This might also be the case in the glomerulus; however this merits further study.

Amann et al. also propose various pathways through which reduced renal function might influence endothelial function. These include the following:

1. Accumulation of toxins that are normally excreted via the kidneys
2. Inability of the kidney to produce active substances, example renalase. Renalase is an enzyme which breaks down catecholamines like adrenaline and noradrenaline in the circulation; its levels are markedly decreased in subjects with end-stage renal disease. In rodents, renalase has been shown to decrease blood pressure, heart rate, heart muscle contractility, and blood vessel resistance.

3. Reduced metabolism of substances normally metabolized by the kidney, example ADMA. The plasma concentration of ADMA are moderately elevated in renal failure, resulting in modification of gene expression patterns in endothelial cells as well as diminished production of nitric oxide secondary to inhibition of NO synthase.

Systemic factors may also play a role. Atmann et al. mention enhanced sympathetic activity at an early stage of renal disease when whole-kidney GFR is still normal. It is thought to be due to increased afferent signals originating from the damaged kidney, possibly contributing to increased incidence of sudden death and mortality secondary to ischaemia in renal patients. However, the triggering intrarenal mechanisms have not yet been identified. In addition, Atmann et al. propose the possibility of inappropriate activation of local RAS of cardiovascular structures in subjects with kidney disease, as suggested by animal studies where local cardiovascular RAS activation was noted in uraemic or subtotally nephrectomised rats.

Genetic influences probably also play a role. It has recently been shown that the P12A and C161T polymorphisms of the PPAR-gamma gene are important predictors of cardiovascular events in patients with diabetic nephropathy. The Pro/Ala genotype of the P12A polymorphism confers a 7.6-fold (95% CI 2.1- to 28.0-fold, $p = 0.002$) excess hazard of developing primary cardiovascular end point as compared to the Pro/Pro genotype, while each T allele at the 161 position confers a 83.4% (95% CI 15.2-291.9%, $p = 0.011$) excess hazard (Szeto et al., 2008). Another interesting polymorphism is the leucine 7 to proline 7 (Leu7Pro) polymorphism, located in the signal peptide part of the human preproneuropeptide Y (Pettersson-Fernholm et al., 2004). In the Finnish Diabetic Nephropathy Study, the Pro7 substitution was more common in patients with proteinuria than in those with normoalbuminuria (16 vs. 11%, $p < 0.05$). Patients with the Pro7 allele had worse glycemic control (HbA(1c) 8.8 vs. 8.5%, $p < 0.005$), more coronary heart disease (CHD) (14 vs. 8%, $p < 0.05$), and higher serum triglycerides (1.65 vs. 1.35 mmol/l, $p < 0.005$) than patients with the wild-type genotype. In multivariate analysis, the Leu7Pro polymorphism was independently associated with HbA(1c) ($p < 0.001$), proteinuria ($p < 0.01$), and CHD ($p < 0.01$), suggesting that the Leu7Pro polymorphism may contribute to the genetic susceptibility to diabetic nephropathy and CHD in type 1 diabetic patients, possibly by influencing glycemic control and triglycerides.

Recently, Takenaka et al. (2010) have shown that short stature is associated with increased mortality in diabetic and non-diabetic subjects with ESRD. Short stature has been linked to nephropathy in both type 1 (Rossing et al., 1995) and type 2 diabetes (Fava et al., 2001); height may therefore partly explain the association between DN and cardiovascular disease. This may be due to common genetic and/or environmental factors predisposing to short stature, DN and cardiovascular disease.

In addition to genetic influences, Brenner et al. (1988) have suggested the hypothesis of "nephron underdosing" whereby aberrant foetal programming secondary to genetic factors, malnutrition, and other insults *in utero* leads to the formation of fewer glomeruli. This results in a diminished ability to excrete sodium and thus predisposes to salt-sensitive hypertension. In favour of this hypothesis is the observation that both diabetic and nondiabetic renal diseases are seen more frequently in families with hypertension. In addition, in normoalbuminuric subjects, the risk for future ESRD is predicted by baseline blood pressure (Hsu et al., 2005). Congenital variability in filtration surface area may explain the varying susceptibility of patients exposed to potentially injurious renal stimuli to eventually manifest chronic nephropathy, as well as the different susceptibility of subsets of type 1 and type 2 diabetics to develop overt glomerulopathy. Ots et al. (2004) have shown that kidney transplantation in 5/6 nephrectomized animals protects against albuminuria and rise in blood pressure. In humans, single kidney GFR declines more rapidly in uninephric individuals compared to binephric ones (Saxena et al., 2006). Undoubtedly, the role of foetal programming on the occurrence of renal and cardiovascular disease needs further study.

7. Therapeutic strategies

A major limitation in the interventions needed to reduce cardiovascular risk in subjects with DN is the fact that in the past renal patients were deliberately excluded from major intervention studies. Hence, current recommendations are mainly based on observational studies or post-hoc analyses of patients with early stages of CKD who had been enrolled in randomized controlled trials. However, information from controlled trials is available for some interventions, as outlined below.

7.1 Blood pressure control

The most important component of treatment is blood pressure (BP) control. Numerous studies have shown that the use of antihypertensive treatment in patients with DN is crucial in the preservation of GFR (Mogensen, 1982; Anderson et al., 1988; Parving et al., 1993) and to reduce mortality in this high-risk group (Parving et al., 1989; Mathiesen et al., 1989). In view of the fact that diabetic patients are a high risk population, the Seventh Report of the Joint National Committee on Prevention, Detection Evaluation and Treatment of High Blood Pressure (JNC 7) (2003) and American Diabetes Association (2004) have recommended a BP target of 130/80 mm Hg in diabetic patients and <125/75 mm Hg (Compendium of ESC Guidelines 2007) in the presence of renal impairment or of significant proteinuria >1 gr/24 hours. Nonetheless, BP lowering should be gradual and monitored closely, especially in haemodialysis patients who often develop hypotensive episodes during fluid removal by ultrafiltration. This is especially important in this high-risk population, keeping in mind that low blood pressure predicts death, particularly in the elderly with high comorbidity and low diastolic blood pressure values.

RAS blockade is the cornerstone of treatment of DN, as discussed below. In addition, diuretics play a crucial role in the treatment of CKD by potentiating the pressure lowering effect of RAS inhibitors. However, diuretics do have adverse effects on the heart and kidneys by triggering counterbalancing antinatriuretic mechanisms, example ACE II, aldosterone, decreased systemic blood pressure, and it is therefore advised that the lowest effective dose should be administered.

Importantly, the combination of RAS inhibitors and low dose thiazide diuretics augments the reduction of albuminuria. Also, RAS inhibitors diminish the thiazide-induced reduction in GFR. As a result, the filtered sodium load is increased, permitting more effective natriuresis. However, in patients with GFR <30mL/min, thiazides cause only a minor increase of natriuresis and they should therefore be exchanged for, or combined with, loop diuretics which are effective even in advanced CKD. In addition, in DN and proteinuric patients, higher diuretic doses are required because in the tubule lumen diuretics are up to 90% protein bound and natriuresis is only determined by the concentration of the free diuretic.

β-blockers, example carvedilol and nebivolol, are useful second-line treatments. Traditionally the use of β-blockers has been discouraged in patients with diabetes because they were associated with adverse effect such as weight gain, reduced peripheral blood flow, pronounced hypoglycemia and nightmares. However, β-blockers help decrease the enhanced sympathetic activity present in kidney disease. In addition, cardioselective β-blockers have less renal circulatory side effects and are associated with less blunting of hypoglycemia awareness and with less elevation of lipid and glucose levels, and are thus preferred to the nonselective type.

Dihydropyridine calcium antagonists should be avoided in hypertensive patients with albuminuria, as suggested by the results of a study conducted by Hummel et al. (2010). The latter have shown that dihydropyridine calcium antagonists are associated with increased albuminuria in patients treated with ACE inhibitors (ACEI)/ angiotensin receptor blockers (ARB). This is an important finding that merits further investigation since it is known that increases in albuminuria even in the low range are associated with increased cardiovascular risk.

7.2 Renin-angiotensin system blockade

Inappropriate activation of the RAS blockadeis a hallmark of CKD and DN. In fact, various studies have shown the beneficial role of ACEI and ARB in the treatment of DM in both type 1 and 2 diabetic subjects. Thus, in the Captopril Collaborative Study Group (Lewis et al., 1993), a significant risk reduction in nephropathy progression was shown in type 1 diabetic patients treated with captopril. Also, a meta-analysis of 12 trials in type 1 diabetic patients with microalbuminuria (The ACE Inhibitors in Diabetic Nephropathy Trialist Group, 2001) revealed that the treatment with ACE inhibitor for two years was associated with a 60% reduction in progression to macroalbuminuria and in threefold increase in regression to normoalbuminuria in comparison with placebo. Mathiesen et al. (1999) has shown that captopril has long lasting (eight years) beneficial renoprotective effect in normotensive patients with type 1 DM and microalbuminuria.

Similar positive results have been demonstrated in type 2 DM. Thus, the Microalbuminuria, Cardiovascular and Renal Outcomes - Heart Outcomes Prevention Evaluation (MICRO-HOPE) study (Gerstein et al., 2000) showed that overt nephropathy was reduced by 24% in type 2 diabetic patients treated with ramipril, resulting in significant protection against cardiovascular events.

ARBs have also been shown to exhibit significant renoprotective effects. In the IRMA II study, Parving et al. (2001) demonstrated that irbesartan had a renoprotective effect in hypertensive patients with type 2 diabetes and microalbuminuria that was independent of its BP lowering effect. Furthermore, the restoration of normoalbuminuria was more evident in the group receiving irbesartan at a dose of 300 mg daily, as compared to the group receiving 150mg daily. Two other studies, IDNT (Lewis et al., 2001) and RENAAL (Brenner et al., 2001) also used ARBs, but they enrolled patients with higher grade of proteinuria and established renal insufficiency. In both studies, the use of ARBs led to lower levels of proteinuria, lower rates of decline in the GFR and later onset of ESRD than the use of control medications.

By contrast, the use of RAS blockade to lower the increased cardiovascular risk in DN has been disappointing. Although valsartan has been reported to decrease arterial stiffness in patients with DN (Karalliedde et al., 2008), there are no data on hard end-points. In a recent meta-analysis, RAS has been shown to improve cardiovascular outcomes in proteinuric CKD of various types (Balamuthusamy et al., 2008). However in another meta-analysis,

Sarafidis et al. (2008) failed to show an effect of RAS inhibition on total mortality in DN patients. In conclusion, though there is strong evidence of renoprotection by both ACEIs and ARBs, evidence for cardiovascular protection in DN patients is still lacking.

7.3 Statins

Altough the effect of statin use on cardiovascular outcomes in patients with DN has not been extensively studied, there is strong evidence for their effectiveness in both diabetes and in CKD. Their effectiveness in reducing cardiovascular events in diabetic subjects was demonstrated in the Collaborative Atorvastatin Diabetes Study (CARDS) (2004) as well as in meta-analysis of all trials having a diabetes subgroup analysis (Costa et al., 2006). Subgroup analysis of the Cholesterol and Recurrent Events (CARE) (Tonelli et al., 2003), Management of Elevated cholesterol in the primary prevention Group of Adult Japanese (MEGA) (Nakamura et al., 2009) and the Scandinavian Simvastatin Survival Study (4S) (Chonchol et al., 2007) studies have all demonstrated significant cardiovascular protection in CKD patients. A meta-analysis by Strippoli et al. found a reduction in fatal and non-fatal cardiovascular events but not in total mortality. Cochrane reviews have concluded that statins significantly reduced the risk of all-cause and cardiovascular mortality in CKD patients who are not receiving renal replacement therapy (Navaneethan et al., 2009a), but there that was insufficient data on renal transplant patients (Navaneethan et al., 2009b).

Statins also play an important role in renoprotection. Several meta-analyses have been performed to assess the effect of statins on renal function and proteinuria. Fried et al. (2001) performed a meta-analysis with 13 controlled prospective studies and concluded that statin use results in a lower rate of decline in eGFR, although the effect was small. In a second meta-analysis of 27 studies, Sandhu et al. (2006) have shown that statin use resulted in an improvement in eGFR and reduction in proteinuria.

The renoprotective effects of statins are probably secondary to an extension of their modulatory effects on inflammation and oxidant stress (reviewed by Kurukulasuriya et al. (2007)). This is achieved through various mechanisms, mainly:

i. Reduction of generation of reactive oxygen species (ROS)
ii. Suppression of activity of pro-oxidant enzyme systems, mainly NADPH oxidase, xanthine oxidase, oxidase activity of endothelial NO-synthase
iii. Inhibition of Rho expression, resulting in up-regulation of eNOS expression, thereby reducing blood pressure and glomerular injury, together with a decrease in the surface protein endothelin-1 levels. The latter is a potent vasoconstrictor and mitogen, and might play a role in delaying glomerulosclerosis
iv. Interference with LDL oxidation via several mechanisms
v. Inhibition of conversion of monocytes to macrophages by inhibiting their uptake of oxidized LDL.

Among their anti-inflammatory and anti-proliferative effects, statins have been shown to reduce levels of monocyte chemo-attractant protein-1, tumor necrosis factor-alpha (TNF-α), transforming growth factor-beta (TGF-β), interleukin-6, platelet-derived growth factor, NFκB, and mesangial proteins. These pleiotropic effects distinguish statins from other lipid-lowering therapies (e.g. resin binders, fibrates, niacin). All the above mechanisms may also contribute to cardiovascular protective properties of statins, although the main mechanism in this case is thought to be through improving lipid profile particularly lowering of LDL-cholesterol.

7.4 Fibrates

Diabetes mellitus is considered a cardiovascular disease risk equivalent. Consequently, subjects with DN are at higher risk than patients suffering from kidney disease secondary to other aetiologies. Statins decrease coronary event rates to the level equal or even greater to that seen in untreated subjects (Costa et al., 2006). Consequently, there is significant substantial residual risk. This may be partly due to the fact that statins have only limited effectiveness on hypertriglyceridemia and low HDL cholesterol, and they do not normalize the abnormal LDL size-distribution pattern seen in DM.
Peroxisome proliferator-activated receptor (PPAR)alpha agonists, which include fibrates, are more effective in lowering triglycerides, in raising HDL and help to improve ratio of small dense: large buoyant LDL particles (Birjmohun et al., 2005; Tokuno A et al., 2007). Outcome trials of PPARalpha agonists have shown decreased cardiovascular morbidity in patients with diabetes and in those with the metabolic syndrome. In addition, plaque progression is diminished, and there is a decrease in both microvascular (including diabetic nephropathy and retinopathy) and macrovascular complications (reviewed by Staels et al., 2008).
Two trials worth mentioning are the FIELD study and the DAIS study. The FIELD study (Keech et al., 2005) was a multinational, randomised controlled trial with about 10,000 patients with type 2 diabetes mellitus, and not taking statin therapy at study entry. 80% of the participants were without previous cardiovascular disease. Participants were randomly assigned to micronised fenofibrate 200 mg daily or matching placebo. In the treatment group, the risk of the primary outcome of coronary events was not significantly reduced. However, fenofibrate did reduce nonfatal MI and revascularization procedures by 24%. Furthermore more controls were on statins, which might have attenuated any beneficial effect of fenofibrate. On the other hand, in the DAIS study (DAIS Group, 2001), fenofibrate reduced angiographic progression of CAD in type 2 diabetic patients. Since the data for reducing CV risk is stronger for statins, fibrates are especially useful as second-line treatment of dyslipidaemia in diabetic patients that cannot tolerate statins. In addition, the combination of fibrates with statins seems to be particularly indicated in diabetic patients with residual hypertriglyceridaemia and/or low HDL despite receiving statin therapy since fibrates help improve overall lipoprotein profile further. However, most fibrates are metabolized by the kidney and, in view of the risk of rhabdomyolysis, careful monitoring and dose adjustment is necessary when statins and fibrates are used as combination treatment in DN patients.

7.5 Correction of anaemia

Anaemia is a common complication of CKD. It is often more severe and occurs at an earlier stage in patients with DN than in patients with CKD secondary to other causes. This anaemia results from erythropoietin (EPO) deficiency. Studies have shown that recombinant human EPO treatment is effective in correcting erythropoietin-deficiency anaemia in patients with DN, besides improving quality of life and well-being in these patients. However, recently, there is increasing concern regarding adverse events caused by EPO treatment when haemoglobin (Hb) concentrations are raised above the recommended target of 11-12g/dL, as outlined below.
The Normal Hematocrit Study, Cardiovascular Risk Reduction by Early Anemia Treatment with Epoetin-beta, Correction of Hemoglobin and Outcomes in Renal Insufficiency, and Trial to Reduce Cardiovascular Events with Aranesp Therapy have shown increased risk of

mortality and/or cardiovascular complications with targeting of a higher Hb in CKD patients. There is increasing debate whether it is the higher Hb level targeted in these trials or the erythropoiesis-stimulating agent (ESA) exposure itself that accounted for the observed increased risk (reviewed by Singh (2010)). This is because, in these trials, achieving a normal or near normal Hb was associated with improved survival and reduced cardiovascular risk while it seems that it was the 'targeting' of a higher Hb with ESA that resulted in increased morbidity. However, the results obtained, by their very nature, cannot prove causality. In addition, several study-inherent and methodological limitations must be considered before simply extrapolating the negative findings of these studies into clinical practice. Therefore, until new evidence becomes available from ongoing and future clinical studies, an upper Hb limit of 12 g/dl should not be exceeded.

The increased morbidity with EPO treatment could be explained by its side effects arising from the vascular system. A frequently seen adverse effect of chronic administration of EPO is an increase in arterial BP; postulated mechanisms for EPO-induced hypertension include enhanced vascular reactivity and vasoconstrictor responses. Scalera et al. (2005) have shown that at concentrations corresponding to plasma levels after EPO therapy in patients with chronic renal failure, EPO and darbepoietin α (NESP) increase endothelial elaboration of ADMA and inhibition of NOS by impairing dimethylarginine dimethylaminohydrolase (DDAH) activity. This is probably mediated by oxidative stress. Scalera et al. thus demonstrate a novel mechanism for EPO-induced downregulation of NO synthesis, which may contribute to explain main side effects observed in patients who are treated with EPO.

Increased blood viscosity also plays a role in EPO-induced hypertension and increases workload on the heart. In addition, increased whole blood viscosity is an important pathophysiological factor in the development of atherothrombosis and appears to be a strong predictor of CVD. In fact, male blood donors and women of premenopausal age with regular menstruation have shown reduced incidence of cardiovascular events such as myocardial infarction, angina, stroke, and the requirement for procedures such as percutaneous transluminal coronary angioplasty and coronary artery bypass graft compared with non-donors and postmenopausal women, respectively. This is possibly related to decreased whole blood viscosity. Consequently, Jeong et al. (2010) have proposed blood viscosity monitoring as part of cardiovascular risk assessment in the context of anaemia correction with ESAs. As discussed above, EPO may also increase platelet number and activation.

The use of intravenous iron in the correction of anaemia in CKD is also uncertain. The vast majority of patients with CKD are iron-deficient secondary to multiple forms of interference with all phases of iron metabolism. Therefore, iron supplementation is given to CKD patients. Intravenous iron was demonstrated to be superior to oral iron in both hemodialysis and nondialysis-dependent CKD patients. Whereas correction of anemia is effective in reducing oxidative stress and, conceptually cardiovascular risk, intravenous iron could promote cytotoxicity and tissue injury, exacerbate oxidative stress and endothelial dysfunction, as well as inflammation and the progression of both CKD and cardiovascular disease (Garneata, 2008). Clinical judgment is thus necessary in each individual case to diagnose iron deficiency and effectively use intravenous iron.

7.6 Antiplatelet agents

Given the high cardiovascular morbidity and mortality associated with DN, it is reasonable to suggest that diabetic subjects suffering from nephropathy should be on regular aspirin treatment. In fact, the American Diabetes Association (2004) suggest that diabetic patients >40years old with ≥1 cardiovascular risk factor should be taking prophylactic aspirin while the ESC guidelines (The Task Force on the Use of Antiplatelet Agents in Patients with Atherosclerotic Cardiovascular Disease, 2004) suggest prophylactic aspirin for diabetic patients with 1-year risk of CHD >1.5%.

However, in diabetic patients, aspirin may be less effective than expected. Thus, in the 1031 diabetic patients enrolled in the Primary Prevention Project (Sacco et al., 2003), the effects of aspirin 100mg daily were surprisingly poor with major vascular events being reduced by only 10% in diabetic individuals versus 31% in nondiabetic individuals. This was confirmed in two recent meta-analyses (De Berardis et al., 2009; Stavrakis et al., 2011). The role of aspirin in diabetic patients who are at increased risk because of renal disease remains inadequately investigated. The Primary Prevention Project Investigators suggest that, in diabetes, platelets may be activated through peculiar aspirin-insensitive mechanisms. This may involve hyperproduction of thromboxane from cells and tissues through aspirin-insensitive COX-2 pathway, or alternative prostanoid producing mechanisms can be activated by hyperglycaemia or insulin resistance. In addition, there is increased turnover of platelets in DM, possibly suggesting the need for higher doses of aspirin than usual in diabetic patients.

In keeping with aspirin resistance, there is increasing interest in picotamide, a dual inhibitor of thromboxane synthase and thromboxane receptor. In the DAVID study (Neri Serneri et al., 2004), >1200 patients with type 2 DM and established PAD were randomly allocated to picotamide 600mg or aspirin 320mg. It was demonstrated that picotamide almost halved general mortality compared with aspirin with a significantly lowered relative risk of death (0.55) and reduced, though not significantly, vascular deaths, from 4.1% to 2.1%. In addition, picotamide caused less bleeding and was better tolerated than aspirin. This study suggests that dual inhibitors of thromboxane synthase and thromboxane receptors may become useful therapies in cardiovascular prevention in diabetic patients. Further studies with picotamide and with other agents of the same class, for example ridogrel and terutroban sodium, are thus desirable.

7.7 Glycosaminoglycans

In view that microalbuminuria, the traditional hallmark of DN, is associated with alterations in endothelial permeability secondary to degradation of heparin-sulphate (a glycosaminoglycan component of the intracellular and basement membrane matrix) increasing attention has been focused on the role of glycosaminoglycans in the treatment of DN and associated cardiovascular complications.

Special attention has been focused on sulodexide, a compound containing 80% slow-moving heparin and 20% dermatan sulphate, both of which have been shown to prevent experimental diabetic nephropathy. In the DINAS study (Gambaro et al., 2002), sulodexide significantly decreased albuminuria by 43% in subjects with DN and the effect persisted at 8-month follow-up with no major adverse events. In addition, sulodexide was effective in both type 1 and type 2 diabetic subjects and it maintained its efficacy during concomitant treatment with ACE inhibitors. The reduction in albuminuria by sulodexide was confirmed in another study by Achour et al. (2005) where albuminuria was significantly decreased at a lower therapeutic dose of sulodexide, independently of diabetes type and baseline presence of micro- or macroalbuminuria. Interestingly, sulodexide has been shown to prevent cardiovascular events in non-diabetic survivors of MI (Condorelli et al., 1994) as well as improving the walking performance of PAD patients, some of whom were diabetic.

Therefore, glycosaminoglycans offer a new perspective in the treatment of diabetic nephropathy. However, further research is needed to investigate how and to what extent these agents influence the course of DN and associated cardiovascular co-morbidities.

7.8 Lifestyle interventions

Lifestyle interventions, mainly regular exercise and diet, play an important role in reducing cardiovascular risk in DN patients. Physical exercise is necessary to improve glycaemic control and decrease cardiovascular risk. Interestingly, in a study by Lazarevic et al. (2007) it was shown that six months of aerobic exercise, without any change in the medication, tended to decrease microalbuminuria in type 2 diabetic subjects, independently of any improvement in insulin resistance and oxidative stress parameters. However, further studies are needed to elucidate the mechanisms underlying the beneficial effects of exercise.

In addition to restricted calorie and fat intake and adequate fibre intake, dietary manipulation, including protein, phosphorus, and sodium restriction, can potentially exert a cardiovascular protective effect in DN patients by decreasing various cardiovascular risk factors. Diminished sodium intake helps in achieving blood pressure control. Increasesd fibre intake plays an important role in lowering serum cholesterol and improving plasma lipid profile. A low protein may help to reduce proteinuria and in decreasing phosphorus intake and preventing and reversing hyperphosphatemia and secondary hyperparathyroidism. These, in turn, may also help ameliorate insulin sensitivity and metabolic control in diabetic patients, as well as increase the responsiveness to erythropoietin therapy, thus enabling correction of anemia. Protein-restricted diets may have also anti-inflammatory and anti-oxidant properties (Cupisti et al., 2007). Nonetheless, even though dietary restriction may be useful to decrease cardiovascular risk in the DN patient, further studies are needed to assess the effect of renal diets on hard outcomes, as cardiovascular events or mortality.

8. Conclusion

The present review underlines the cardiovascular risk to which patients with diabetic nephropathy are exposed and summarizes some of the mechanisms that lead to the increased risk of adverse cardiovascular events. Some of the risk factors are modifiable and can be improved with currently available therapy including aggressive treatment of dyslipidemia, antiplatelet treatment, restriction of protein intake together with adequate exercise. Nonetheless, further research is needed to unravel the pathophysiology underlying cardiovascular complications associated with diabetic nephropathy as well as to investigate novel therapies to enable a decrease in the morbidity and mortality associated with this serious diabetes-related complication. These may require new approaches including the management of the increased oxidative stress and low-grade inflammation.

9. References

Achour A, Kacem M, Dibej K, Skhiri H, Bouraoui S, El May M (2005). One year course of oral sulodexide in the management of diabetic nephropathy. *J Nephrol* 18:568-74.

Adler AI, Stevens RJ, Manley SE, Bilous RW, Cull CA, Holman RR (2003). Development and progression of nephropathy in type 2 diabetes: The United Kingdom Prospective Diabetes Study (UKPDS 64). *Kidney Int* 63: 225 -232.

Ahmed S, Cannon CP, Giugliano RP, Murphy SA, Morrow DA, Antman EM, Braunwald E, Gibson CM (2003). The independent and combined risk of diabetes and non-endstage renal impairment in non-ST-segment elevation acute coronary syndromes. *J Natl Med Assoc.* 2003 Nov; 95(11): 1042-7.

Alebiosu CO, Odusan O, Familoni OB, Jaiyesimi AE (2004). Cardiovascular risk factors in type 2 diabetic Nigerians with clinical diabetic nephropathy. *Cardiovasc J S Afr.* 2004 May-Jun; 15(3): 124-8.

Alebiosu CO, Odusan O, Jaiyesimi A (2008). Morbidity in relation to stage of diabetic nephropathy in type 2 diabetic patients. *Int J Cardiol.* 2008 Dec 17; 131(1): 105-12.

Alwakeel JS, Al-Suwaida A, Isnani AC, Al-Harbi A, Alam A (2009). Concomitant macro and microvascular complications in diabetic nephropathy. *Saudi J Kidney Dis Transpl.* 2009 May; 20(3): 402-9.

Amann K, Ritz E, Wiest G, Klaus G, Mall G (1994). A role of parathyroid hormone for the activation of cardiac fibroblasts in uremia. *J Am Soc Nephrol* 4: 1814–1819.

Amann K, Wanner C, Ritz E (2006). Cross-talk between the kidney and the cardiovascular system. *J Am Soc Nephrol.* 2006 Aug; 17(8): 2112-9.

American Diabetes Association (2004). Aspirin therapy in diabetes. *Diabetes Care* 27: S72-3.

American Diabetes Association Position Statement (2004). Hypertension management in adults with diabetes. *Diabetes Care* 27:S65–S67

Anavekar NS, Gans DJ, Berl T, Rohde RD, Cooper W, Bhaumik A, Hunsicker LG, Rouleau JL, Lewis JB, Rosendorff C, Porush JG, Drury PL, Esmatjes E, Raz I, Vanhille P, Locatelli F, Goldhaber S, Lewis EJ, Pfeffer MA (2004). Predictors of cardiovascular events in patients with type 2 diabetic nephropathy and hypertension: A case for albuminuria. *Kidney Int.* 66 (suppl 92): S50–S55.

Anavekar NS, Solomon SD, McMurray JJ, Maggioni A, Rouleau JL, Califf R, White H, Kober L, Velazquez E, Pfeffer MA (2008). Comparison of renal function and cardiovascular risk following acute myocardial infarction in patients with and without diabetes mellitus. *Am J Cardiol.* 2008 Apr 1;101(7):925-9.

Anderson S, Brenner BM (1988). Influence of antihypertensive therapy on development and progression of diabetic glomerulopathy. *Diabetes Care* 11: 846-9.

Aso Y, Yoshida N, Okumura K, Wakabayashi S, Matsutomo R, Takebayashi K, Inukai T (2004). Coagulation and inflammation in overt diabetic nephropathy: association with hyperhomocysteinemia. *Clin Chim Acta.* 2004 Oct; 348(1-2): 139-45.

Astrup AS, Tarnow L, Rossing P, Hansen BV, Hilsted J, Parving HH (2006). Cardiac autonomic neuropathy predicts cardiovascular morbidity and mortality in type 1 diabetic patients with diabetic nephropathy. *Diabetes Care* 2006 Feb; 29(2): 334-9.

Astrup AS, Nielsen FS, Rossing P, Ali S, Kastrup J, Smidt UM, Parving HH (2007). Predictors of mortality in patients with type 2 diabetes with or without diabetic nephropathy: a follow-up study. *J Hypertens* 2007 Dec; 25(12):2479-85.

Block GA, Hulbert-Shearon TE, Levin NW, Port FK (1998). Association of serum phosphorus and calcium x phosphate product with mortality risk in chronic hemodialysis patients: A national study. *Am J Kidney Dis* 31: 607–617.

Balamuthusamy S, Srinivasan L, Verma M, Adigopula S, Jalandhara N, Hathiwala S, Smith E (2008). Renin angiotensin system blockade and cardiovascular outcomes in patients with chronic kidney disease and proteinuria: a meta-analysis. *Am Heart J.* 2008 May; 155(5): 791-805.

Beck MO, Silveiro SP, Friedman R, Clausell N, Gross JL (1999). Asymptomatic coronary artery disease is associated with cardiac autonomic neuropathy and diabetic nephropathy in type 2 diabetic patients. *Diabetes Care* 1999 Oct; 22(10): 1745-7.

Berl T, Hunsicker LG, Lewis JB, Pfeffer MA, Porush JG, Rouleau JL, Drury PL, Esmatjes E, Hricik D, Parikh CR, Raz I, Vanhille P, Wiegmann TB, Wolfe BM, Locatelli F, Goldhaber SZ, Lewis EJ; Irbesartan Diabetic Nephropathy Trial. Collaborative Study Group (2003). Cardiovascular outcomes in the Irbesartan Diabetic Nephropathy Trial of patients with type 2 diabetes and overt nephropathy. *Ann Intern Med* 138: 542–9.

Bianchi C, Penno G, Pancani F, Civitelli A, Piaggesi A, Caricato F, Pellegrini G, Del Prato S, Miccoli R (2007). Non-traditional cardiovascular risk factors contribute to peripheral arterial disease in patients with type 2 diabetes. *Diabetes Res Clin Pract.* 2007 Nov; 78(2):246-53. Epub 2007 May 10.

Birjmohun RS, Hutten BA, Kastelein JJ, Stroes ES (2005). Efficacy and safety of high-density lipoprotein cholesterol-increasing compounds: a meta-analysis of randomized controlled trials. J Am Coll Cardiol 45: 185–197.

Bouchi R, Babazono T, Nyumura I, Toya K, Hayashi T, Ohta M, Hanai K, Kiuchi Y, Suzuki K, Iwamoto Y (2009). Is a reduced estimated glomerular filtration rate a risk factor for stroke in patients with type 2 diabetes? *Hypertens Res.* 2009 May; 32(5): 381-6. Epub 2009 Mar 27.

Bouchi R, Babazono T, Yoshida N, Nyumura I, Toya K, Hayashi T, Hanai K, Tanaka N, Ishii A, Iwamoto Y (2010). Relationship between chronic kidney disease and silent cerebral infarction in patients with Type 2 diabetes. *Diabet Med.* 2010 May; 27(5): 538-43.

Boulanger CM, Amabile N, Guérin AP, Pannier B, Leroyer AS, Mallat CN, Tedgui A, London GM (2007). In vivo shear stress determines circulating levels of endothelial microparticles in end-stage renal disease. *Hypertension.* 2007 Apr; 49(4): 902-8.

Brenner BM, Garcia DL, Anderson (1988). Glomeruli and blood pressure. Less of one, more the other? *Am J Hypertens* 1: 335–347.

Brenner BM, Cooper ME, De Zeeuw D, Mitch WE, Parving HH, Remuzzi G, Snapinn SM, Zhang ZX, Shahinfar S, RENAAL Study (2001). Effects of losartan on renal and cardiovascular outcomes in patients with type 2 diabetes and nephropathy. *N Engl J Med.* 345: 861–869.

Busch M, Franke S, Wolf G, Brandstadt A, Ott U, Gerth J, Hunsicker LG, Stein G; Collaborative Study Group (2006). The advanced glycation end product N(epsilon)-carboxymethyllysine is not a predictor of cardiovascular events and renal outcomes in patients with type 2 diabetic kidney disease and hypertension. *Am J Kidney Dis* 48: 571–9.

Busch M, Franke S, Rüster C, Wolf G (2010). Advanced glycation end-products and the kidney. *Eur J Clin Invest.* 2010 Aug; 40(8): 742-55.

Chonchol M, Cook T, Kjekshus J, Pedersen TR, Lindenfeld J (2007). Simvastatin for secondary prevention of all-cause mortality and major coronary events in patients with mild chronic renal insufficiency. *Am J Kidney Dis.* 2007 Mar; 49(3): 373-82.

Clausen P, Jacobsen P, Rossing K, Jensen JS, Parving HH, Feldt-Rasmussen B (2000). Plasma concentrations of VCAM-1 and ICAM-1 are elevated in patients with Type 1 diabetes mellitus with microalbuminuria and overt nephropathy. *Diabet Med.* 2000 Sep; 17(9): 644-9.

Collins AJ, Li S, Gilbertson DT, Liu J, Chen SC, Herzog CA (2003). Chronic kidney disease and cardiovascular disease in the Medicare population. *Kidney Int Suppl.* 87: S24-S31.

Compendium of ESC Guidelines 2007, Section III: Diabetic Heart Disease. Lippincott Williams and Wilkins; 2007. pp. 33–52

Condorelli M, Chiarello M, Dagianti A, Penco M, Dalla Volta S, Pengo V, Schivazappa L, Mattioli G, Mattioli AV, Brusoni B, et al. (1994). IPO-V2: a prospective multicenter, randomized, comparative clinical investigation of effects of sulodexide in preventing cardiovascular accidents in the first year after acute myocardial infarction. *J Am Coll Cardiol* 23: 27-34.

Corrêa Leite ML (2011). Fibrinogen, hematocrit, platelets in mild kidney dysfunction and the role of uric acid: an Italian male population study. *Clin Appl Thromb Hemost.* 2011 Feb; 17(1): 58-65. Epub 2009 Oct 13.

Costa J, Borges M, David C, Vaz Carneiro (2006). Efficacy of lipid lowering drug treatment for diabetic and non-diabetic patients: meta-analysis of randomised controlled trials. *BMJ* 2006 May 13; 332(7550): 1115-24. Epub 2006 Apr 3

Cupisti A, Aparicio M, Barsotti G (2007). Potential benefits of renal diets on cardiovascular risk factors in chronic kidney disease patients. *Ren Fail.* 29(5): 529-34.

DAIS Group (2001). Effect of fenofibrate on progression of coronary-artery disease in type 2 diabetes: the Diabetes Atherosclerosis Intervention Study, a randomised study. *Lancet* 2001 Mar 24; 357(9260): 905-10.

Davis WA, Norman PE, Bruce DG, Davis TM (2006). Predictors, consequences and costs of diabetes-related lower extremity amputation complicating type 2 diabetes: the Fremantle Diabetes Study. *Diabetologia.* 2006 Nov; 49(11): 2634-41.

De Berardis G, Sacco M, Strippoli GF, Pellegrini F, Graziano G, Tognoni G, Nicolucci A (2009). Aspirin for primary prevention of cardiovascular events in people with diabetes: meta-analysis of randomised controlled trials. *BMJ* 2009 Nov 6; 339:b4531.

Deckert T, Feldt-Rasmussen B, Borch-Johnsen K, Jensen T, Kofoed-Enevoldsen A (1989). Albuminuria reflects widespread vascular damage. The Steno hypothesis. *Diabetologia* 32: 219–226.

Dinneen SF, Gerstein HC (1997). The association of microalbuminuria and mortality in non-insulin-dependent diabetes mellitus: a systematic overview of the literature. *Arch Intern Med.* 157(13): 1413-1418.

Fava S, Azzopardi J, Watkins PJ, Hattersley AT (2001). Adult height and proteinuria in type 2 diabetes. *Nephrol Dial Transplant.* 2001 Mar; 16(3): 525-8.

Fliser D (2010). Perspectives in renal disease progression: the endothelium as a treatment target in chronic kidney disease. *J Nephrol.* 2010 Jul-Aug; 23(4): 369-76.

Foley RN, Murray AM, Li S, Herzog CA, McBean AM, Eggers PW, Collins AJ (2005). Chronic kidney disease and the risk for cardiovascular disease, renal replacement, and death in the United States Medicare population, 1998 to 1999. *J Am Soc Nephrol.* 2005 Feb; 16(2): 489-495.

Fox CS, Larson MG, Vasan RS, Guo CY, Parise H, Levy D, Leip EP, O'donnell CJ, D'Agostino RB Sr, Benjamin EJ (2006). Cross-sectional association of kidney function with valvular and annular calcification: the Framingham heart study. *J Am Soc Nephrol.* 2006 Feb; 17(2): 521-7. Epub 2005 Dec 28.

Gambaro G, Kinalska I, Oksa A, Pont'uch P, Hertlová M, Olsovsky J, Manitius J, Fedele D, Czekalski S, Perusicová J, Skrha J, Taton J, Grzeszczak W, Crepaldi G (2002). Oral sulodexide reduces albuminuria in microalbuminuric type 1 and type 2 diabetic patients: the Di.N.A.S. randomized trial. *J Am Soc Nephrol* 13:1615-25.

Garneata L (2008). Intravenous iron, inflammation, and oxidative stress: is iron a friend or an enemy of uremic patients? *J Ren Nutr.* 2008 Jan; 18(1): 40-5.

Gerstein HC, Yusuf S, Mann JFE, et al (2000). Effects of ramipril on cardiovascular and microvascular outcomes in people with diabetes mellitus: results of the HOPE study and MICRO–HOPE substudy. *Lancet* 355: 253–259.

Gerstein HC, Mann JF, Yi Q, Zinman B, Dinneen SF, Hoogwerf B, Hallé JP, Young J, Rashkow A, Joyce C, Nawaz S, Yusuf S; HOPE Study Investigators (2001). Albuminuria and risk of cardiovascular events, death, and heart failure in diabetic and nondiabetic individuals. *JAMA* 286(4): 421-426.

Go AS, Chertow GM, Fan D, McCulloch CE, Hsu CY (2004). Chronic kidney disease and the risks of death, cardiovascular events, and hospitalization. *N Engl J Med.* 351(13): 1296-1305.

Gouverneur M, Berg B, Nieuwdorp M, Stroes E, Vink H (2006). Vasculoprotective properties of the endothelial glycocalyx: Effects of fluid shear stress. *J Intern Med* 259: 393–400.

Groop L, Ekstrand A, Forsblom C and Widen E, Groop P-H, Teppo A-M, Eriksson J (1993): Insulin resistance, hypertension and microalbuminuria in patients with type 2 (non-insulin-dependent) diabetes mellitus. *Diabetologia* 36: 642-7

Henry CB, Duling BR (1999). Permeation of the luminal capillary glycocalyx is determined by hyaluronan. *Am J Physiol* 277: H508–H514.

Hernández C, Chacón P, Martí R, García-Pascual L, Mesa J, Simó R (2000). Relationship of lipoprotein(a) and its phenotypes with the albumin excretion rate in diabetic patients: a multivariate analysis. *Nephron* 2000 May; 85(1): 27-33.

Hsieh MC, Tien KJ, Perng DS, Hsiao JY, Chang SJ, Liang HT, Chen HC, Tu ST (2009). Diabetic nephropathy and risk factors for peripheral artery disease in Chinese with type 2 diabetes mellitus. *Metabolism* 2009 Apr; 58(4): 504-9.

Hsu CY, McCulloch CE, Darbinian J, Go AS, Irbarren C (2005). Elevated blood pressure and risk of end-stage renal disease in subjects without baseline kidney disease. *Arch Intern Med* 165: 923-925.

Hummel D, Raff U, Schwarz TK, Schneider MP, Schmieder RE, Schmidt BM (2010). Dihydropyridine calcium antagonists are associated with increased albuminuria in treatment-resistant hypertensives. *J Nephrol* 2010 Sep-Oct; 23(5):563-8.

Ismail N, Cornell S. Epidemiology of type 2 diabetes and diabetic nephropathy in different ethnicities. In *Nephropathy in Type 2 Diabetes*, Ritz E , Rychlik I (eds). Oxford University Press: Oxford, 1999; 11-24.

Jeong SK, Cho YI, Duey M, Rosenson RS (2010). Cardiovascular risks of anemia correction with erythrocyte stimulating agents: should blood viscosity be monitored for risk assessment? Cardiovasc Drugs Ther. 2010 Apr; 24(2): 151-60.

Jones CA, Krolewski AS, Rogus J, Xue JL, Collins A, Warram JH (2005). Epidemic of end-stage renal disease in people with diabetes in the United States population: Do we know the cause? *Kidney Int* 67: 1684 -1691.

Kang D-H, Park S-K, Lee I-K, Johnson RJ (2005). Uric acid-induced C-reactive protein expression: Implication on cell proliferation and nitric oxide production of human vascular cells. *J Am Soc Nephrol* 16(12): 3553-3562.

Karalliedde J, Smith A, DeAngelis L, Mirenda V, Kandra A, Botha J, Ferber P, Viberti G (2008). Valsartan improves arterial stiffness in type 2 diabetes independently of blood pressure lowering. *Hypertension*. 2008 Jun; 51(6): 1617-23. Epub 2008 Apr 21.

Keech A, Simes RJ, Barter P, Best J, Scott R, Taskinen MR, Forder P, Pillai A, Davis T, Glasziou P, Drury P, Kesäniemi YA, Sullivan D, Hunt D, Colman P, d'Emden M, Whiting M, Ehnholm C, Laakso M; FIELD study investigators (2006). Effects of long-term fenofibrate therapy on cardiovascular events in 9795 people with type 2 diabetes mellitus (the FIELD study): randomised controlled trial. *Lancet*. 2005 Nov 26; 366(9500): 1849-61. Erratum in: Lancet. 2006 Oct 21;368(9545):1415. *Lancet*. 2006 Oct 21; 368(9545):1420.

Khosla UM, Zharikov S, Finch JL, Nakagawa T, Roncal C, Mu W, Krotova K, Block ER, Prabhakar S, Johnson RJ (2005). Hyperuricemia induces endothelial dysfunction. *Kidney Int*. 67(5): 1739-1742.

Kidney Disease Outcomes Quality Initiative (K/DOQI) (2004). K/DOQI clinical practice guidelines on hypertension and antihypertensive agents in chronic kidney disease. *Am J Kidney Dis*. 2004 May; 43(5)(suppl 1): S1-S290.

Kielstein JT, Böger RH, Bode-Böger SM, Schaffer J, Barbey M, Koch KM, Frölich JC (1999). Asymmetric dimethylarginine plasma concentrations differ in patients with end-stage renal disease: relationship to treatment method and atherosclerotic disease. *J Am Soc Nephrol* 10: 594–600.

Klausen K, Borch-Johnsen K, Feldt-Rasmussen B, Jensen G, Clausen P, Scharling H, Appleyard M, Jensen JS (2004). Very low levels of microalbuminuria are associated with increased risk of coronary heart disease and death independently of renal function, hypertension, and diabetes. *Circulation* 2004 Jul 6; 110(1):32-35.

Krzyzanowska K, Mittermayer F, Shnawa N, Hofer M, Schnabler J, Etmüller Y, Kapiotis S, Wolzt M, Schernthaner G (2007). Asymmetrical dimethylarginine is related to renal function, chronic inflammation and macroangiopathy in patients with Type 2 diabetes and albuminuria. *Diabet Med*. 2007 Jan; 24(1): 81-6.

Lazarevic G, Antic S, Vlahovic P, Djordjevic V, Zvezdanovic L, Stefanovic V (2007). Effects of aerobic exercise on microalbuminuria and enzymuria in type 2 diabetic patients. *Ren Fail* 29(2): 199-205.

Leiper JM, Vallance P (2006). The synthesis and metabolism of asymmetric dimethylarginine (ADMA). *Eur J Clin Pharmacol* 62: 33–38.

Levey AS, Coresh J, Balk E, Kausz AT, Levin A, Steffes MW, Hogg RJ, Perrone RD, Lau J, Eknoyan G; National Kidney Foundation (2003). National Kidney Foundation practice guidelines for chronic kidney disease: evaluation, classification, and stratification [published correction appears in Ann Intern Med. 2003; 139(7):605]. *Ann Intern Med.* 2003; 139(2): 137-147.

Lewis EJ, Hunsicker LG, Bain RP, Rohde RD (1993). The effect of angiotensin converting enzyme inhibition on diabetic nephropathy. *N Engl J Med* 329: 1456–1462

Lewis EJ, Hunsicker LG, Clarke WR, Berl T, Pohl MA, Lewis JB, Ritz E, Atkins RC, Rohde R, Raz I, Collaborative Study Group (2001). Renoprotective effect of the angiotensin-receptor antagonist irbesartan in patients with nephropathy due to type 2 diabetes. *N Engl J Med* 345: 851–860.

Li J, Luo Y, Xu Y, Yang J, Zheng L, Hasimu B, Yu J, Hu D (2007). Risk factors of peripheral arterial disease and relationship between low ankle-brachial index and mortality from all-cause and cardiovascular disease in Chinese patients with type 2 diabetes. *Circ J.* 2007 Mar; 71(3): 377-81.

Lindsay RS, Little J, Jaap AJ, Padfield PL, Walker JD, Hardy KJ (1999). Diabetic nephropathy is associated with an increased familial risk of stroke. *Diabetes Care* 1999 Mar; 22(3): 422-5.

Lindsey JB, Cipollone F, Abdullah SM, McGuire DK (2009). Receptor for advanced glycation end-products (RAGE) and soluble RAGE (sRAGE): cardiovascular implications. *Diab Vasc Dis Res.* 2009 Jan; 6(1): 7-14.

Liu H, Shi H, Yu J, Chen F, Jiang Q, Hu D (2010). Is Chronic Kidney Disease Associated with a High Ankle Brachial Index in Adults at High Cardiovascular Risk? *J Atheroscler Thromb.* 2010 Nov 25. [Epub ahead of print]

Magri CJ, Calleja N, Buhagiar G, Fava S, Vassallo J. Ankle-brachial index in a type 2 diabetic population with proliferative retinopathy: associated risk factors and complications. *Int Angiology.* In press.

Mann JFE, Yi QL, Gerstein HC (2004). Albuminuria as a predictor of cardiovascular and renal outcomes in people with known atherosclerotic cardiovascular disease. *Kidney Int* 66: S59–S62

Mathiesen ER, Borch Johnsen K, Jensen DV, Deckert T (1989). Improved survival in patients with diabetic nephropathy. *Diabetologia* 32: 884-6.

Mathiesen R, Hommel E, Hansen HP, Smidt UM, Parving HH (1999).Randomised controlled trial of long term efficacy of captopril on preservation of kidney function in normotensive patients with insulin dependent diabetes and microalbuminuria. *BMJ* 319: 24–25.

Mattock MB, Barnes DJ, Viberti G, Keen H; Burt D, Hughes JM; Fitzgerald AP, Sandhu B, Jackson PG (1998). Microalbuminuria and coronary heart disease in NIDDM: an incidence study. *Diabetes* 47: 1786–1792

McQuarrie EP, Patel RK, Mark PB, Delles C, Connell J, Dargie HJ, Steedman T, Jardine AG (2010). Association between proteinuria and left ventricular mass index: a cardiac

MRI study in patients with chronic kidney disease. *Nephrol Dial Transplant.* 2010 Jul 12. [Epub ahead of print]

Miettinen H, Haffner SM, Lehto S, Rönnemaa T, Pyörälä K, Laakso M (1996). Proteinuria predicts stroke and other atherosclerotic vascular disease events in nondiabetic and non-insulin-dependent diabetic subjects. *Stroke* 27(11): 2033-2039.

Miyazato J, Horio T, Takiuchi S, Kamide K, Sasaki O, Nakamura S, Nakahama H, Inenaga T, Takishita S, Kawano Y (2005). Left ventricular diastolic dysfunction in patients with chronic renal failure: impact of diabetes mellitus. *Diabet Med.* 2005 Jun; 22(6): 730-6.

Mogensen CE (1982). Long-term antihypertensive treatment inhibiting progression of diabetic nephropathy. *BMJ* 285: 685-8.

Mogensen CE, Christensen CK, Vittinghus E (1983). The stages in diabetic renal disease: with emphasis on the stage of incipient diabetic nephropathy. *Diabetes* 32 (Suppl. 2): 64–78

Molitch ME, Rutledge B, Steffes M, Cleary P (2006). Renal insufficiency in the absence of albuminuria among adults with Type 1 diabetes in the Diabetes Control and Complications Trial (DCCT)/Epidemiology of Diabetes Interventions and Complications (EDIC) Study. ADA Annual Meeting 2006 (Abstract 23-OR).

Mostaza JM, Suarez C, Manzano L, Cairols M, García-Iglesias F, Sanchez-Alvarez J, Ampuero J, Godoy D, Rodriguez-Samaniego A, Sanchez-Zamorano MA; MERITO Study Group (2006). Relationship between ankle-brachial index and chronic kidney disease in hypertensive patients with no known cardiovascular disease. *J Am Soc Nephrol.* 2006 Dec; 17(12 Suppl 3): S201-5.

Nag S, Bilous R, Kelly W, Jones S, Roper N, Connolly V (2007). All-cause and cardiovascular mortality in diabetic subjects increases significantly with reduced estimated glomerular filtration rate (eGFR): 10 years' data from the South Tees Diabetes Mortality study. *Diabet Med.* 2007 Jan; 24(1): 10-7

Nakamura H, Mizuno K, Ohashi Y, Yoshida T, Hirao K, Uchida Y; MEGA Study Group (2009). Pravastatin and cardiovascular risk in moderate chronic kidney disease. *Atherosclerosis.* 2009 Oct; 206(2): 512-7. Epub 2009 Apr

Navaneethan SD, Pansini F, Perkovic V, Manno C, Pellegrini F, Johnson DW, Craig JC, Strippoli GF (2009a). HMG CoA reductase inhibitors (statins) for people with chronic kidney disease not requiring dialysis. *Cochrane Database Syst Rev.* 2009 Apr 15; (2): CD007784.

Navaneethan SD, Perkovic V, Johnson DW, Nigwekar SU, Craig JC, Strippoli GF (2009b). HMG CoA reductase inhibitors (statins) for kidney transplant recipients. *Cochrane Database Syst Rev.* 2009 Apr 15; (2): CD005019.

Navarro JF, Mora C, Gómez M, Muros M, López-Aguilar C, García J (2008). Influence of renal involvement on peripheral blood mononuclear cell expression behaviour of tumour necrosis factor-alpha and interleukin-6 in type 2 diabetic patients. *Nephrol Dial Transplant.* 2008 Mar; 23(3): 919-26. Epub 2007 Oct 2.

Nelson RG, Pettitt DJ, Baird HR, Charles MA, Liu QZ, Bennett PH, Knowler WC (1993): Pre-diabetic blood pressure predicts urinary albumin excretion after the onset of type 2 (non-insulin-dependent) diabetes mellitus in Pima Indians. *Diabetologia* 36: 998-1001.

Nelson RG, Pettitt DJ, de Courten MP, Hanson RL, Knowler WC, Bennett PH (1996). Parental hypertension and proteinuria in Pima Indians with NIDDM. *Diabetologia.* 1996 Apr; 39(4): 433-8

Nemes A, Takács R, Gavallér H, Várkonyi TT, Wittmann T, Forster T, Lengyel C (2010). Correlations between aortic stiffness and parasympathetic autonomic function in healthy volunteers. *Can J Physiol Pharmacol.* 2010 Dec; 88 (12): 1166-71.

Neri Serneri GC, Coccheri S, Marubini E , et al., on behalf of the Drug evaluation in Atherosclerotic Vascular disease in Diabetics (DAVID) Study Group (2004). Picotamide, a combined inhibitor of thromboxane A2 synthase and receptor, reduces 2-year mortality in diabetics with peripheral arterial disease: the DAVID Study. *Eur Heart J* 25: 1845-52.

Nin JW, Jorsal A, Ferreira I, Schalkwijk CG, Prins MH, Parving HH, Tarnow L, Rossing P, Stehouwer CD (2010). Higher plasma soluble receptor for advanced glycation end products (sRAGE) levels are associated with incident cardiovascular disease and all-cause mortality in Type 1 diabetes: a 12-year follow-up study. *Diabetes* 59(8), 2027–2032.

Nishimura M, Hashimoto T, Kobayashi H, Fukuda T, Okino K, Yamamoto N, Nakamura N, Yoshikawa T, Takahashi H, Ono T (2004). Association between cardiovascular autonomic neuropathy and left ventricular hypertrophy in diabetic haemodialysis patients. *Nephrol Dial Transplant.* 2004 Oct; 19(10): 2532-8. Epub 2004 Jul 13.

Noordzij MJ, Lefrandt JD, Smit AJ (2008). Advanced glycation end products in renal failure: an overview. *J Ren Care.* 2008 Dec ;34(4): 207-12.

O'Hare AM, Glidden DV, Fox CS, Hsu CY (2004). High prevalence of peripheral arterial disease in persons with renal insufficiency: results from the National Health and Nutrition Examination Survey 1999-2000. *Circulation* 109: 320-323.

Ots M, Troy JL, Rennke HG, Mackenzie HS, Brenner BM (2004). Impact of the supplementation of kidney mass on blood pressure and progression of kidney disease. *Nephrol Dial Transplant.* 2004 Feb; 19(2): 337-41.

Parving HH, Hommel E (1989). Prognosis in diabetic nephropathy. BMJ 299: 230-3.

Parving HH, Smidt UM, Hommel E, Mathiesen ER, Rossing P, Nielsen F, Gall MA (1993). Effective antihypertensive treatment postpones renal insufficiency in diabetic nephropathy. *Am J Kidney Dis* 22: 188-95.

Parving HH, Lehnert H, Bröchner-Mortensen J, Gomis R, Andersen S, Arner P; Irbesartan in Patients with Type 2 Diabetes and Microalbuminuria Study Group (2001). The effect of irbesartan on the development of diabetic nephropathy in patients with type 2 diabetes. *N Engl J Med* 345: 870–876.

Pettersson-Fernholm K, Karvonen MK, Kallio J, Forsblom CM, Koulu M, Pesonen U, Fagerudd JA, Groop PH; FinnDiane Study Group (2004). Leucine 7 to proline 7 polymorphism in the preproneuropeptide Y is associated with proteinuria, coronary heart disease, and glycemic control in type 1 diabetic patients. *Diabetes Care* 2004 Feb; 27(2): 503-9.

Ragosta M, Samady H, Isaacs RB, Gimple LW, Sarembock IJ, Powers ER (2004). Coronary flow reserve abnormalities in patients with diabetes mellitus who have end-stage renal disease and normal epicardial coronary arteries. *Am Heart J* 2004 Jun; 147(6): 1017-23.

Ritz E, Stefanski A (1996). Diabetic nephropathy in type 2 diabetes. *Am J Kidney Dis* 27: 167-194.

Ritz E, Orth SR (1999a). Nephropathy in patients with type 2 diabetes mellitus. *N Engl J Med* 341: 1127-1133.

Ritz E, Rychlik I, Locatelli F, Halimi S (1999b). End-stage renal failure in type 2 diabetes: a medical catastrophe of worldwide dimensions. *Am J Kidney Dis* 34: 795-808.

Ritz E (2010). Hypertension and kidney disease. *Clin Nephrol.* 2010 Nov; 74 Suppl 1: S39-43.

Rossing P, Tamow L, Nielson FS, Boelskifte S, Brenner BM, Parving HH (1995). Short stature and diabetic nephropathy. *Br Med J* 310: 296–297.

Sacco M, Pellegrini F, Roncaglioni MC, et al. on behalf of the PPP Collaborative Group (2003). Primary prevention of cardiovascular events with low-dose aspirin and vitamin E in type 2 diabetic patients: results of the Primary Prevention Project (PPP) trial. *Diabetes Care* 26: 3264-72.

Sarafidis PA, Stafylas PC, Kanaki AI, Lasaridis AN (2008). Effects of renin-angiotensin system blockers on renal outcomes and all-cause mortality in patients with diabetic nephropathy: an updated meta-analysis. *Am J Hypertens.* 2008 Aug;21(8):922-9. Epub 2008 Jun 5.

Saxena AB, Myers BD, Derby G, Blouch KL, Yan J, Ho B, Tan JC (2006). Adaptive hyperfiltration in the aging kidney after contralateral nephrectomy. *Am J Physiol Renal Physiol.* 2006 Sep; 291(3):F629-34. Epub 2006 Mar 8.

Scalera F, Kielstein JT, Martens-Lobenhoffer J, Postel SC, Täger M, Bode-Böger SM (2005). Erythropoietin increases asymmetric dimethylarginine in endothelial cells: role of dimethylarginine dimethylaminohydrolase. *J Am Soc Nephrol.* 2005 Apr; 16(4): 892-8. Epub 2005 Feb 23.

Schiffrin EL, Touyz RM (2004). From bedside to bench to bedside: role of renin-angiotensin-aldosterone system in remodeling of resistance arteries in hypertension. *Am J Physiol Heart Circ Physiol* 287: H435–H446

Schnabel R, Blankenberg S, Lubos E, Lackner KJ, Rupprecht HJ, Espinola-Klein C, Jachmann N, Post F, Peetz D, Bickel C, Cambien F, Tiret L, Münzel T (2005). Asymmetric dimethylarginine and the risk of cardiovascular events and death in patients with coronary artery disease: results from the AtheroGene Study. *Circ Res* 97: e53– 59.

Schukla N, Thompson CS, Angelini GD, Mikhailidis DP, Jeremy JY (2002). Homocysteine enhances impairment of endothelium-dependent relaxation and guanosine cyclic monophosphate formation in aortae from diabetic rabbits. *Diabetologia* 45:1325-31.

Shoji T, Emoto M, Kawagishi T, Kimoto E, Yamada A, Tabata T, Ishimura E, Inaba M, Okuno Y, Nishizawa Y (2001). Atherogenic lipoprotein changes in diabetic nephropathy. *Atherosclerosis.* 2001 Jun; 156(2): 425-33.

Singh AK (2010). What is causing the mortality in treating the anemia of chronic kidney disease: erythropoietin dose or hemoglobin level? *Curr Opin Nephrol Hypertens* 2010 Sep; 19(5): 420-4.

Sobotka PA, Liss HP, Vinik AI (1986). Impaired hypoxic ventilatory drive in diabetic patients with autonomic neuropathy. *J Clin Endocrinol Metab* 62:658–663.

Soedamah-Muthu SS, Chaturvedi N, Teerlink T, Idzior-Walus B, Fuller JH, Stehouwer CD; Eurodiab ProspectivE Complications Study Group (2005). Plasma homocysteine and microvascular and macrovascular complications in type 1 diabetes: a cross-sectional nested case-control study. *J Intern Med.* 2005 Nov ;258(5): 450-9.

Staels B, Maes M, Zambon A (2008). Fibrates and future PPARalpha agonists in the treatment of cardiovascular disease. *Nat Clin Pract Cardiovasc Med.* 2008 Sep; 5(9): 542-53. Epub 2008 Jul 15.

Stavrakis S, Stoner JA, Azar M, Wayangankar S, Thadani U (2011). Low-dose aspirin for primary prevention of cardiovascular events in patients with diabetes: a meta-analysis. *Am J Med Sci.* 2011 Jan; 341(1): 1-9.

Strippoli GF, Navaneethan SD, Johnson DW, Perkovic V, Pellegrini F, Nicolucci A, Craig JC (2008). Effects of statins in patients with chronic kidney disease: meta-analysis and meta-regression of randomised controlled trials. *BMJ* 2008 Mar 22; 336(7645): 645-51. Epub 2008 Feb 25.

Surdacki A, Nowicki M, Sandmann J, Tsikas D, Boeger RH, Bode-Boeger SM, Kruszelnicka-Kwiatkowska O, Kokot F, Dubiel JS, Froelich JC (1999). Reduced urinary excretion of nitric oxide metabolites and increased plasma levels of asymmetric dimethylarginine in men with essential hypertension. *J Cardiovasc Pharmacol* 33: 652–658.

Suzuki E, Egawa K, Nishio Y, Maegawa H, Tsuchiya M, Haneda M, Yasuda H, Morikawa S, Inubushi T, Kashiwagi A (2003). Prevalence and major risk factors of reduced flow volume in lower extremities with normal ankle-brachial index in Japanese patients with type 2 diabetes. *Diabetes Care* 2003 Jun; 26(6): 1764-9.

Suzuki K, Kato K, Hanyu O, Nakagawa O, Aizawa Y (2001). Left ventricular mass index increases in proportion to the progression of diabetic nephropathy in Type 2 diabetic patients. *Diabetes Res Clin Pract.* 2001 Dec; 54(3): 173-80.

Szeto CC, Chow KM, Poon PY, Kwan BC, Li PK (2008). Peroxisome proliferator-activated receptor-gamma gene polymorphism and risk of cardiovascular disease in patients with diabetic nephropathy. *Am J Nephrol.* 2008; 28(5): 715-22. Epub 2008 Apr 17.

Takenaka T, Sato T, Hoshi H, Kato N, Sueyoshi K, Tsuda M, Watanabe Y, Takane H, Ohno Y, Suzuki H (2010). Height constitutes an important predictor of mortality in end-stage renal disease. *Cardiol Res Pract.* 2010 Nov 11; 2011: 242353.

USRDS 2004 Annual Data Report, Bethesda, National Institutes of Health, National Institute of Diabetes and Digestive and Kidney Diseases, 2004.

Tarnow L, Hovind P, Teerlink T, Stehouwer CD, Parving HH (2004). Elevated plasma asymmetric dimethylarginine as a marker of cardiovascular morbidity in early diabetic nephropathy in type 1 diabetes. *Diabetes Care* 27: 765–769.

Tessari P, Kiwanuka E, Barazzoni R, Vettore M, Zanetti M (2006). Diabetic nephropathy is associated with increased albumin and fibrinogen production in patients with type 2 diabetes. *Diabetologia* 2006 Aug; 49(8): 1955-61. Epub 2006 May 16.

The ACE Inhibitors in Diabetic Nephropathy Trialist Group (2001). Should all patients with type 1 diabetes mellitus and microalbuminuria receive angiotensin-converting enzyme inhibitors? A meta-analysis of individual patient data. *Ann Intern Med.* 34: 370–379.

The CARDS Investigators (2004). Primary prevention of cardiovascular disease with atorvastatin in type 2 diabetes in the Collaborative Atorvastatin Diabetes Study (CARDS): multicentre randomised placebo-controlled trial. *Lancet* 2004; 364: 685–696.

The seventh report of the Joint National Committee on Prevention, Detection, Evaluation and Treatment of High Blood Pressure (2003). *JAMA* 289:2560–2572.

The Task Force on the Use of Antiplatelet Agents in Patients with Atherosclerotic Cardiovascular Disease of the European Society of Cardiology (2004). Expert consensus document on the use of antiplatelet agents. *Eur Heart J* 25:166-81.

Thorn LM, Forsblom C, Fagerudd J, Pettersson-Fernholm K, Kilpikari R, Groop PH; FinnDiane Study Group (2007). Clustering of risk factors in parents of patients with type 1 diabetes and nephropathy. *Diabetes Care* 2007 May; 30(5): 1162-7. Epub 2007 Mar 2.

Tokuno A, Hirano T, Hayashi T, Mori Y, Yamamoto T, Nagashima M, Shiraishi Y, Ito Y, Adachi M (2007). The effects of statin and fibrate on lowering small dense LDL-cholesterol in hyperlipidemic patients with type 2 diabetes. *J Atheroscler Thromb.* 2007 Jun; 14(3): 128-32.

Tonelli M, Moyé L, Sacks FM, Kiberd B, Curhan G; Cholesterol and Recurrent Events (CARE) Trial Investigators (2003). Pravastatin for secondary prevention of cardiovascular events in persons with mild chronic renal insufficiency. *Ann Intern Med.* 2003 Jan 21; 138(2): 98-104.

Veglio M, Sivieri R, Chinaglia A, Scaglione L, Cavallo-Perin P (2000). QT interval prolongation and mortality in type 1 diabetic patients: a 5-year cohort prospective study. *Diabetes Care* 23:1381–1383.

Weiner DE, Tighiouart H, Stark PC, Amin MG, MacLeod B, Griffith JL, Salem DN, Levey AS, Sarnak MJ (2004). Kidney disease as a risk factor for recurrent cardiovascular disease and mortality. *Am J Kidney Dis* 44(2): 198-206.

Weinrauch LA, Berger AJ, Aronson D, Gleason RE, Lee AT, D'Elia JA (2006). Regression of left ventricular hypertrophy in diabetic nephropathy: loss of parasympathetic function predicts response to treatment. *J Clin Hypertens (Greenwich).* 2006 May; 8(5): 330-5.

Whitsel EA, Boyko EJ, Siscovick DS (2000). Reassessing the role of QTc in the diagnosis of autonomic failure among patients with diabetes: a meta-analysis. *Diabetes Care* 23: 241–247.

Yilmaz MI, Saglam M, Qureshi AR, Carrero JJ, Caglar K, Eyileten T, Sonmez A, Cakir E, Oguz Y, Vural A, Yenicesu M, Stenvinkel P, Lindholm B, Axelsson J (2008). Endothelial dysfunction in type-2 diabetics with early diabetic nephropathy is associated with low circulating adiponectin. *Nephrol Dial Transplant.* 2008 May; 23(5):1621-7. Epub 2008 Jan 5.

Yokoyama H, Aoki T, Imahori M, Kuramitsu M (2004). Subclinical atherosclerosis is increased in type 2 diabetic patients with microalbuminuria evaluated by intima-media thickness and pulse wave velocity. *Kidney Int.* 2004 Jul; 66(1): 448-54.

Yoshimura T, Suzuki E, Ito I, Sakaguchi M, Uzu T, Nishio Y, Maegawa H, Morikawa S, Inubushi T, Hisatomi A, Fujimoto K, Takeda J, Kashiwagi A (2008). Impaired peripheral circulation in lower-leg arteries caused by higher arterial stiffness and greater vascular resistance associates with nephropathy in type 2 diabetic patients with normal ankle-brachial indices. *Diabetes Res Clin Pract.* 2008 Jun; 80(3): 416-23. Epub 2008 Mar 11.

Zander E, Heinke P, Reindel J, Kohnert KD, Kairies U, Braun J, Eckel L, Kerner W (2002). Peripheral arterial disease in diabetes mellitus type 1 and type 2: are there different risk factors? *Vasa.* 2002 Nov; 31(4): 249-54.

Zoccali C, Benedetto FA, Maas R, Mallamaci F, Tripepi G, Malatino LS, Böger R; CREED Investigators (2002). Asymmetric dimethylarginine, C-reactive protein, and carotid intima-media thickness in end-stage renal disease. *J Am Soc Nephrol* 13: 490–496.